THEORY OF
CORTICAL PLASTICITY

THEORY OF
CORTICAL PLASTICITY

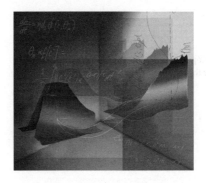

Leon N Cooper
Brown University, USA

Nathan Intrator
Tel-Aviv University, Israel & Brown University, USA

Brian S Blais
Bryant College & Brown University, USA

Harel Z Shouval
The University of Texas Medical School at Houston
& Brown University, USA

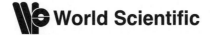 **World Scientific**

NEW JERSEY • LONDON • SINGAPORE • BEIJING • SHANGHAI • HONG KONG • TAIPEI • CHENNAI

Published by

World Scientific Publishing Co. Pte. Ltd.

5 Toh Tuck Link, Singapore 596224

USA office: Suite 202, 1060 Main Street, River Edge, NJ 07661

UK office: 57 Shelton Street, Covent Garden, London WC2H 9HE

British Library Cataloguing-in-Publication Data
A catalogue record for this book is available from the British Library.

ISBN 981-238-746-3
ISBN 981-238-791-9 (pbk)

Desk Editor: Tan Rok Ting
Artist: Loo Chuan Ming
Graphic Image Designers: Maria Dyer, Richard Fishman, Ali Zarrabi

Printed in Singapore by World Scientific Printers (S) Pte Ltd

Dedication Page

We dedicate this work to our experimental and theoretical comrades-in-arms who, over many years, have helped us produce the results on which this book is based.

Preface

Is theory possible in neuroscience? Not only possible, in our opinion, necessary. For a system as complex as the brain it is obvious that we cannot just make observations. (The number of possible observations is substantially larger than the available number of scientist-hours, even projecting several centuries into the future.) Without a theoretical structure to connect diverse observations with one another, the result would be a listing of facts of little use in understanding what the brain is about.

The eminent biochemist Edmond Fischer has said* "Biochemistry provides us with words – what is missing is language." It is theory that provides us with language-language that shapes the direction of analysis, that guides us toward significant experiments; language that provides a framework within which questions become relevant and leads us from assumptions to conclusions.

But what kind of language or theory is necessary? If one or two steps is all that is required to make connections between assumptions and conclusions, little mathematics is needed. However, if what is required is a long chain of reasoning with a quantitative dependence on parameters, mathematics, while possibly not required, helps. (It is important to distinguish such mathematical structures from computer simulations, where connections between assumptions and conclusions are often lost in mountains of printouts.) In this respect experiments that are theory driven may be regarded as extensions of hypothesis driven experiments in situations in which the path between hypothesis and experiment is too long or too complex to be followed without a mathematical structure. Examples of such theory driven experiments will be given later in this book.

A "correct" theory is not necessarily a good or a useful theory. It is presumably correct to say that the brain, is one consequence of the Schrödinger

---

*Private Communication

equation (the basic equation of quantum physics) applied to some very large number of electrons and nuclei. In analyzing a system as complicated as the brain, we must avoid the trap of trying to include everything too soon. Theories involving vast numbers of neurons in all their complexity can lead to systems of equations that defy analysis. Their fault is not that what they contain is incorrect, but that they contain too much. A theory that predicts everything predicts nothing.

The usefulness of a theoretical framework lies in its concreteness and in the precision with which questions can be formulated. The more precise the questions, the easier it is to compare theoretical consequences with experience. An approach that has been successful is to find the minimum number of assumptions that imply as logical consequences the qualitative features of the system that we are trying to describe. If we pose the question this way, it means that we agree to simplify. As Albert Einstein once said, "Make things as simple as possible, but no simpler." Once the major qualitative features are understood, complexity can be added as indicated by experiment.

The task, then, is first to limit the domain of our investigation, to introduce a set of assumptions concrete enough to give consequences that can be compared with observation. We must be able to see our way from assumptions to conclusions. The next step is experimental: to assess the validity of the underlying assumptions, if possible, and test their predicted consequences.

In the work that follows, we present the Bienenstock, Cooper and Munro (BCM) theory of synaptic plasticity. The theory is sufficiently concrete so that it can be and, as is discussed below, has been compared with experiment. The theory has suggested experiments that have uncovered new phenomena such as Long Term Depression (LTD), bi-directional synaptic modification dependent on the depolarization of the post-synaptic cell and the sliding modification threshold. These are in agreement with BCM synaptic modification function and provide experimental verification of the postulates of the BCM theory. Theory has suggested experiments to test various subtle and counter-intuitive consequences such as the noise dependence of the loss of response of the closed eye in monocular deprivation and has clarified connections between seemingly unrelated observations in different brain regions such as LTD and Long Term Potentiation (LTP) in hippocampus to reverse suture results in visual cortex. In addition, as is shown in Chapter 3 (Objective Function Formulation), there is a connection between the BCM unsupervised learning algorithm and the statistical method of projection pursuit – a procedure that seeks interesting projections in high dimensional spaces of data points. This suggests the possibility that the biological neuron has evolved in such a way as to perform a sophisticated statistical procedure.

The BCM theory should be regarded as a phenomenological theory in the sense that its basic variables and assumptions are expected to be defined and refined when it becomes possible to construct them from underlying cellular and molecular mechanisms. (This is analogous to the ideal gas equation PV=nRT with its variables defined from underlying kinetic theory or statistical mechanics and the equation itself modified for real gases by additions such as the van der Waals forces and the sizes of real molecules.)

Most of the connections between the BCM theory and experiments that we discuss in this book require complex simulations. A special feature of this work is the accompanying software package (built by one of our authors, Brian Blais) that will allow the reader to repeat these simulations varying both parameters and assumptions, with many different learning algorithms. Thus through mathematical analysis as well as the ability to repeat and change the simulations, we hope readers will be able to obtain hands-on knowledge of the structure of this theory and the connections between assumptions and consequences as well as the possibility of creating variations of their own.

Acknowledgements

We would like to thank our many coworkers, especially our colleagues in the Brown University Institute for Brain and Neural Systems, whose research has made this book possible. In particular we express our gratitude to Mark Bear and the members of his laboratory for the pioneering experimental work that has confirmed both postulates and consequences of our theory.

We also would like to acknowledge the following who at one time or another have participated in our efforts: Claire Adams, Ömer Artun, Elie Bienenstock, Pete Bilderback, Roger Blumberg, Gastone Castellani, Eugene Clothieux, Maria Cuartas, Serena Dudek, David Goldberg, Xin Huang, Alfredo Kirkwood, Charles Law, Christian Latino, Ann Lee, Hey-Kyoung Lee, Fishel Liberman, Yong Liu, Paul Munro, Menasche Nass, Erkki Oja, Michael Paradiso, David Poznik, Elizabeth Quinlan, Cynthia Rittenhouse, Alan Saul, Chris Scofield, Bradley Seebach, Wes Wallace, and Yeung Luk Chong, as well as Maria Dyer, Richard Fishman, and Ali Zarrabi who designed the cover image.

In addition we acknowledge the government agencies and private foundations for support of the research on which this book is based: the Army Research Office, the Office of Naval Research, the National Scientific Foundation, the National Institute of Health, the Ittleson Foundation, the Alfred P. Sloan Foundation, and the Dana Foundation.

Contents

Leon N Cooper, Nathan Intrator, Brian S. Blais, Harel Z. Shouval

The Software Package, *Plasticity*

This book comes with a software package designed by one of the authors, Brian Blais. Entitled *Plasticity*, this package allows the user to reproduce any of the results quoted in the book[†]. It is a research tool, an education tool, as well as a reference for anyone reading the book. The source code for the package is provided, and is open to anyone who wants to look at it or modify it. It is the feeling of the authors that scientific understanding comes from the free and open exchange of ideas, and that such a package lays bare all of the implementation details.

[†]Some of the development of the package *Plasticity* was supported by NIH Grant Number P20 RR16457-01 from the BRIN Program of the National Center for Research Resources

Notation

$\mathbf{m} = (m_1 \ldots m_i \ldots m_N)^T$ -modifiable synaptic weight vector.

m_i is the synaptic weight between input neuron i and the output neuron.

M - the synaptic weight matrix when there is more than one output neuron. $[M_{ij}]$ represents the connection between LGN neuron j and cortical neuron i.

$\mathbf{m} = (\mathbf{m}^l, \mathbf{m}^r)$ when there are inputs from two eyes, $\mathbf{m}^{l(r)}$ represents the weight vector to input neurons from the left (right) eye channel.

$\mathbf{d} = (d_1 \ldots d_N)^T$ Is the a vector of input activities to a single cortical neuron. d_i represents the activity of input neuron i.

$\mathbf{d}^i$, an upper index $\mathbf{d}^i$ denotes that this is the i'th vector of input activity. If there are K different input vectors $i = 1 \ldots K$.

$\mathbf{d} = (\mathbf{d}^l, \mathbf{d}^r)$ when there are inputs from two eyes, $\mathbf{d}^{l(r)}$ represents the input vector to the left (right) eye channel.

$\mathbf{n}$ the vector of uncorrelated random activity, or noise

c The activity level of a single cortical neuron.

$\mathbf{c}$ Cortical cell activity vector $\mathbf{c} = (c_1, \ldots, c_N)^T$, when there are N cortical neurons.

c^i is the activity of a cortical neurons given input pattern i. In the linear region by $c^i = \mathbf{m}^i \cdot \mathbf{d}$. In the nonlinear case $c_i = \sigma(\mathbf{m}^i \cdot \mathbf{d})$.

σ Transfer function.

L The lateral connections matrix between cortical neurons: L_{ij} is the synapse connection between the ith neuron to the jth neuron.

ϕ The BCM synaptic modification function, which depends on the postsynaptic activity and on the sliding modification threshold θ_M, thus $\phi = \phi(c, \theta_M)$.

θ_M The sliding modification threshold in the BCM theory.

$\theta_M{}^*$ The sliding modification threshold value at a fixed point

p_i , the probability of input pattern i.

η , the learning rate, which sets the speed of weight modification

τ , the memory constant, which sets the temporal window size over which the modification threshold is averaged (see $\bar{\bar{x}}$) below

$E[x]$, denotes an ensemble average of x. For example $E[\mathbf{d}] = \sum_i p_i \mathbf{d}^i$.

$<x> = E[x]$

$\bar{x}$, ensemble average of x. $\bar{x} = E[x]$

$\bar{\bar{x}}$ Temporal average given by $\frac{1}{\tau} \int_{-\infty}^{t} x(t') e^{-\frac{(t-t')}{\tau}} dt'$. For example

$\bar{\bar{c}}$ Temporal average of cell activity.

$\theta_M = \bar{\bar{c}}^2$, the sliding modification threshold.

Q The Covariance matrix or function.

$Q_{ij} = E[(d_i - \bar{d}_i)(d_j - \bar{d}_j)]$, is the covariance matrix of cortical inputs $\mathbf{d}$, .

$Q(\mathbf{x}, \mathbf{x}') = E[(d(\mathbf{x}) - \bar{\mathbf{x}})(d(\mathbf{x}') - \bar{\mathbf{x}}')]$, the covariance function for inputs in continuous space

∇_x The gradient with respect to x, $\nabla_x F(\mathbf{x}) = (\frac{dF}{dx_1} \cdots \frac{dF}{dx_N})$

Common Acronyms and Abbreviations

AMPA a-amino-3-hydroxy-5-methyl-4-isoxazoleproprionate, agonist for the glutamate receptor AMPAR

AMPAR a glutamate receptor

BCM Bienenstock, Cooper, and Munro Learning Rule

BD Binocular Deprivation

BR Binocular Recovery

CDF Cumulative distribution function

DC Direct Current, referring to the average (non-zero) component of a solution

DOG Difference of Gaussians

DS Direction Selectivity

HFS High Frequency Stimulation

ICA Independent Component Analysis

i.i.d. Independent Identically Distributed

$\mathbf{K_1}$ Multiplicative form of Kurtosis

$\mathbf{K_2}$ Subtractive form of Kurtosis

LFS Low Frequency Stimulation

LGN Lateral Geniculate Nucleus

LTD Long Term Depression

LTP Long Term Potentiation

MD Monocular Deprivation

MR Monocular Rearing

NMDA N-methyl-D-aspartate, agonist for the glutamate receptor NMDAR

NMDAR a glutamate receptor

NR Normal Rearing

OD Ocular Dominance

OR Orientation Selectivity

PC Principle Components

PCA Principle Component Analysis

QBCM Quadratic form of BCM

RF Receptive Field
RS Reverse Suture
S_1 Multiplicative form of Skewness
S_2 Subtractive form of Skewness
TTX tetrodotoxin, a sodium channel blocker

Chapter 1

Introduction

It is widely believed that much of the learning and resulting organization of the central nervous system occurs due to modification of the efficacy or strength of at least some of the synaptic junctions between neurons, thus altering the relation between presynaptic and postsynaptic potentials. The vast amount of experimental work done in visual cortex – particularly area 17 of cat and monkey – strongly indicates that one is observing a process of synaptic modification dependent on the information locally and globally available to the cortical cells. Furthermore, it is known that small but coherent modifications of large numbers of synaptic junctions can result in distributed memories [Cooper, 1973; McClelland et al., 1986] Whether and how such synaptic modification occurs, what precise forms it takes, and what the physiological and/or anatomical bases of this modification are, the questions we would most like to answer.

There is no need to assume that such mechanisms operate in exactly the same manner in all portions of the nervous system or in all animals. However, one would hope that certain fundamental similarities exist so that a detailed analysis of the properties of these mechanisms in one preparation would lead to conclusions that are generally applicable.

Because of its great complexity, visual cortex would not seem to be an auspicious region of the brain to carry out an investigation of synaptic plasticity or of the mechanisms and sites of memory storage. It is almost certain that much of the architecture of visual cortex is preprogrammed genetically, leaving a relatively minor percentage to be shaped or modified by experience. However besides being accessible to single-cell electrophysiology, so that the output of individual cells can be measured, the inputs to visual cortex can be controlled by varying the visual experience of the animal. This has made visual cortex a preferred area for experimentation and analysis. Over a half-century, a great deal of work has been done, to investigate the responses of visual cortical cells, as well as the alterations in these responses under different visual rearing conditions.

Efforts to provide an understanding of the development of primary visual cortex - its natural development as well as its development under various unusual visual environments go back at least two generations. Hubel and Wiesel investigated the effects of what we now call monocular deprivation to better understand the problems of amblyopia. Theoretical efforts to understand the development of selective (Hubel-Wiesel) cells go back to the early seventies, with the work of von der Malsburg [von der Malsburg, 1973; Perez et al., 1975; Nass and Cooper, 1975].

Early experiments that indicated visual environment dependence of the development of the response properties of cells in visual cortex were highly controversial. Even today (as we will discuss further in this chapter), there is not complete agreement as to the respective role of genetic and environmental factors. We take the point of view that there is at least some dependence on environmental factors and that these can be used to study the more general phenomena of cellular modification (synaptic modification) – that whatever percentage of visual cortical organization is due to environmental factors can be used to illuminate the more general phenomenon of learning and memory storage. This view is reinforced by the recent unification of various putative memory phenomena (LTP and LTD) with visual cortical development (as will be discussed both later in this chapter, and again Chapter 9).

In this monograph we present a systematic development of the BCM theory[Bienenstock et al., 1982] of cortical plasticity, compare this with other cortical plasticity theories and make comparisons with experimental results. It is our hope that a general form of modifiability manifests itself for at least some cells of visual cortex that are accessible to experiment. If so, one then may be able to distinguish between different cortical plasticity theories with theoretical tools and the aid of sophisticated experimental techniques.

Along with our theoretical discussion, we will attempt to indicate experiments that can test particular ideas in detail. Although the phenomena of visual cortex modification as well as LTP have been intensively explored for more than a generation, new techniques are now available so that the various theoretical ideas can be tested in much more detail. In spite of the fact that a great number of experiments have been done in visual cortex, many of the questions we would most like to answer have not been addressed directly. The most subtle consequences of theory, the ones that will restrict the underlying biological mechanisms are not yet adequately tested. Most visual cortex experimental work are population studies. While these results are very suggestive, they often do not give the detailed information required. We now have available experimental technologies that make possible chronic studies in which we can follow individual cells over an extended period of time. In addition, our mathematical analysis has reached a point where we are capable of much deeper analysis of the statistics of natural scenes, an essential component in making subtle comparisons between theoretical predictions and experimental results.

1.1 Visual Cortex Plasticity

Light bouncing off objects in the world is focused by the lens in our eye onto the retina. It is then sampled and transduced by receptors in the retina where the retinal circuitry transforms these signals. The ganglion cells which are the output neurons of the retina transmit this information through the optic nerve via the optic chiasm, where the inputs from both eyes cross, onto the Lateral Geniculate Nucleus (LGN). From the LGN the signal are projected to the primary visual cortex. The cortex in turn projects back to the LGN (Figure 1.1a).

Ganglion cells in the retina, and cells in the LGN respond to spots of light on a screen. The shape of this response region and the magnitude of response within this region is usually referred to as the receptive field. The shape of receptive fields in the retina and the LGN is circular; typically they have a center region in which responses are increased (ON cells) or decreased (OFF cells) and an antagonist surround area [Kuffler, 1953; Wiesel and Hubel, 1962]. Cells in both the retina and the LGN are monocular, that is they respond to inputs only from one eye .

In contrast, neurons in the primary visual cortex (area 17) of normal adult cats are sharply tuned to the orientation of an elongated slit of light and most are activated by stimulation of either eye (Hubel & Wiesel, 1960). In the cat, both of these properties – orientation selectivity and binocularity are exhibited already in the spiny stellate neurons in layer IV B, the layer into which LGN neurons project (Figure 1.1b).

The majority of binocular neurons in the striate cortex of normal adult cat do not respond equally to stimulation of either eye; instead they typically display an eye preference. To quantify this observation Hubel and Wiesel (1962) originally separated the population of recorded neurons into seven ocular dominance (OD) categories. The OD distribution in a normal kitten or adult cat shows a broad peak at group 4, which reflects a high percentage of binocular neurons in area 17 (Figure 1.1c).

The are several deprivation experiments that can alter the normal OD pattern of cats. The most dramatic is that called monocular deprivation (MD). This is done by eye patching, lid suture [Wiesel and Hubel, 1962] or the use of a diffuse lens to cover one eye [Blakemore, 1976]. During a critical period [Frégnac and Imbert, 1984; Sherman and Spear, 1982], MD causes a shift in the OD pattern toward the dominant eye; that is cells become more strongly driven by the open eye. This is the most robust and non-controversial form of functional plasticity in the visual cortex. The normal OD pattern is also strikingly altered if the two eyes do not view the same image (strabismus) and the effect on individual cells is similar to that of MD.[van Sluyters, 1977; van Sluyters and Levitt, 1980]

Cells which have been disconnected from the closed eye through MD can reconnect to it by using a procedure called reverse suture (RS) [Blakemore and van Sluyters, 1974; Mioche and Singer, 1989]. In RS the eye that was open during MD is sutured closed and the closed eye is opened. This procedure reconnects cells to the previously closed eye but does not, in general, create binocular cells.

It is now generally accepted that receptive fields in the visual cortex of cats are dramatically influenced by the visual environment (for a comprehensive review see, Frégnac and Imbert, 1984). However, the precise effect of visual deprivation on orientation selectivity is more controversial, and there is a debate on whether the requirement for a patterned visual environment is instructive or permissive: whether patterned input is used directly to produce orientation selective (instructive), or whether it signals another process to produce orientation selectivity (permissive). It is clear that some cells have weak orientation tuning before eye-opening [Hubel and Wiesel, 1963; Frégnac and Imbert, 1984]. However prolonged periods of binocular deprivation (BD) performed either by suturing both eyes, or by dark rearing can stop the development of normal sharply tuned receptive fields, and even abolish their weak, pre-eye-opening, orientation bias [Imbert and Buisseret, 1975; Frégnac and Imbert, 1978; Levental and Hirsh, 1980; Chapman et al., 1999]. It is generally believed that the degradation of orientation selectivity due to BD is much slower than MD [Wiesel and Hubel, 1965]. However there is some evidence [Freeman et al., 1981], that the effect of BD may be faster than expected.

There have been many experiments that seem to support the claim that rearing in restricted environments e.g., environments with only vertical stripes or only circular blobs have a profound effect on orientation selectivity in visual cortex [Blakemore and Van-Sluyters, 1975; Rauschecker and Singer, 1981; Frégnac and Imbert, 1984; Stryker et al., 1978; Sengpiel et al., 1999]. These experiments however are difficult to interpret and their effect is not as robust as the ocular dominance shift during MD, although most evidence shows a significant shift in orientation selectivity[Sherk and Stryker, 1975].

Thus, in spite of some differences in interpretation, there is strong experimental evidence in support of the view that receptive fields are plastic after eye opening, that both their Ocular Dominance and Orientation Selectivity depend on the visual environment and that a patterned environment is necessary for formation of normal mature receptive fields. Furthermore, the vast majority of experiments in which animals were reared in a restricted visual environment indicate that the distribution of preferred orientations changes as well. This indicates that the post-eye-opening plasticity of orientation selectivity is not only permissive but also instructive.

1.2 Theoretical background

Theoretical attempts to understand experience dependent development of visual cortex date back to the early seventies with the work of von der Malsburg (1973), Perez et al (1975) and Nass and Cooper (1975). Nass and Cooper (1975) focused on the environmentally driven development of Hubel-Wiesel-type feature detectors, showing that with Hebbian-type modification, exposure of the cells to repeated patterns would result in cells strongly responsive to those patterns. They encountered the usual, now well-known problems with Hebbian mechanisms. A maximum synaptic value was required in order that the system not run away. In addition, they introduced the idea of lateral inhibition between the cells so that they didn't all acquire the same pattern.

Similar attempts were made at approximately the same time by von der Malsburg and Perez et al. They ran into the same problems. (As early as 1956 [Rochester et al., 1956] one sees the introduction of various ideas to prevent the Hebbian growth of synapses from running away). von der Malsburg and Perez introduced the idea that, somehow, the sum of synaptic strengths would remain constant. Nass and Cooper used the device of ending the modification of synaptic strengths when the cell response reached a maximum level (depending on the precise formulation, these are not unrelated.).

At about the same time in the laboratory of Michel Imbert at the College de France in Paris, experimental results were obtained showing that the tuning properties of visual cortical cells depended strongly on the environment in which the young kittens were reared [Buisseret and Imbert, 1976]. If the kittens were reared in a normal environment the cells were sharply tuned. If they were dark reared, the cells were broadly tuned; very few of the normal Hubel-Wiesel cells appeared, and most striking, the situation could be reversed by very short exposure to the normal visual environment at the height of the critical period. This environmental dependence of selectivity cried to be explained.

Cooper et al. [Cooper et al., 1979](CLO) proposed that one could generalize the rule of Nass and Cooper to another in which synapses increased if the post-synaptic cell response was above what came to be known the modification threshold and decreased if the response was below. They found that, with some rather artificial assumptions, they could obtain selectivity in patterned environments but not in noise-like environments.

The threshold modification algorithm of CLO has the form

$$\dot{m} = \phi_{CLO}d.$$

where m is the synaptic weight, d is the input, and $\dot{m}$ denotes the *change* in the weights. The ϕ function, which specifies the change in the weights, is shown in Figure 1.2.

Although this work seemed promising, there were several obvious flaws. First, it dealt with a single cortical cell, neglecting the fact that visual cortex is extraordinarily rich and complex with many cells receiving input from LGN and from each other. Second, modeling of the external visual environment, while plausible, was artificial. Third, the modification algorithm itself had what seemed to be a serious problem. The threshold had to be set very carefully, with the cell response to only one pattern above threshold and the response to all of the others below threshold. In many ways, work in this area since that time has been designed to correct these flaws.

The first problem addressed was that of the artificiality of setting the modification threshold. If it was set too high, the response of all patterns would be below threshold and the cell would lose its responsiveness to all patterns. If it was set too low then more than one pattern responded above threshold, and the cell would become responsive to more than one pattern and thus be less selective.

In 1982, Bienenstock Cooper and Munro (BCM) proposed that the value of the modification threshold is not fixed, but instead varies as a nonlinear function of the average output of the postsynaptic neuron. This feature provided stability properties in such a way that the threshold set itself to separate one pattern from the rest leading to selective cell in pattered environment. In addition, it explained various other features of the deprivation experiments, for example, why the low level of postsynaptic activity caused by binocular deprivation does not drive the strengths of all cortical synapses to zero.

The BCM paper [Bienenstock et al., 1982] is the basic paper in which the algorithm is explored in its almost completely developed form, discussing the fixed points and their stability. It is shown that, in a patterned environment, the cell becomes selective; in a noisy environment the cell loses selectivity, all in a very robust fashion. In addition, under various deprivation conditions, in particular monocular deprivation, the response of the cells is in agreement with what is observed experimentally. This has come to be known as the BCM algorithm. Later, we demonstrate that this algorithm has powerful statistical properties. We are thus tempted to conjecture that the algorithm evolved in such a way as to enable cortical neurons to process early information in a manner that was valuable statistically.

This form of synaptic modification can be written as:

$$\dot{m}_j = \phi(c, \theta_M)d_j \tag{1.1}$$

where m_j is the efficacy of the jth lateral geniculate nucleus (LGN) synapse onto a cortical neuron, d_j is the level of presynaptic activity of the jth LGN afferent, c is the activity of the postsynaptic neuron (spiking or depolarization), that is given (in the linear approximation), by $m \cdot d$, and θ_M is a nonlinear function of some average of cell activity. The change in the synaptic weight ($\dot{m}_j$) is a function of the shape of the ϕ function, dependent on the modification threshold, which itself is a function of the history of activity of the cell. In some simplified situations, the averaged activity of the cell over all input patterns, $\bar{c}$, is used to approximate the history of activity of the cell $\bar{\bar{c}}$, thus, the temporal average is replaced by a spatial average. The shape of the function ϕ is given in Figure 1.3 for two different θ_M thresholds.

1.3　Comparison of Theory and Experiment

In general, there are two ways to test theories and/or to distinguish among them. One is to compare their consequences with experiment; the other is to directly verify their underlying assumptions. Recently two such avenues of research have supported the BCM theory. Physiological experiments have verified some of its basic assumptions, while analysis and simulations have shown that the theory can explain existing experimental observations of selectivity and ocular dominance plasticity in kitten visual cortex in a wide variety of visual environments and make testable predictions.

In order to make comparison between theory and experiment, various simplifying assumptions must be made. In general these involve

- The synaptic modification postulate.
- The network architecture.
- The nature of the visual environment.

Throughout this book we make analyses at different levels of complexity to elucidate the underlying principles and to make comparison with experimental observations. We start with simple low dimensional single neuron examples, in order to gain intuition and conclude with networks of interacting neurons in a natural image environment.

First we will describe results obtained with sets of linearly independent inputs in a single neuron setting [Bienenstock et al., 1982; Intrator and Cooper, 1992], we then examine the case of overlapping input vectors [Clothiaux et al., 1991] and finally we use sets of pre-processed natural images [Law and Cooper, 1994; Shouval et al., 1996b]. Furthermore we have extended our single cell results [Bienenstock et al., 1982; Clothiaux et al., 1991; Law and Cooper, 1994; Shouval et al., 1996b] to networks of interconnected neurons [Cooper and Scofield, 1988; Castellani et al., 1999; Shouval et al., 1997a].

Results at all levels of complexity that have been examined are in good agreement with experiment. Highly selective oriented receptive fields evolve for natural image environments [Law and Cooper, 1994; Shouval et al., 1996b]. When a two eye visual environment is used receptive fields with varying degrees of ocular dominance evolve [Shouval et al., 1996b; Shouval et al., 1997a]. The effect of network interactions has been analyzed [Cooper and Scofield, 1988] and simulated [Shouval et al., 1997a]. Simulations reveal the same type of receptive fields as in the single cell case but with ocular dominance patches and slowly varying orientation selectivity. Deprivation experiments have been simulated as well[Clothiaux et al., 1991; Blais et al., 1996; Blais et al., 1999] and also the development of direction selectivity[Blais et al., 2000]. All types of experimental results can be replicated by BCM neurons for the same set of parameters.

Throughout these simulations we have assumed that the input channel (or channels) originating from the closed eye (or eyes) provides an input of uncorrelated noise to the cortical cell. The results obtained are critically dependent on the level of this noise. The time it takes oriented receptive fields to decay in deprivation experiments such as MD, RS and BD all depend on the level of noise – the higher the noise level the faster the decay time. This happens because noise from the deprived eye seldom create activities that are higher than the threshold θ_M and thus mostly contribute to the decay; the stronger they are the faster the decay. Such results are contrary to what would be obtained using models that employ explicit competition between the eyes (See Chapter 7) where the decay time, typically, increases as the level of noise increases.

The level of noise can be experimentally manipulated in deprivation experiments. This can be achieved by using different methods of deprivation. Retinal activity in lid sutured animals should be higher than in those with a dark patch placed on the eyes and should be reduced close to zero in animals that have TTX (a sodium channel blocker) injected to the eye. The relevant parameter, for the models, is LGN activity. If the level of LGN activity indeed depends on the retinal activity we could use these different protocols to manipulate the noise level in the LGN and thus to determine experimentally which of the different proposed models agrees better with experimental results.

A set of experiments performed by Rittenhouse et. al. (1999) have shown that the level of the noise in the deprived eye could be manipulated by comparing normal MD with lid suture to MD in which TTX was injected into the eye. TTX abolishes action potentials in the retina and significantly reduces the spontaneous rate in LGN. In these experiments it was found that the shift in MD was faster in the lid suture case than in the TTX case. These results are in agreement with predictions of the BCM theory.

1.4   Cellular Basis for the Postulates of the BCM Theory

The BCM theory of synaptic plasticity, as described briefly in the previous sections, and in more detail in the chapters below, is based on three postulates:

(1) The change in synaptic weights $(\dot{m}_j)$ is proportional to presynaptic activity (d_j).

(2) The change in synaptic weights is proportional to a non-monotonic function (denoted by ϕ) of the postsynaptic activity (c). For low c, the synaptic weight decreases $(\dot{m}_j < 0)$ while for larger c it increases $(\dot{m}_j > 0)$. The cross over point between $\dot{m}_j < 0$ and $\dot{m}_j > 0$ is denoted by θ_M.

(3) The modification threshold (θ_M) is itself an increasing function of the history of postsynaptic activity.

When the BCM theory was proposed there was little support for any of these postulates. Today, in contrast, these postulates have significant support. Recent experimental work suggests that the well known phenomena of long term potentiation (LTP), long term depression (LTD) and the BCM synaptic modification theory of cortical plasticity, are manifestations of the same underlying learning mechanism under different experimental conditions.

Postulate 1, states that plasticity will occur only in synapses that are stimulated presynaptically. This is what biologists refer to as synapse specificity. Synapse specificity has strong support for both LTP and LTD [Dudek and Bear, 1992]. In addition this assumption is consistent with the observation that more presynaptic activity results in a higher degree of plasticity, although this might not be linear.

There is now substantial evidence both in hippocampus and neocortex [Dudek and Bear, 1992; Mulkey and Malenka, 1992; Artola and Singer, 1992; Kirkwood and Bear, 1994a; Mayford et al., 1995] in support of postulate 2. There is significant evidence that active synapses undergo LTD or LTP depending on the level of postsynaptic spiking or depolarization in a manner that is consistent with the BCM theory, as shown in Figure 1.4. The reasoning behind the experiment is as follows. If the cell activity is some integrated activity, over a small time window, then it would be proportional to the input frequency. If also, in the short time of the input stimulus we assume that the threshold doesn't move much, then the $\phi(\cdot)$ function would be approximately constant. The total weight change for N

input spikes at a particular frequency would be

$$\Delta m = \sum_{i=1}^{N} \phi(c, \theta_M) d_i \approx \phi(d, \theta_M) \sum_{i=1}^{N} d_i \qquad (1.2)$$

$$= \phi(c, \theta_M) \times (\text{total input}) \qquad (1.3)$$

Since the total input into the cell is kept constant (N spikes for all input frequencies), the measured change in synaptic efficacy, or equivalently, the amount of LTP/LTD is proportional to $\phi(c, \theta_M)$.

Furthermore, in many regions of the cerebral cortex, Ca^{2+} fluxes through N-methyl-D-aspartate-gated ion channels (NMDA receptors) can trigger these two forms of synaptic plasticity [Bear and Malenka, 1994]. A smooth transition from net LTD to net LTP may be observed by systematically varying the amount of postsynaptic NMDA receptor activation, usually by altering the frequency or pattern of conditioning stimulation [Dudek and Bear, 1992; Kirkwood and Bear, 1994a; Mayford et al., 1995]. Another paradigm in which the level of NMDA receptor activation can be controlled is a pairing protocol. Here a low frequency presynaptic stimulus is delivered while the postsynaptic cell is clamped to a fixed voltage, which controls the level of NMDA receptor activation [Stevens and Wang, 1994; Cummings et al., 1996; Crair et al., 1998; Feldman, 2000].

The third key postulate of the BCM theory: that the value of θ_M (the crossover point between LTD and LTP) varies with post synaptic activity, has been tested in several ways. Previous studies had shown that the sign and magnitude of a synaptic modification in both hippocampus [Huang et al., 1992] and the Mauthner cell of goldfish [Yang and Faber, 1991] depends on the recent history of synaptic activation.

A more direct test of the postulate of the moving threshold – that after a period of increased activity θ_M increases, promoting synaptic depression while after a period of decreased activity θ_M decreases, promoting synaptic potentiation has been tested by studying LTD and LTP of layer III synaptic responses in slices of visual cortex prepared from 4-6 week-old light-deprived and control rats [Kirkwood et al., 1996]. This experiment (Figure 1.5) shows that in deprived animals θ_M is lower than in normal animals. In control slices from the hippocampus no change in θ_M is observed.

An additional experiment by Wang and Wagner in 1999 has produced similar results in hippocampal slices in which the postsynaptic activity was controlled directly by different stimulation protocols (that did not induce plasticity) directly in the slice. Here too they observed that the threshold in highly stimulated slices is higher than in control slices.

1.5   A Model of Inputs to Visual Cortex Cells

The inputs projected onto layer IV-B from the LGN depend on the visual environment, the eye movements, and the preprocessing of the images which occurs in the retina and the LGN. There are different types of ganglion cells in the retina [Orban, 1984]. They differ both in their spatial and temporal filtering properties and their properties vary from species to species. Most ganglion cells are center surround and they are split evenly between ON and OFF subtypes. In cats a further subdivision is between X, Y and W cells. About 50% of the cells are X cells, which are smaller, with receptive field centers of $\approx .2 - 1$ degrees, and they exhibit linear summation of their inputs. Y cells are larger, non-linear, more transient, and have higher conduction velocities. W cells have much slower conduction velocities, have heterogeneous properties and often do not project to LGN.

Primarily we are interested in postnatal development of receptive fields in both normal and deprived conditions. We therefore often use natural images is simulations of natural postnatal development. We have chosen to model the spatial properties of the retinal preprocessing by convolving the natural images with a difference of Gaussians filter (DOG). The ratio between the widths of the central and surround Gaussians is usually assumed to be 1:3, although we do examine the effect of altering this ratio. The different values used are motivated by experimental results[Linsenmeier et al., 1982].

Some retinal ganglion cells are highly transient while others have a more stationary response. We have assumed throughout this paper a stationary temporal filter. This is appropriate since this book describes only rate based models of synaptic plasticity, which are not very sensitive to the temporal properties of their inputs.

The LGN has a complex machinery, including a massive feedback from the cortex. Recently it was shown that this back projection has a significant impact on the temporal correlation in LGN[Sillito et al., 1994] and that it increases the correlations between LGN layers from different eyes [Weliky and Katz, 1999]. However, there is no consensus on how this circuitry effects the spatio-temporal properties of LGN cells, which in many respects resemble those of retinal ganglion cells. We have chosen, for simplicity, to model the LGN as a simple relay station which does not alter the response properties of the retinal ganglion cells.

Broadly speaking there are two major classes of eye movements: slow smooth movements, termed *smooth pursuit* and fast movements called *saccades*. Smooth pursuit compensates for head movements or movements in the image by smooth movements of the eyes. Its goal is to stabilize the image on the retina. Smooth pursuit tracks the object or visual flow field, but it is slow and saturates at 10-100 degree/sec and takes approximately 200 ms to initiate. The effect of this type of movement is to reduce temporal changes in the visual environment, thus stretching out the temporal correlations. This type of eye movement exists throughout the animal kingdom from invertebrates to humans.

Saccades are very quick stereotyped movements, in which the eyes abruptly jump from one position to another. The speed of a saccade could be up to 1000 degree/sec but have latencies of $\approx 200ms$. The large initial saccade is often followed by small corrective saccades due to an undershoot of the initial saccade.

There is another class of miniature eye movements for which there is no obvious use [Carpenter, 1977](Ch 6). There are three distinct types of such eye movements: tremor, drift and micro saccades. A tremor is the smallest of these movements, has an amplitude of $\approx 10 - 20''$, of the order of magnitude of the size of the smallest cone. In frequency domain it has a low pass characteristic, flat to 10Hz and dropping to zero at 150-200 Hz. Drift movements are larger than tremors and are also very slow. The velocities are in the region of $1'sec^{-1}$, with median amplitudes of $2 - 5'$. Micro saccades often occur at the end of a drift and on average returns the visual target to the center of the fovea. The amplitude of the smallest micro saccades is $1 - 2'$. There is a wide variation in micro saccade latency, which depends on other factors such as drift. It is debatable if micro-saccades occur in natural viewing.

In most of our work we model viewing of a stationary environment. Saccades are modeled by randomly picking a new patch from our input environment, either from the same or another image. In order to model the development of direction selectivity we also incorporated slow drift into our model. This is implemented by choosing a random direction, velocity and duration of drift. During this drift consecutive image patches from the environment are chosen for creating the inputs.

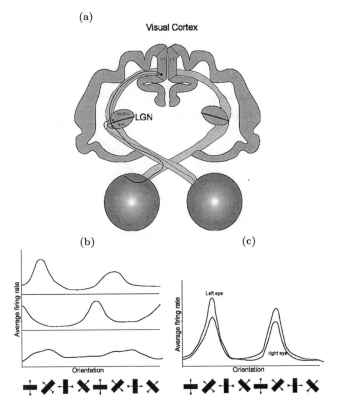

Figure 1.1: Visual cortex plasticity. (a) The visual pathway. Ganglion cells from left and right project to separate layers in the LGN. Ganglion cells and cells in LGN have center surround receptive fields. From LGN cells project onto the primary visual cortex. Cells in visual cortex normally respond to both eyes (binocular) and are orientation selective. (b) Most cells in visual cortex are orientation selective; they respond differently to moving bars or gratings of different orientations. Visual experience is necessary for the normal development of orientation selectivity. Immediately after eye opening (bottom panel), neurons exhibit only a weak orientation bias. When animals are raised in a normal patterned environment (middle and top panels), sharp orientation selectivity develops. If animals are raised in the dark cells fail to develop sharp orientation selectivity and lose their initial weak bias. (c) Cells in visual cortex respond to inputs from both eyes. The relative magnitude of these responses determines the ocular dominance class of each cell.

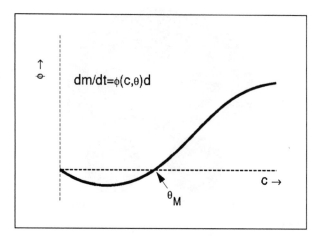

Figure 1.2: The CLO synaptic modification function, ϕ. It has two zero crossings, as well as synaptic depression below θ_M, and enhancement above. θ_M does not move.

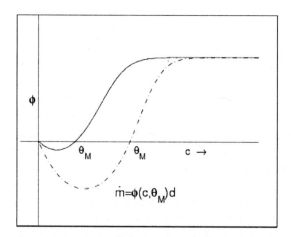

Figure 1.3: The modification function for two values of the threshold.

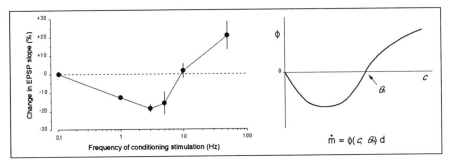

Figure 1.4: Comparison of experimental observations with BCM ϕ function for synaptic modification. Data replotted from Dudek and Bear (1992).

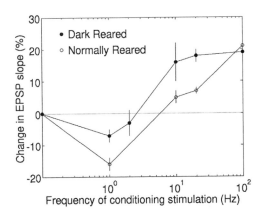

Figure 1.5: The sliding modification threshold (experimental), reproduced from [Kirkwood, et.al. 1996]

Chapter 2

Single Cell Theory

"Things should be made as simple as possible, but no simpler."

Albert Einstein

2.1 Introduction

One of the most important features of the BCM theory, is the *sliding modification threshold*, θ_M, the cross-over point at which synaptic modification changes sign. Cooper, Liberman and Oja (1979) (CLO) introduced the idea that synaptic modification changes sign at a cross-over point they called the modification threshold. According to CLO, for cell activity above threshold, modification follows a classical Hebbian rule; for cell activity below threshold, modification is anti-Hebbian. This means that only patterns that elicit high post-synaptic activity (beyond the threshold θ_M) will have their concurrently active synapses strengthened (the Hebbian region), while active synapses which elicit post-synaptic activity, but fail to elicit strong enough activity, will have their synapses weakened (non-Hebbian region). BCM added the idea that this modification threshold moves as some function of cell activity. If this function is properly non-linear, the theory is stabilized, because the threshold moves quickly enough to catch up to the cell activity caused by increasing or decreasing weights.

Extensive simulations are usually required to compare this theory with experiment in real world situations. In these simulations, the logical connections between assumptions and conclusions are sometimes obscured by the many parameters and the complexity of the data. Thus it is of great value to analyze systems that are simple enough so that this path can be made clear. In this chapter, the consequences of the BCM theory are explored in the simplified situation of a single cell in various simple environments. Many of the characteristic features of the theory revealed in this analysis are preserved in the more complex situations investigated in later chapters.

2.2   Definitions and Notation

Visual cortex is very complex; there are many layers, different neuron types
with many interactions between neurons. A typical neuron in this region
(striate cortex) receives thousands of afferents from other cells. Most of
these come from the lateral geniculate nucleus (LGN) and from other cortical neurons. The transfer function that leads to these afferents is nonlinear
and may include complex time dependencies.

In order to display the qualitative properties of the BCM neuron in as
transparent a manner as possible, we analyze a very simplified situation:
a single neuron with inputs from both eyes (i.e., LGN) but without intra-
cortical interactions (Figure 2.1), with a very simplified representation of
the visual environment. We make a variety of other simplifying assumptions on averages and time dependencies – all with the object of displaying
qualitative properties. In later sections we will gradually add complications
and discuss the consequences.

The output of this simplified neuron (in the linear approximation) is
written

$$c = \mathbf{m}^l \cdot \mathbf{d}^l + \mathbf{m}^r \cdot \mathbf{d}^r = \sum_j m_j^l d_j^l + \sum_j m_j^r d_j^r, \qquad (2.1)$$

where $\mathbf{d}^l$ ($\mathbf{d}^r$) are the LGN inputs coming from the left (right) eye to the
vector of synaptic junctions $\mathbf{m}^l$ ($\mathbf{m}^r$).

In general, synaptic weight changes over time
$\dot{m}_j$ can be written

$$\dot{m}_j = F(d_j, m_j; d_k \ldots, m_k \ldots, c; \bar{\bar{c}}; X, Y, Z). \qquad (2.2)$$

which states that the change in the synaptic weight ($\dot{m}_j$) is a function (F)
of the input to that synapse (d_j), the other inputs and weights ($d_k \ldots$,
, $m_k \ldots$), the output of the postsynaptic neuron (c) and its history ($\bar{\bar{c}}$), and
other factors (X, Y, Z). Here variables such as d_j, m_j are designated local. These represent information (such as the incoming signal, d_j, and the
strength of the synaptic junction, m_j) available locally at the j'th synaptic junction. Variables such as $d_k, \ldots, c$ are designated quasi-local. These
represent information (such as c, the depolarization or *activity* of the postsynaptic cell, or d_k, the incoming signal to another synaptic junction) that
is not locally available to the j'th junction but is physically connected to
the junction by the cell body itself–thus necessitating some form of internal communication between various parts of the cell and its synaptic
junctions. Global variables are designated $X, Y, Z, \ldots$. These latter represent information (e.g. presence or absence of neuro-modulators such as
nor-epinephrine or acetylcholine or the average activity of large numbers of

cortical cells) that is present in a similar fashion for all or a large number of cortical neurons (distinguished from local or quasi-local variables presumably carrying detailed information that varies from synapse to synapse or cell to cell). The quantity, $\bar{\bar{c}}$ represents time averaged post-synaptic activity. The appropriate definition of averaged pre- or post-synaptic cell activity very likely depends on the situation being analyzed; In some situations [Abeles, 1981; Markram et al., 1997], the precise timing of each spike may be essential. For example, if one is interested in information conveyed by the detailed timing of neuronal spikes as in synfire chains [Abeles, 1981] timing on the order of milliseconds is important and, as has recently been shown [Abbott et al., 1997; Tsodyks and Markram, 1996], the equilibrium response of the post-synaptic neuron is related in a somewhat more complicated manner to the input – a key issue may be whether equilibrium or transient properties are most relevant.

At the other extreme, global variables are likely determined by the activity of groups of neurons producing some slow varying quantity of neuromodulators and would be averaged over relatively long periods of time – seconds or even longer.

Pre-synaptic activity appropriate to produce cell depolarization that results in synaptic modification in visual cortex is likely to be of the order of some reasonable part of a second. Variations that are too short [Mioche and Singer, 1989], do not produce effects, whereas averages over more than a second, would clearly lose information. Our definition of d is input integrated over a time period that characterizes the resulting synaptic depolarization that is appropriate for the information communication (very likely transient behavior) relevant to synaptic modification in visual cortex.

The time period over which **m** is modified must be some part of a second in order that relevant information not be lost. (The actual modification does not have to occur in the same time period as that over which information is stored.) Any time period much larger would not preserve information about individual patterns. If our later identification of LTD and LTP as different manifestations of the same process of synaptic modification is correct, then experimental measurement shows that the time for such modifications to be in place is relatively short – of the order of seconds.

The appropriate physiological equivalent for c is not yet known. It is fundamental to the theoretical argument that c express the integrated activity of a group of synapses. This could be all of the synapses on a cell, some dendritic component of a cell or even a small group of cells depending on what is the fundamental processing unit. It is possible that different processing units exist in different regions of cortex.

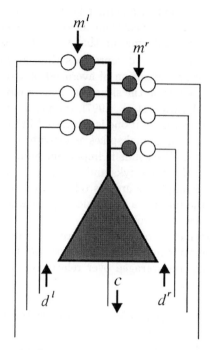

Figure 2.1: Illustrated schematically are pyramidal neurons and the proximal segments of their apical dendrites. In the single cell theory, input is considered only from LGN. d^l, d^r, m^l, m^r are inputs from LGN and synaptic junctions between LGN and cortex.

The time period over which c is averaged, for the reasons given above, is likely some part of a second. It is still not clear whether c is best considered the post-synaptic cell firing rate, integrated post-synaptic depolarization or some other related cell property such as Ca^{++} concentration.

While these are an important experimental questions, our theory is not critically dependent on the interpretation of c (whether, for example, c represents post-synaptic cell depolarization or firing rate). The properties of c that we assume (a continuous, possibly nonlinear, function of the sum of the inputs (previous layer cell activities) times the synaptic efficacies of the relevant synapses) are general enough to fit any reasonable definition of the cell activity.

The appropriate time intervals for the definition of $\mathbf{d}$, c, or for the modification of $\mathbf{m}$, must be clearly distinguished from that for the modification threshold θ_M. As we will discuss in detail below, θ_M varies depending on cell activity. However, the characteristic time for the variation of θ_M is of the order of minutes to hours. Thus, it is very likely that the underlying physiological mechanisms for the variation of θ_M are different from those for modifications of synaptic strengths.

2.3 BCM Synaptic Modification

BCM synaptic modification for active synapses [Bienenstock et al., 1982] is characterized by a negative (depression) region for small values of c, a positive (potentiation) region for large values of c as well as a cross-over point that separates these regions. This cross-over point, called the modification threshold, θ_M, moves as a function of $\bar{\bar{c}}$ and stabilizes the system. All of this can be written*

$$\dot{m}_j = \eta\phi(c, \bar{\bar{c}}; X, Y, Z, \ldots)d_j, \tag{2.3}$$

so that the jth synaptic junction, m_j, changes its value in time as the product of the input activity (the local variable d_j) and a function ϕ of quasi-local and time-averaged quasi-local variables, c and $\bar{\bar{c}}$, as well as global variables X, Y, X. In addition, there is a learning rate, η, which modulates the speed of the weight change but does not change any other property of the learning. Neglecting global variables, one arrives at the following form of synaptic modification equation:

$$\dot{m}_j^{l(r)} = \eta\phi(c, \theta_M)d_j^{l(r)}, \tag{2.4}$$

Where $m^{l(r)}$ and $d^{l(r)}$ are the synaptic efficacies and inputs connecting to the left (right) eye and θ_M is a nonlinear function of some time averaged measure of cell activity, and the constant η is the learning rate.

Since our initial interest is in learning that takes place due to the visual environment, we ignore many other factors that affect learning and memory. These include state of arousal, attention, beginning or end of the critical period and so forth. We believe that these factors, appear as global modulators, or changes in cortical circuitry [Kirkwood and Bear, 1994b], but do not affect the general form of the learning rule. As such, they can be taken out of the learning rule and absorbed into the learning rate, η. The shape of the function ϕ is given in Figure 2.2 for two different values of the threshold θ_M.

What is of particular significance is the change of sign of ϕ at the modification threshold θ_M and the nonlinear variation of θ_M with the average

---

*One can of course envisage a more general dependence on d_j, $\hat{\phi}(c, \bar{\bar{c}}; X, Y, Z, \ldots; d_j)$. Equation 2.3 might be regarded as the lowest order term of a Taylor expansion; the one that most easily can be compared with the pure Hebbian form $\dot{m}_j = cd_j$

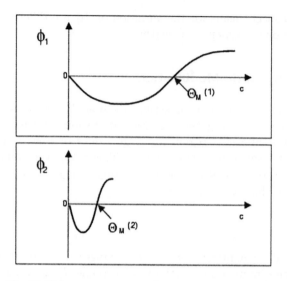

Figure 2.2: The BCM synaptic modification function ϕ plotted against the output of the post-synaptic cell, c, for two values of the modification threshold θ_M. The bottom plot corresponds to lower post-synaptic cell activity. These curves can be compared with the experimental curves in [Kirkwood, et.al. 1996]

output of the cell $\bar{\bar{c}}$. In the form originally proposed by BCM, this was written

$$\theta_M = (\bar{\bar{c}})^2, \tag{2.5}$$

where the average of cell activity is given by a temporal average over the past history of cell activity of the following form:

$$\bar{\bar{c}} = \frac{1}{\tau} \int_{-\infty}^{t} c(t')e^{-\frac{(t-t')}{\tau}} dt'. \tag{2.6}$$

which is the activity integrated over an exponential time window, τ.

A more stable form was given later by Intrator and Cooper[Intrator and Cooper, 1992]:

$$\theta_M = \overline{\overline{c^2}} = \frac{1}{\tau} \int_{-\infty}^{t} c^2(t')e^{-\frac{(t-t')}{\tau}} dt'. \tag{2.7}$$

which is the *squared* activity integrated over an exponential time window, τ.

2.4 One Dimensional Analysis

Although a realistic treatment of synaptic plasticity requires many inputs, and possibly many neurons, it is useful to explore a simple (almost trivial) system that very clearly and succinctly explains some of the properties of the BCM neuron. For this reason we explore a system with one input, denoted by d. The output of the neuron is given by the weight, m, times the input, $c = m \cdot d$. We will assume that the $\phi(c, \theta_M)$ function takes the simplest, parabolic form, with a learning rate $\eta = 1$.

$$\phi(c, \theta_M) = c(c - \theta_M)$$

Thus we have the change in the weights is given by Equation 2.4

$$\dot{m} = c(c - \theta_M)d$$

2.4.1 *Fixed threshold*

In the case of a non-sliding, fixed threshold, $\theta_M \equiv \theta_o$, we have

$$\dot{m} = c(c - \theta_o)d$$

which has fixed points when $c = 0$ and $c = \theta_o$. For input, $d > 0$, we can divide the response, c, into three regions, from which we can infer their stability:

(1) $c < 0$: $\dot{m} > 0$, *c increases*
(2) $c > 0$ and $c < \theta_o$: $\dot{m} < 0$, *c decreases*
(3) $c > \theta_o$: $\dot{m} > 0$, *c increases*

Pictorially, this can be represented as follows.

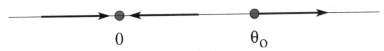

$$0 \qquad\qquad\qquad \theta_o$$

It is clear that the only stable fixed point in this case is the trivial $c = 0$ fixed point. In a multi-pattern environment, this would be an unselective fixed point.

2.4.2 *Instantaneously sliding threshold*

For an instantaneously sliding threshold ($\tau \to 0$ in Equation 2.6), $\theta_M \equiv c^2$, we have

$$\dot{m} = c(c - c^2)d$$
$$\dot{m} = c^2(1 - c)d$$

which has fixed points when $c = 0$ and $c = 1$ (which is also the value of the threshold at the fixed point). Again, for input $d > 0$, we can divide the response, c, into three regions, from which we can infer their stability:

(1) $c < 0$: $\dot{m} > 0$, *c increases*
(2) $c > 0$ and $c < 1$: $\dot{m} > 0$, *c increases*
(3) $c > 1$: $\dot{m} < 0$, *c decreases*

Pictorially, this can be represented as follows.

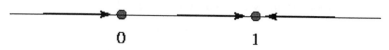

$$0 \qquad\qquad\qquad 1$$

It is clear that the only stable fixed point in this case is the $c = 1$ fixed point. In a multi-pattern environment, this could be (and is almost always) a selective fixed point.

The stability in this case arises from the fact that the threshold adjusts itself. When the output is high, the threshold rises and brings the weights back down. When the output is low, the threshold falls and brings the weights back up. The BCM neurons adjusts the weights to *keep the output constant*. One by-product of this is that the weights will grow to be proportional to $1/d$: the larger the input, the smaller the final weight value, and vice versa.

2.4.3   *Instantaneously sliding threshold with a Probabilistic Input*

In the case of a probabilistic input, namely one that is only presented to the neuron some of the time and a zero input value presented the rest of the time, the fixed point is modified. To see this we make the following observations about Equation 2.8:

- in the case where 0 is presented as input, the weights do not modify (but the threshold does!)
- in the case where d is presented as input, the weights modify exactly the same as before, using Equation 2.8
- if the threshold is the *average* value of c^2, and p is the probability that the input value d is presented (and 0 is presented with probability $(1 - p)$), we obtain $\theta_M = p(m \cdot d)^2 + (1 - p)(m \cdot 0)^2 = pc^2$

The new modification equations are

$$\dot{m} = c(c - pc^2)d$$
$$\dot{m} = c^2(1 - pc)d$$

which has the same stability as the previous example, except that the output (and also the threshold, θ_M), converge to $c = 1/p$, or the inverse of the probability of the input pattern in the environment. The more frequent the pattern, the smaller the overall output of the neuron is.

2.4.4 *Summary of the One Dimensional Case*

In summary, we make the following observations on the one dimensional case, which also translates to all higher dimensions

(1) When there is a *fixed* threshold, the system is unstable, or trivially stable at $c = 0$
(2) The sliding threshold provides stability
(3) The weights change to *keep the output of the neuron constant*
(4) A consequence of the last point is that, for smaller input patterns, the weights grow larger to keep the output constant
(5) The output fixed point converges to a value proportional to (and in many cases equal to) the inverse of the probability of the input pattern in the environment

2.5 The Nonlinear Sliding Threshold

BCM's original choice for θ_M was

$$\theta_M = (\bar{c})^p, \quad p > 1 \tag{2.8}$$

where c is post-synaptic cell activity. For simplicity, they chose $p = 2$ (The consequences of $p \neq 2$ are discussed later.) $\bar{c}$ means an average over the input environment (in early simulations, θ_M was updated with each presentation of the entire input environment – thus, very rapidly adjusting to changes in synaptic strength as well as to changes in the environment. If θ_M is updated instantaneously (say after each input pattern, $\tau \to 0$ in Equation 2.6) θ_M undergoes large and rapid fluctuations. This is unlikely from a physiological point of view and is undesirable mathematically.)

For simplicity, $\bar{c}$ was assumed to be a good approximation to $\bar{\bar{c}}$ the temporal average of the cell's activity.

One problem with Equation 2.8 is that it may become zero for non zero cell activity. This happens when $\bar{d}$, the average over the input activity, is zero. This can be remedied by letting

$$\theta_M = \overline{[c^2]}. \tag{2.9}$$

as was proposed [Intrator, 1990b; Intrator and Cooper, 1992]. A detailed discussion of these various forms will be given in Chapter 3.

From Equation 2.9 we see that θ_M will change gradually through "normal" changes in synaptic strength or perhaps more rapidly due to sudden changes in the visual environment. If θ_M changes too slowly (τ too large in 2.6) it can take too long to catch up with c resulting in large oscillations of cell response and synaptic strength even under normal rearing conditions with no changes in the environment. The non-linear dependence of θ_M on $\bar{\bar{c}}$ guarantees that eventually θ_M will catch up with c. Allowing θ_M to change more rapidly, eliminates large oscillations[†]. Thus, for a given learning rate, η, there is a mathematically reasonable range of τ. An example with a single input neuron with $d = 2$ is shown in Figure 2.3. For the neuron to experience damped oscillations, and converge to the fixed point, the learning rate (η), memory constant (τ) and the input value (d) must be related by $\eta \tau d^2 < 1$. The details are omitted here, but can be found in [Blais, 1998].

However, there are experimental bounds on how rapidly θ_M can change. These are explored in detail in Chapter 7 where simulations using real image inputs are discussed. There it is seen that reasonable values of τ range from a few seconds to an hour. This allows us to infer that the molecular mechanisms that underlie θ_M can be quite different from those responsible for modifications in synaptic strength and might involve gene expression and protein synthesis. This is a particularly attractive hypothesis since θ_M is thought to be a cell property. [We note that when the underlying cellular mechanisms are elucidated, it might turn out that θ_M could change in a more complex manner; for example, the threshold might increase at a rate different from the one at which it decreases.]

Independent of how rapidly θ_M adjusts to new environments, it is clear that the value of θ_M should be quite different in different visual environments (e.g., NR or MD environments as opposed to a BD or RS environment).

As we will see later this accounts for the very different responses of the closed eye(s) in these different environments.

In reverse suture, for example, there can be no recovery of the newly opened eye until θ_M drops to a level low enough so that the cell output ($c = \mathbf{m}^l \cdot \mathbf{d}^c + \mathbf{m}^r \cdot \mathbf{d}^o$)[‡] at least occasionally is larger than θ_M. According to Mioche and Singer (1989), the recovery of the newly opened eye in RS takes several days. How this comes about will be discussed in Chapter 7 where the actual kinetics of such changes are examined in realistic visual

---

[†]However small oscillations can occur and may be measurable.

[‡]which is low initially as the strong weights ($\mathbf{m}^l$) are now connected to the closed eye ($\mathbf{d}^c$) and the small weights of the previously closed eye ($\mathbf{m}^r$) are connected to the open eye ($\mathbf{d}^o$).

environments.

In BD, the initial response of the post-synaptic cell

$$c = \mathbf{m}^l \cdot \mathbf{n}^l + \mathbf{m}^r \cdot \mathbf{n}^r \qquad (2.10)$$

is similar to that in RS, where $\mathbf{n}$ is a vector of noise (from the closed eyes). In Chapter 7 it will be seen that the rate of decrease of the response to the two closed eyes is very sensitive to the rate of decrease of θ_M. There is some experimental suggestion that this rate of fall of cell response is more rapid than is generally believed. [Freeman et al., 1981]

2.6 Analysis of a Two Dimensional Neuron

As was pointed out by BCM, the modification Equation 2.4 results in a temporal competition between patterns, rather than a spatial competition between synapses. This means that only patterns that elicit high post-synaptic activity (beyond the threshold θ_M) will have their concurrently active synapses strengthened (the Hebbian region), while active synapses which elicit post-synaptic activity, but fail to elicit strong enough activity, will have their synapses weakened (anti-Hebbian region).

The occurrence of negative and positive regions for ϕ results in the cell becoming selectively responsive to subsets of stimuli in what we might call a 'normal' visual environment. This happens because the response of the cell is diminished to those patterns for which the output, c, is below threshold (ϕ negative) while the response is enhanced to those patterns for which the output, c, is above threshold (ϕ positive). The non-linear variation of the threshold θ_M with the average output of the cell contributes to the development of selectivity and the stability of the system [Bienenstock et al., 1982; Intrator and Cooper, 1992]. We will demonstrate these and other features of the BCM theory using some very simple examples, below. This will be done by investigating the fixed points of equations 2.3, 2.4 as well as Equation 2.9 as appropriate.

When $\dot{m} = 0$, on average, the weights stop changing. These values of $\mathbf{m}$ are called fixed or critical points. If a small perturbation is added to a weight vector at a fixed point the dynamics may cause the weight vector to either move back to the same fixed point or to move farther away from it. A stable critical or fixed point is one that is stable to such perturbations: the weight vector moves back to the same point after a perturbation. For a non-stable fixed point, the dynamics moves $\mathbf{m}$ from that point after a small perturbation. At a critical point of Equation 2.4, $\dot{m} = 0$ for all inputs, (more precisely, given all input patterns in the environment, the average change in the weights is zero, or $E[\dot{m}] = 0$). The properties of such fixed points (if they do exist) depend upon the input environment $\{\mathbf{d}\}$. Examples of this dependence are discussed in the following sections.

To illustrate this and other qualitative properties as clearly as possible, we analyze the behavior of a single neuron with two synaptic junctions (Figure 2.4) in various environments.

We use a modification threshold in the instantaneous limit ($\tau \rightarrow 0$) in which ($\bar{\bar{c}}$) of Equation 2.6 is replaced by an average over the environment

$$\bar{\bar{c}} \rightarrow \bar{c} = \mathbf{m} \cdot \bar{\mathbf{d}}. \tag{2.11}$$

The importance of non-zero values of τ is been discussed above (Section 2.5).

2.6.1   *Two input environment*

We consider first an environment consisting of two non-parallel input vectors $\mathbf{d}^1$ and $\mathbf{d}^2$ (Figure 2.5) with probability p_1 and p_2 respectively. These vectors span the two-dimensional space. We have chosen the points to lie in the first quadrant, since it represents positive activity levels

In this situation there are two stable solutions (projection directions) $\mathbf{m}^1$ and $\mathbf{m}^2$; each has the property of being orthogonal to one of the inputs (Figure 2.5). In a higher dimensional space, for n linearly independent inputs, a stable solution is one that it is orthogonal to all but one of the inputs.

For analysis of the stability of the solution we replace Equation 2.4, the stochastic differential equation, by the same equation averaged over the input environment, resulting in the deterministic differential equation:

$$\dot{\mathbf{m}} = \eta[p_1\phi(c(\mathbf{d}^1), \theta_M)\mathbf{d}^1 + p_2\phi(c(\mathbf{d}^2), \theta_M)\mathbf{d}^2], \tag{2.12}$$

This equation is just Equation 2.4 summed over the two different input patterns, $\mathbf{d}^1$ and $\mathbf{d}^2$, weighted by their probability of occurring in the input environment, p_1 and p_2 respectively. This equation represents the averaged or the expected value of Equation 2.4. This environment would represent two distinct input patterns entering a single eye. Detailed mathematical conditions and equivalence between the two dynamical systems is discussed in Appendix 3A. For now, we concentrate on the study of Equation 2.12.

There are four critical points to this equation, we denote them by pairs of $\mathbf{m}^i, \theta_M{}^i$, where we use a superscript on $\mathbf{m}$ and θ to denote the fixed point number. At a critical point $\dot{\mathbf{m}}^i = 0$, thus

$$\phi(c(\mathbf{d}^1), \theta_M) = \phi(c(\mathbf{d}^2), \theta_M) = 0. \tag{2.13}$$

This holds if $c(\mathbf{d}^i) = 0$, or $c(\mathbf{d}^i) = \theta_M$, for $i = 1, 2$ and leads to four possible critical points:

(1) $\mathbf{m}^1$ such that $\mathbf{m}^1 \cdot \mathbf{d}^2 = 0$, and $\mathbf{m}^1 \cdot \mathbf{d}^1 = \theta_M^1$.
(2) $\mathbf{m}^2$, such that $\mathbf{m}^2 \cdot \mathbf{d}^1 = 0$, and $\mathbf{m}^2 \cdot \mathbf{d}^2 = \theta_M^2$.
(3) $\mathbf{m}^3 = 0$, so that $\mathbf{m}^3 \cdot \mathbf{d}^1 = \mathbf{m}^3 \cdot \mathbf{d}^2 = 0$.
(4) $\mathbf{m}^4$ such that $\mathbf{m}^4 \cdot \mathbf{d}^1 = \mathbf{m}^4 \cdot \mathbf{d}^2 = \theta_M^4$ [§].

We call the critical points, $\mathbf{m}^1$ and $\mathbf{m}^2$ selective fixed points, because the neuron has a positive response ($c = \theta_M^1$ or $c = \theta_M^2$, respectively) to only one of the patterns and a response of zero to the other pattern. Fixed points $\mathbf{m}^3$ and $\mathbf{m}^4$ are not selective because the neuron responds to both patterns with the same response, $c = 0$ and $c = \theta_M^4$ respectively.

2.6.2 Stability analysis

A fundamental property of the BCM critical points is that only those that are selective are stable. This is illustrated in the two input example for $p_1 = p_2 = 1/2$ below.

Selective Critical Points

Consider the selective critical point

$$\mathbf{m}^1 \cdot \mathbf{d}^1 = \theta_M^1$$
$$\mathbf{m}^1 \cdot \mathbf{d}^2 = 0, \tag{2.14}$$

where $\theta_M^1 = E[c^2] = \frac{1}{2}[(\mathbf{m}^1 \cdot \mathbf{d}^1)^2 + (\mathbf{m}^1 \cdot \mathbf{d}^2)^2] = \frac{1}{2}(\theta_M{}^1)^2$ so that $\theta_M^1 = 2$.
For a small perturbation such that

$$\mathbf{m} = \mathbf{m}^1 + \mathbf{x}.$$

The two inputs give

$$\mathbf{m} \cdot \mathbf{d}^1 = \theta_M^1 + \mathbf{x} \cdot \mathbf{d}^1$$
$$\mathbf{m} \cdot \mathbf{d}^2 = \mathbf{x} \cdot \mathbf{d}^2, \tag{2.15}$$

so that

$$\theta_M = \theta_M^1 + 2\mathbf{x} \cdot \mathbf{d}^1 + \text{(terms of order } x^2). \tag{2.16}$$

(In this analysis we allow θ_M to adjust instantaneously. Slower adjustment may result in oscillations, as described in Section 2.5 and require more complicated analysis.)

[§] such that $\mathbf{m}^4 = 0.5(\mathbf{d}^1 + \mathbf{d}^2)$.

At $c \simeq 0$ and $c \simeq \theta_M$ we make linear approximations: the slope of ϕ at those stable points. We apply this linear expansion of ϕ to obtain

$$\phi \simeq -\epsilon_2 c, \qquad c \simeq 0,$$
$$\phi \simeq \epsilon_1(c - \theta_M), \quad c \simeq \theta_M. \qquad (2.17)$$

where ϵ_1 and ϵ_2 are the slopes of the modification function about θ_M and 0, respectively, as shown in Figure 2.6 (Note that for the Quadratic BCM, $\epsilon_1 = \epsilon_2 = \theta_M$.) When a pattern is presented and it yields a response around θ_M, we refer to this pattern as *preferred*. When a pattern is presented and it yields a response around 0, we refer to this pattern as *non-preferred*. In the present situation, the environment consists of only two cases: preferred and non-preferred patterns.

In order to examine whether the fixed point is stable we examine if on average the norm of the perturbation $\| \mathbf{x} \|$ increases or decreases in time. If $\| \mathbf{x} \|$ decreases then the point is stable, if it increases then the point it is non stable.

For the preferred input, $\mathbf{d}^1$,

$$\dot{\mathbf{x}} = -\epsilon_1(c - \theta_M)\mathbf{d}^1$$
$$= -\epsilon_1[(\mathbf{m}^1 + \mathbf{x}) \cdot \mathbf{d}^1 - \theta_M^* - 2\mathbf{x} \cdot \mathbf{d}^1 + O(\| \mathbf{x} \|^2)]\mathbf{d}^1$$
$$\simeq -\epsilon_1(\mathbf{x} \cdot \mathbf{d}^1)\mathbf{d}^1 \qquad (2.18)$$

For the non-preferred input, $\mathbf{d}^2$,

$$\dot{\mathbf{x}} = -\epsilon_2(\mathbf{x} \cdot \mathbf{d}^2)\mathbf{d}^2. \qquad (2.19)$$

using $\frac{1}{2}\frac{d}{dt} \| \mathbf{x} \|^2 = \mathbf{x} \cdot \dot{\mathbf{x}}$, we obtain

$$\frac{d}{dt}E[\| \mathbf{x} \|^2] = \frac{1}{2}\left[\frac{1}{2}\mathbf{x} \cdot \left(-\epsilon_1 \left(x \cdot \mathbf{d}^1\right)\mathbf{d}^1 - \epsilon_2(x \cdot \mathbf{d}^2)\mathbf{d}^2\right)\right] \qquad (2.20)$$

$$= -\frac{1}{4}\left[\epsilon_1(\mathbf{x} \cdot \mathbf{d}^1)^2 + \epsilon_2(\mathbf{x} \cdot \mathbf{d}^2)^2\right] \leq 0, \qquad (2.21)$$

so that $\| \mathbf{x} \|^2 \to 0$; and the selective critical point is stable.

Non-selective critical points

(1) For critical point (3) where $\mathbf{m}^3 = 0$ and $\theta_M^3 = 0$[¶]

$$\mathbf{m}^3 \cdot \mathbf{d}^1 = \mathbf{m}^3 \cdot \mathbf{d}^2 = 0. \qquad (2.22)$$

[¶]Unlike the modification form presented in [Bienenstock et al., 1982], the quadratic modification form [Intrator and Cooper, 1992] can not have $\theta_M = 0$ as a critical point, unless all the weights are zero.

At this point, all the synaptic weights are zero so that

$$\theta_M = E[c^2] = \frac{1}{2}[((\mathbf{m}^3 + \mathbf{x}) \cdot \mathbf{d}^1)^2 + ((\mathbf{m}^3 + \mathbf{x}) \cdot \mathbf{d}^2)^2],$$
$$= \frac{1}{2}[(\mathbf{x} \cdot \mathbf{d}^1)^2 + (\mathbf{x} \cdot \mathbf{d}^2)^2]. \tag{2.23}$$

This is smaller than $(\mathbf{x} \cdot \mathbf{d}^i)$ $(i = 1, 2)$ for $\mathbf{x}$ small enough. Thus for input $\mathbf{d}_1 > 0$, $\dot{x} = d_1\phi(\mathbf{d}_1) > 0$ and similarly for input $\mathbf{d}_2 > 0$, $\dot{x} = d_1\phi(\mathbf{d}_1) > 0$. Therefore, since $\frac{1}{2}\frac{d}{dt} \parallel \mathbf{x} \parallel^2 = \mathbf{x} \cdot \dot{\mathbf{x}}$ we have that $\frac{d}{dt}E[\parallel \mathbf{x} \parallel^2] \geq 0$ Therefore this critical point is not stable.

(2) For the critical point $\mathbf{m}^4$,

$$\mathbf{m}^4 \cdot \mathbf{d}^1 = \mathbf{m}^4 \cdot \mathbf{d}^2 = \theta_M^4,$$

In this case $\theta_M^4 = 1$. Again, let $\mathbf{m} = \mathbf{m}^4 + \mathbf{x}$, then

$$\theta_M = \theta_M^4 + \mathbf{x} \cdot (\mathbf{d}^1 + \mathbf{d}^2) + O(\parallel \mathbf{x} \parallel^2). \tag{2.24}$$

thus for $\mathbf{d}_1$: $\dot{x} = \epsilon_1 (\mathbf{x} \cdot \mathbf{d}_1 - \mathbf{x} \cdot (\mathbf{d}_1 + \mathbf{d}_2)(\mathbf{x} + \mathbf{d}_1))$
and for $\mathbf{d}_2$: $\dot{x} = \epsilon_2 (\mathbf{x} \cdot \mathbf{d}_1 - \mathbf{x} \cdot (\mathbf{d}_1 + \mathbf{d}_2)(\mathbf{x} + \mathbf{d}_2))$
so that

$$\frac{d}{dt}E[\parallel \mathbf{x} \parallel^2] = -\epsilon_1(\mathbf{x} \cdot \mathbf{d}^1)(\mathbf{x} \cdot \mathbf{d}^2), \tag{2.25}$$

It is sufficient that there is one direction of $\mathbf{x}$ for which Equation 2.25 is positive for the critical point to be unstable, and it can easily be made positive (for example by setting $\mathbf{x} \propto -(\mathbf{d}^1 + \mathbf{d}^2)$). Thus, this critical point is unstable.

A property of the fixed points easily seen in the 2D analysis reveals a very important feature of BCM modification. Using the selective fixed point $\mathbf{m}^1$ such that $\mathbf{m}^1 \cdot \mathbf{d}^1 = \theta_M$, and $\mathbf{m}^1 \cdot \mathbf{d}^2 = 0$, and the definition of θ_M as the spatial average of the squared of the activity we get:

$$\mathbf{m}^1 \cdot \mathbf{d}^1 = E[(\mathbf{m}^1 \cdot \mathbf{d})^2] = p_1(\mathbf{m}^1 \cdot \mathbf{d}^1)^2. \tag{2.26}$$

Thus, it follows that

$$c(\mathbf{d}^1) = \mathbf{m}^1 \cdot \mathbf{d}^1 = 1/p_1, \tag{2.27}$$

so that the non-zero activity is proportional to the inverse of the probability of that non-zero activity. This is in sharp contrast to other feature extraction methods, most notably Principal Component Analysis (PCA). In PCA, for example, the length of the vector of weights is either kept fixed at a certain value (say 1) or becomes proportional to the variance of the projections onto that vector. The variance of the activity of that neuron accounts for a fraction of the variance in the environment and the principal components are ordered in descending order of the variance of their activity. In BCM modification, the magnitude of the weight vector is scaled so that maximum activity becomes proportional to the inverse probability of the event to which the cell becomes selective. Thus, the receptive field obtained by BCM modification learning rule, can both signal the presence of a certain feature as well as give an estimate of the probability of that event. As will be seen later (Section 3.3.1), this can be used to detect suspicious coincidences.

2.6.3   *Single input environment*

We next consider an environment consisting of a single input pattern $\{d\} = d^1$. In this case the two dimensional synaptic space is not spanned; The deterministic differential Equation 2.12 becomes

$$\dot{m} = \eta[\phi(c(\mathbf{d}^1), \theta_M)\mathbf{d}^1]. \tag{2.28}$$

The set of critical points is now composed of two lines: $m \cdot \mathbf{d}^1 = \theta_M$ and $m \cdot \mathbf{d}^1 = 0$.

For $\mathbf{m} \cdot \mathbf{d}^1 = \theta_M$ which of the critical points (lying along the dotted line in Figure 2.7 will be reached depends on the initial value of $\mathbf{m}$ (since changes in $\mathbf{m}$ can only be along the direction of $\mathbf{d}^1$).

This very simple example leads us to an important and general observation. Suppose that the real visual environment was best represented by $\{\mathbf{d}^1, \mathbf{d}^2\}$ while $\{\mathbf{d}^1\}$ represents a restricted visual environment – for example only vertical edges. If the animal is reared in the restricted environment, we would expect *reduced selectivity* since the vectors along the fixed line $(\mathbf{m} \cdot \mathbf{d}^1 = \theta_M)$ are not necessarily perpendicular to $\mathbf{d}^2$ (Section 2.6.1). The additional input $\mathbf{d}^2$ is thus required to produce maximum selectivity. There is some experimental evidence suggesting that this may indeed be the case [Blakemore and van Sluyters, 1974; Rauschecker and Singer, 1981].

2.6.4   *Many input environment*

We now consider an environment consisting of a large (possibly infinite) number of vectors $\{\mathbf{d}^1, \mathbf{d}^2, \mathbf{d}^3, \ldots\}$. This is the extreme, opposite to the previous one dimensional case; here the space is over spanned (linearly dependent inputs). We consider two cases; (i) Inputs composed of independent vectors with noise around each. (Figure 2.8) (ii) Inputs randomly spread over the input space – essentially noise.

In the latter situation, the environment is unstructured and therefore there are no stable fixed points. In the former situation, the solution is stable and selective as in the two input case. These very simple examples illustrate some of the main features of the BCM theory. Most of these features are qualitatively preserved even when more complex environments are considered such as K linearly independent input vectors, or even visual environments composed of natural images. However some quantitative properties such as the value of θ_M or its rate of change depend the details of the assumptions:

Among the key features of the BCM theory are the following:

(1) The critical points depend on the environment
(2) In a "normal" or rich environment only selective critical points are stable. In such an environment, this leads to selective (Hubel-Wiesel cells).
(3) A restricted environment generally leads to less selective critical points.
(4) The rate at which θ_M adjusts to changes in post-synaptic cell activity is critical in determining the stability properties of the theory as well as detailed agreement with experiment.

2.7   Some Experimental Consequences

A key feature of the BCM theory is its ability to account for the development of receptive fields in various visual environments. In what follows, we illustrate some of the main qualitative features using a binocular generalization of the above 2 dimensional neuron, as well as a very simple representation of the visual environment.

2.7.1   *Normal Rearing*

The normal visual environment is represented by patterned input to both eyes

$$\mathbf{d} = \{\mathbf{d}^r, \mathbf{d}^l\}.$$

where $\mathbf{d}^r = (d_1^r, d_2^r, \cdots, d_K^r)$ and $\mathbf{d}^l = (d_1^l, d_2^l, \cdots, d_K^l)$ are the right and left eye input vectors.

For such inputs (as illustrated in the 2 dimensional example) we obtain selective fixed points. In addition, if $\mathbf{d}^r = \mathbf{d}^l$ (both eyes see the same patterns at the same time) the visual cortical cells become binocular (misalignment of the eyes will be discussed later). Thus, we obtain $\mathbf{m} \cdot \mathbf{d}^i = \mathbf{m}^l \cdot \mathbf{d}^{li} + \mathbf{m}^r \cdot \mathbf{d}^{ri}$

$$\mathbf{m} \cdot \mathbf{d}^i = \begin{cases} \theta_M & \text{for } i = 1 \text{ (preferred pattern) with probability } \rho_1 \\ 0 & \text{for } i > 1 \text{ (non-preferred pattern) with probability } \rho_2 \end{cases} \tag{2.29}$$

2.7.2 *Monocular deprivation*

One of the most robust and frequently employed alterations of the visual environment is that called *monocular deprivation* (MD). In this manipulation, one eye is closed (either by lid suture, occlusion with an eye patch or silenced in a more dramatic fashion, such as pharmacological blockade) while the other is open and exposed to a normal visual environment. (In a variation, the open eye might be exposed to a restricted or altered visual environment [Rauschecker and Singer, 1981].) The essential and striking experimental result is that for most cells, the response of the closed eye is reduced rapidly [Duffy et al., 1976] to zero. In contrast when both eyes are closed (in the same manner as above) the response to both eyes is reduced, however this effect is probably much slower (how rapidly is not yet clear [Freeman et al., 1981]) and some responsiveness probably remains. An immediate question is why responsiveness is greater when both eyes (rather than only one) are closed. One possible explanation is that there is some form of competition between the two eyes. This might (for example) be due (as was once suggested) to inhibitory connections – a possibility not regarded as likely at present.

Following the argument first given in BCM, we present an analysis of these phenomena from the point of view of the BCM theory. In addition to providing a clear understanding of these experimental results, there are several striking consequences that can be tested further.

The modification of synaptic weights driven by input from the left and right eye (i.e. a binocular neuron) is given by

$$\dot{\mathbf{m}}^{l(r)} = \phi \mathbf{d}^{l(r)}. \tag{2.30}$$

Now consider monocularly deprived visual environment in which the open (left) eye receives normal visual experience while the closed (right) eye is sutured or patched. This environment is represented by

$$\{\mathbf{d}^l, \mathbf{d}^r\} = \{\mathbf{d}^{open}, \mathbf{d}^{closed}\} \rightarrow \{\mathbf{d}, \mathbf{n}\}.$$

where $\mathbf{d}$ represents patterned input from the open eye and $\mathbf{n}$ represents "noise" from the closed eye. We use the symbol $\rightarrow$ to make note of a convention we employ for convenience. Sometimes we differentiate in the equations between the left and right-eye vectors, $\mathbf{d}^l$ and $\mathbf{d}^r$, and sometimes we group them together as one input vector, $\mathbf{d}$, when the distinction is not necessary and we wish to refer to the entire input to the neuron.

We assume now that the deprivation is started after the normal rearing so the receptive field has already reached its fixed point. Further we assume that θ_M is updated very quickly, thus we can assume (without loss of generality) that for the open (left) eye

$$\mathbf{m}^l \cdot \mathbf{d}^{li} = \theta_M \quad i = 1 \quad \text{(preferred input)}$$
$$\mathbf{m}^l \cdot \mathbf{d}^{li} = 0 \quad i > 1 \quad \text{(non} - \text{preferred inputs).} \tag{2.31}$$

where $\mathbf{d}^{li}$ is the *ith* input vector to the left eye. (In a realistic environment, the actual responses fall with some distribution peaking near zero.). Now denote synapses to the closed eye by

$$\mathbf{m}^r = \mathbf{x},$$

and make a linear expansion of ϕ in the region near $c = 0$ and $c = \theta_M$, as shown in Figure 2.6.

Thus

$$\phi \simeq -\epsilon_2 c; \text{ where } c \text{ is near zero}$$
$$\phi \simeq +\epsilon_1(c - \theta_M); \text{ where } c \text{ is near } \theta_M \tag{2.32}$$

The output, c, of the neuron is a function of the weighted inputs from the left, open eye and the weighted noisy input of the right, closed eye and is given by

$$c = \mathbf{m}^l \cdot \mathbf{d}^{li} + \mathbf{x} \cdot \mathbf{n}$$

so that the output for preferred and non-preferred input patterns to the open eye becomes

$$c \simeq \begin{cases} \theta_M + \mathbf{x} \cdot \mathbf{n} & \text{for } i = 1 \\ \mathbf{x} \cdot \mathbf{n} & \text{for } i > 1. \end{cases}$$

the change in the weights from the closed eye is given by

$$\dot{\mathbf{x}} \simeq \begin{cases} +\epsilon_1(\theta_M + \mathbf{x} \cdot \mathbf{n} - \theta_M)\mathbf{n} & \text{for } i = 1 \\ -\epsilon_2(\mathbf{x} \cdot \mathbf{n})\mathbf{n} & \text{for } i > 1 \end{cases}$$

Averaging over the noise input and assuming, for simplicity, that the average noise ($\bar{n}$) is zero, we obtain

$$\dot{\mathbf{x}} \simeq -\epsilon_2 \overline{n^2} \mathbf{x} \text{ for } i > 1. \tag{2.33a}$$

$$\dot{\mathbf{x}} \simeq \epsilon_1 \overline{n^2} \mathbf{x} \text{ for } i = 1. \tag{2.33b}$$

For neurons with dimensionality > 2, most of the patterns would elicit a response $c \approx 0$; this is also the case for more realistic environments (Chapter 6). Therefore Equation 2.33a will dominate the dynamics and will cause a decay of the closed eye weights, thus effectively disconnecting the closed eye from the cell.

Inspection of Equations 2.33a and 2.33b reveals a remarkable counter-intuitive dependence of the rate of disconnection of the closed eye with the noise level from that eye. The larger the noise level ($\overline{n^2}$) the quicker the disconnection. From this we infer that in two comparable MD situations (e.g., lid suture vs. dark patch ||) that differ only in the amount of noise from the closed eye, the case in which the noise is larger (e.g., sutured eye) would disconnect more rapidly. Recent experiments[Rittenhouse et al., 1999] confirm that lid sutured eye does in fact disconnect more rapidly than one with TTX applied. The results are shown in Figure9.6.

Combining Equations 2.33b and 2.33a with the probabilities of the preferred (p_1) and non-preferred patterns ($\sum_{i=2}^{N} p_i$) we get

$$\dot{x} \simeq (\epsilon_1 p_1 - \epsilon_2 \sum_{i=2}^{N} p_i)\overline{n^2}x \qquad (2.34)$$

We observe from Equation 2.34 that the rate at which the closed eye is disconnected depends on the probability that the preferred patterns appear to the open eye compared to the rest of the environment (all of the non-preferred patterns). Normally, for a selective cell, we expect that the probability of the preferred pattern is less than the sum of the probabilities for the rest of the patterns in the environment, $p_1 \ll \sum_{i=2}^{N} p_i$. Before the cell becomes selective to the open eye this argument does not apply.

Thus, in a MD protocol beginning with non-selective cells (e.g., before normal rearing) selectivity for the open eye should develop *before* the closed eye is disconnected. This correlation between selectivity and ocular dominance is clearly seen in our simulations and is suggested in various experimental results [Rauschecker and Singer, 1979; Rauschecker and Singer, 1981; Ramoa et al., 1988; Bear et al., 1990].

Summarized below are some of the interesting features from simulations using K input patterns $\mathbf{d}^1 \ldots \mathbf{d}^K$ distorted by noise.

(a)   Normal rearing: The inputs $\mathbf{d}$ to the cortical cell are a stochastic sequence of patterns $\mathbf{d}^1 \ldots \mathbf{d}^K$ (these patterns represent the response of LGN cells to images presented to the retina). It is assumed that

---

|| It seems reasonable to assume that reducing the noise level in the closed eye by using a dark patch or a TTX injection, would also reduce the noise level in the corresponding layers of LGN which provide the input to the cortical cell (for example see [Rittenhouse et al., 1999].)

under conditions of normal rearing, certain patterns such as edges are a repeated part of the environment. The patterns may be corrupted by noise, but they are statistically independent.

(b) Restricted environment: The pattern space is restricted to one or a few patterns. This is intended to represent the effects of rearing in an environment consisting of perhaps only vertical or horizontal edges.

(c) Dark reared environment: The environment consists of just random noise vectors, which represent the dark discharges of retinal cells.

then various binocular rearing conditions can be represented as follows:

(i) Normal Binocular Rearing (NR): $\mathbf{d}^l(t) = \mathbf{d}^r(t)$ for all time, t.

(ii) Monocular Deprivation (MD): $\mathbf{d}^r$ is a noise term, $\mathbf{d}^r = n$.

(iii) Reverse Suture (RS): $\mathbf{d}^l$ is a noise term, $\mathbf{d}^l = n$.

(iv) Binocular Deprivation (BD): All components of $\mathbf{d}^l$ and $\mathbf{d}^r$ are i.i.d.: $\mathbf{d}^l$ and $\mathbf{d}^r$ are uncorrelated noise terms.

(v) Strabismic Rearing(UR): $\mathbf{d}^l$ and $\mathbf{d}^r$ are independent identically distributed (i.i.d): they have the same distribution, but no statistical relationship exists between them.

(vi) Binocular Recovery (BR): Same input structure as Normal Binocular Rearing, but the initial conditions are set by the fixed point of Monocular Deprivation (MD).

The evolution of the cell's response under these rearing conditions is summarized in Figure 2.9. It is found that simulation of the behavior of the system under these rearing conditions give the following:

(1) NR. All asymptotic states are selective and binocular, with matching preferred orientations for stimulation through each eye.

(2) MD and RS. The only stable asymptotic states are selective and monocular. The cell will converge to one of these states whatever the initial conditions. In particular, this accounts for reverse suture experiments. [Blakemore and van Sluyters, 1974; Movshon, 1976].

(3) BD. The state of the cell undergoes a random walk in phase space. The two tuning curves therefore undergo random fluctuations. These fluctuations may result sometimes in a weak orientation preference or unbalanced ocular dominance. However, the system never stays in such states very long; its average state on the long run is perfectly binocular and non-oriented. Moreover, whatever the second order statistics of $\mathbf{d}$ and the circular environment in which tuning curves are assessed, a regular unimodal orientation tuning curve is rarely observed, and selectivity as observed in the NR case (both experimental and theoretical) cannot be obtained from purely random synaptic weights.

(4) UR. This rearing environment causes the cell to converge to equilibrium

states that are like those found in MD: the state of the cell converges to selective and monocular equilibria. However, unlike MD there are intermediate states that are selective and binocular, with mismatched and orientation preferences in the two eyes.

(5) BR. This rearing environment causes the cell to recover from MD, with selective fixed points identical to NR.

These results are in agreement with the experimental data in the domain of visual cortex development, and generalize to more complex environments such as natural images (see Figure 7.5) discussed later.

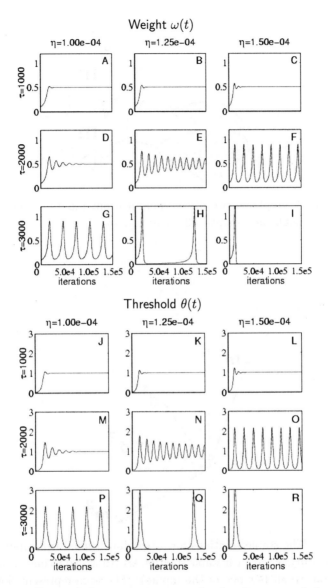

Figure 2.3: Effects of the parameters on the development of the one dimensional neuron. The value of the weight, m, and the threshold, θ, are shown as functions of time for different values of the learning rate, η, and the memory constant, τ. The value of the input here is $d = 2$, so the fixed point should be $m = 1/2$ and $\theta = 1$. For the neuron to experience damped oscillations, and converge to the fixed point, the learning rate (η), memory constant (τ) and the input value (d) must be related by $\eta\tau d^2 < 1$.

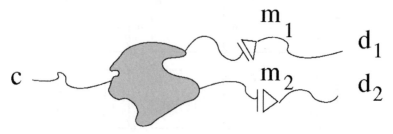

Figure 2.4: A simplified two dimensional neuron: inputs d_1, d_2 affect the output c through the synaptic efficacies m_1, m_2.

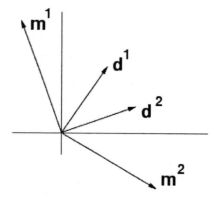

Figure 2.5: The stable solutions for a two dimensional two input problem are m_1 and m_2. Each such stable solution is orthogonal to one of the inputs (in general, to all but one of the inputs). The axes represent both input magnitude (for the **d** vectors) and weight magnitude (for the **m** vectors). It is conceptually simpler to view the mathematical orthogonality on the same plot, even though in reality these quantities would be measured in different units.

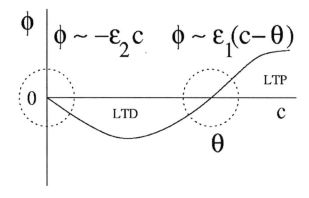

Figure 2.6: Linear approximation of ϕ for a selective neuron

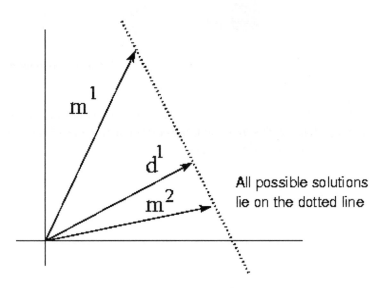

Figure 2.7: Under a restricted (one input environment) of a 2 dimensional neuron, all possible solutions for $\mathbf{m} \cdot \mathbf{d}^1 = \theta_M$ lie on the dotted line which is perpendicular to the single input $\mathbf{d}^1$.

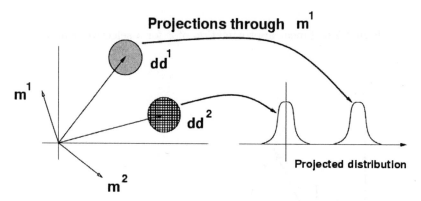

Figure 2.8: The stable solutions for a two dimensional two input problem are m_1 and m_2. Each such stable solution is orthogonal to one of the inputs (in general, to all but one of the inputs).

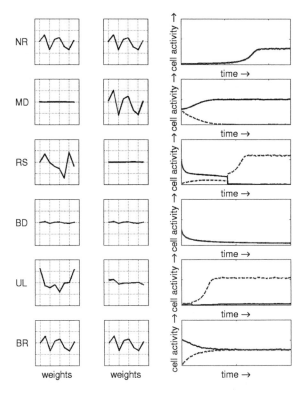

Figure 2.9: BCM Simulations in an Environment of 8 Linearly Independent Vectors. Left: Final weight configuration, left and right eyes. Right: Maximum response to patterns in the environment through the left eye (solid line) and the right eye (dashed line), as a function of time. Simulations from top to bottom are as follows. Normal Rearing (NR): both eyes presented with patterned input. Monocular Deprivation (MD): following NR, one eye is presented with noisy input and the other with patterned input. Reverse Suture: following MD, the eye given noisy input is now given patterned input, and the other eye is given noisy input. Binocular Deprivation (BD): following NR, both eyes are given noisy input. **It is important to note that for BCM if Binocular Deprivation is run longer, selectivity will eventually be lost.**. Strabismus (UR): both eyes are presented with patterned input, but the patterns presented to each eye are uncorrelated eith each other. Binocular Recovery: following MD, both eyes presented with patterned input.

Appendix 2A

Stability of BCM with a Weight Decay Term, in a Linearly Independent Environment

Although the BCM equations do not require any weight decay term for stability, it is likely that weight decay mechanisms exist biologically. In this appendix we explore some of the initial consequences of introducing a weight decay term.

2A.1 Initial Fixed Points

We start with the quadratic BCM equations, with a decay term:

$$c = \mathbf{m} \cdot \mathbf{d} \qquad (2A.1)$$

$$\dot{\mathbf{m}} = c(c - \theta)\mathbf{d} - \lambda\mathbf{m} \qquad (2A.2)$$

$$\theta = E\left[c^2\right] \qquad (2A.3)$$

Multiply both sides of Equation 2A.2 by $\mathbf{d}$, and define θ in terms of the output values and the probability of each pattern (this limits the decay to active synapse $(d > 0)$):

$$\dot{c}_i = c_i \left(c_i - \sum_j p_j c_j^2 \right) d_i^2 - \lambda c_i$$

Define the norm of the input vector for pattern i as $n_i \equiv d_i^2$, factor the λ in, and define $\epsilon_i = \lambda/n_i$.

$$\dot{c}_i = n_i c_i \left(c_i - \epsilon_i - \sum_j p_j c_j^2 \right) \qquad (2A.4)$$

We have a set of fixed points with all combinations of the following:

$$c_i = 0$$

$$c_i = \epsilon_i + \sum_j p_j c_j^2$$

We look only at two sets of fixed points:

1   $c_i = 0$ for all i (zero fixed point)
2   $c_i = 0$ for all $i > 1$, $c_1 = \epsilon_1 + \sum_j p_j c_j^2 = \epsilon_1 + p_1 c_1^2$ or (selective fixed point)

$$c_1 = \frac{1}{2p_1}\left(1 \pm \sqrt{1 - 4\epsilon_1 p_1}\right) \equiv \frac{\gamma_{1\pm}}{2p_1}$$

$$c_i = 0 \text{ for all } i > 1$$

For the others it is difficult to determine the stability.

2A.1.1   *Consistency*

If $\lambda = 0$, then $\gamma_+ = 2$ and $\gamma_- = 0$. This leads to the familiar fixed points $c_1 = 1/p_1, c_2 = 0$ and $c_1 = 0, c_2 = 0$.

2A.2   Stability

To determine the stability, we look at the Jacobian of the Equation(s) 2A.4:

$$J_{ij} \equiv \frac{\partial \dot{c}_i}{\partial c_j}$$

For $i = j$ this becomes

$$J_{ii} = n_i \left(2c_i - \epsilon_i - 3p_i c_i^2 - \sum_{j \neq i} p_j c_j^2\right)$$

For $i \neq j$ this becomes

$$J_{ij}|_{i \neq j} = n_i \left(-2p_j c_j c_i\right)$$

For the two sets of fixed points, we have:

1 $c_i = 0$ for all i

$$J = \begin{pmatrix} -\epsilon_1 & 0 & 0 & \cdots \\ 0 & -\epsilon_2 & 0 & \cdots \\ 0 & 0 & \ddots & \end{pmatrix}$$

2 $c_i = 0$ for all $i > 1$, $c_1 = \epsilon + \sum_j p_j c_j^2 = \epsilon_1 + p_1 c_1^2$

$$J = \begin{pmatrix} n_1\left(\frac{\gamma_{1\pm}}{p_1} - \epsilon_1 - \frac{3p_1}{4p_1^2}\gamma_{1\pm}^2\right) & 0 & 0 & 0 \cdots \\ 0 & n_2\left(-\epsilon_2 - \frac{p_1}{4p_1^2}\gamma_{1\pm}^2\right) & 0 & 0 \cdots \\ 0 & 0 & n_3\left(-\epsilon_3 - \frac{p_1}{4p_1^2}\gamma_{1\pm}^2\right) & 0 \\ 0 & 0 & 0 & \ddots \end{pmatrix}$$

For stability, the eigenvalues all have to be negative. If all of the off diagonal terms are zero, then this amounts to all of the diagonal terms being negative. For the two sets of fixed points, we have:

1 $c_i = 0$ for all i: The diagonals are all negative, so this point is stable.
2 $c_i = 0$ for all $i > 1$, $c_1 = \epsilon + \sum_j p_j c_j^2 = \epsilon_1 + p_1 c_1^2$

Like above, the Jacobian is diagonal. The diagonal terms are:

$$J_{11} = \underbrace{n_1\left(\frac{\gamma_{1\pm}}{p_1} - \epsilon_1 - \frac{3p_1}{4p_1^2}\gamma_{1\pm}^2\right)}_{\text{needs to be } <0}$$

$$J_{22} = \underbrace{n_2\left(-\epsilon_2 - \frac{p_1}{4p_1^2}\gamma_{1\pm}^2\right)}_{\text{already } <0}$$

$$J_{33} = \underbrace{n_3\left(-\epsilon_3 - \frac{p_1}{4p_1^2}\gamma_{1\pm}^2\right)}_{\text{already } <0}$$

$$\vdots$$

Expand the $\gamma_{1\pm}$ we get:

$$\gamma_{1\pm} \equiv 1 \pm \sqrt{1 - 4\epsilon_1 p_1}$$
$$\approx 1 \pm (1 - 2\epsilon_1 p_1)$$

$$= \begin{cases} (+) & 2 - 2\epsilon_1 p_1 \\ (-) & +2\epsilon_1 p_1 \end{cases}$$

$$\gamma_{1\pm}^2 = 1 \pm 2\sqrt{1 - 4\epsilon_1 p_1} + (1 - 4\epsilon_1 p_1)$$

$$\approx 2 - 4\epsilon_1 p_1 \pm 2\left(1 - 2\epsilon_1 p_1 + 4\epsilon_1^2 p_1^2\right)$$

$$= \begin{cases} (+) & 4 - 8\epsilon_1 p_1 + 8\epsilon_1^2 p_1^2 \approx 4 - 8\epsilon_1 p_1 \\ (-) & -8\epsilon_2^2 p_1^2 \approx 0 \end{cases}$$

The Jacobian, first element, less than zero reduces to

$$n_1\left(\frac{\gamma_{1\pm}}{p_1} - \epsilon_1 - \frac{3p_1}{4p_1^2}\gamma_{1\pm}^2\right) < 0$$

$$\frac{\gamma_{1\pm}}{p_1} - \epsilon_1 - \frac{3}{4p_1}\gamma_{1\pm}^2 < 0$$

(+)

$$\frac{2 - 2\epsilon_1 p_1}{p_1} - \epsilon_1 - \frac{3(4 - 8\epsilon_1 p_1)}{4p_1} < 0 \qquad (2A.5)$$

$$-\frac{1}{p_1} + 3\epsilon_1 < 0 \qquad (2A.6)$$

$$\epsilon_1 < \frac{1}{3p_1} \qquad (2A.7)$$

(-)

$$\frac{+\epsilon_1 p_1}{p_1} - \epsilon_1 - \frac{3}{4p_1}\left(-8\epsilon_1^2 p_1^2\right) = \epsilon_1 + 3p_1\epsilon_1^2$$

$$> 0 \Rightarrow \text{ (unstable)}$$

$\gamma_\pm$ must be real

$$\gamma_{1\pm} \equiv 1 \pm \sqrt{1 - 4\epsilon_1 p_1} \qquad (2A.8)$$

$$\Rightarrow 1 - 4\epsilon_1 p_1 > 0 \qquad (2A.9)$$

$$\Rightarrow \epsilon_1 < \frac{1}{4p_1} \qquad (2A.10)$$

2A.2.1 *Consistency*

If $\lambda = 0$, the (+) solution is simply $-1/p_1$, so the fixed point is stable.

2A.2.2 *Consequences*

The consequence of Equations 2A.7 and 2A.10 is that for stability it is required that

$$\epsilon_1 < \frac{1}{4p_1} \qquad (2A.11)$$

$$\lambda < \frac{n_1}{4p_1} \qquad (2A.12)$$

This means that the weight decay selectively makes unstable the fixed points for *common* patterns ($p_1 \gg 1$) or *weak* patterns ($n_1 \ll 1$).

Chapter 3

Objective Function Formulation

3.1 Introduction

In this chapter, we present an objective function formulation of the BCM theory that enables us to demonstrate the connection between unsupervised BCM learning and various statistical methods, in particular, that of Projection Pursuit. It provides a general method for stability analysis of the fixed points of the theory and enables us to analyze the behavior and the evolution of the network under various visual rearing conditions. It also allows comparison with many existing unsupervised methods.

In this framework, we extend the single-neuron learning rule to nonlinear neurons and to a network of laterally connected neurons. The formulation via objective function gives a natural form for the learning rule as gradient descent optimization. The objective function formulation of the BCM theory has led us to modify slightly our learning rule resulting in improved stability and statistical properties (Appendix 3A presents some mathematical results concerning the convergence and characterization of the fixed points.) This variant of the BCM rule has some advantages over the original exploratory projection pursuit model [Friedman, 1987]. Due to its computational efficiency, it can extract several features in parallel, taking into account the interaction between the different extracted features via a lateral inhibition network. Feature extraction based on this model has been applied to various real-world problems [Intrator et al., 1996; Huynh et al., 1996; Tankus et al., 1997; Dotan and Intrator, 1998].

3.2 Formulation of the BCM Theory Using an Objective Function

The objective function formulation of the synaptic modification theory of Bienenstock, Cooper and Munro (BCM) yields a statistically plausible objective function whose minimization finds those projections having a single dimensional projected distribution that is far from Gaussian.

This formulation allows us to interpret the biological neuron's behavior from a statistical point of view. In addition, it provides a more powerful means of investigating the kinetics of synaptic development as well as the location and stability of the fixed points under various environmental conditions.

3.2.1 *Single Neuron*

We first informally describe the statistical formulation that leads to this objective function. Using a metaphor motivated by statistical decision theory, a neuron is considered as capable of making a certain binary decision (possibly firing) given a level of internal activity that can be associated with some neuro-transmitter activation. This decision is dependent on the input and synaptic weight vectors. A loss function is attached to each decision. The neuron's task is then to make the decision that minimizes the loss. Since the loss function depends on the synaptic weight vector in addition to the input vector, it is natural to seek a synaptic weight vector that will minimize the sum of the losses associated with all inputs, or more precisely, the expected loss (also called the risk). The search for such a vector, which yields an optimal synaptic weight vector in this formulation, can be viewed as learning or parameter estimation. In those cases where the risk is a smooth function, its minimization can be accomplished by gradient descent (keeping in mind that the procedure can get stuck in a local minimum).

The ideas presented so far make no specific assumptions about the loss function, and it is clear that different loss functions may yield different learning procedures. For example, if the loss function is related to the inverse of the projection variance (including some normalization) then minimizing the risk finds directions that maximize the variance of the projections, i.e., the principal components.

Before presenting a loss function, let us more precisely define the neuronal input, and two useful functions: We consider a neuron with input vector $\mathbf{d} = (d_1, \ldots, d_n)$, synaptic weight vector $\mathbf{m} = (m_1, \ldots, m_n)$, both in R^n, and activity (in the linear region) $c = (\mathbf{m} \cdot \mathbf{d})$. The input $\mathbf{d}$ is assumed to be a bounded, and piece-wise constant stochastic process. We allow some time dependence in the presentation of the training patterns*. These assumptions are plausible, since they represent the closest continuous approximation to the usual training algorithms, in which training patterns are presented at random. They are needed for the approximation of the resulting deterministic gradient descent by a stochastic one [Intrator, 1990a,

---

*Formally, we require that d is Type II mixing which allows some dependence of the future of the process on its past (Further details are in Appendix 3A.)

See Appendix 3A]. For this reason we use a *learning rate* μ that has to decay in time so that this approximation is valid.

Our projection index is aimed at finding directions for which the projected distribution is far from Gaussian (See discussion in Section 3.4); more specifically, since high dimensional clusters have a multi-modal projected distribution, our aim is to find a projection index (loss function) that emphasizes multi-modality. For computational efficiency, we would like to base the projection index on polynomial moments of low degree. Using second degree polynomials, one can get measures of the mean and variance of the distribution; these, however, do not give information on multi-modality; therefore, higher order polynomials are necessary. Further, the projection index should exhibit the fact that bimodal distribution is already interesting, and any additional mode should make the distribution even more interesting. A discussion and comparison with other projection index methods is given in Section 3.5

With this in mind, consider the following family of loss functions that depend on the synaptic weight vector and on the input $\mathbf{d}$. Define the threshold $\theta_M = E[(\mathbf{m} \cdot \mathbf{d})^2]$, and the functions $\hat{\phi}(c, \theta_M) = c^2 - \frac{1}{2} c \theta_M$, $\phi(c, \theta_M) = c^2 - c \theta_M$.

$$
\begin{aligned}
L_m(\mathbf{d}) &= -\mu \int_0^{(\mathbf{m} \cdot \mathbf{d})} \hat{\phi}(s, \theta_M) ds \\
&= -\mu \{ \frac{1}{3} (\mathbf{m} \cdot \mathbf{d})^3 - \frac{1}{4} E[(\mathbf{m} \cdot \mathbf{d})^2](\mathbf{m} \cdot \mathbf{d})^2 \}
\end{aligned}
\tag{3.1}
$$

The motivation for this loss function can be seen in Figure 3.1, which represents the ϕ function and the associated loss function $L_m(\mathbf{d})$. For simplicity the loss for a fixed threshold θ_M and synaptic vector $\mathbf{m}$ can be written as $L_m(c) = -\mu c^2 (\frac{c}{3} - \frac{\theta_M}{4})$, where c represents the linear projection of $\mathbf{d}$ onto $\mathbf{m}$. [The loss can also be viewed as measuring the amount of energy dissipation or neuro-transmitter release for a given neuronal activity level $(\mathbf{m} \cdot \mathbf{d})$ and an instantaneous nonlinear transmitter release $\hat{\phi}$ that depends on the activity history θ_M.]

The graph of the loss function shows that for any fixed m and Θ_m, the loss is small for a given input $\mathbf{d}$, when either $c = (\mathbf{m} \cdot \mathbf{d})$ is close to zero, or when $(\mathbf{m} \cdot \mathbf{d})$ is larger than Θ_m. Moreover, the loss function remains negative for $(\mathbf{m} \cdot \mathbf{d}) > \theta_M$, therefore any kind of distribution at the right hand side of θ_M is possible, and the preferred ones are those which are concentrated further from θ_M.

The sliding threshold θ_M is dynamic and depends on $(\mathbf{m} \cdot \mathbf{d})$ in a non-linear way. It follows that $\theta_M = E(\mathbf{m} \cdot \mathbf{d})^2$ always moves itself to a position such that the distribution will never be concentrated at only one of its sides. This is because $(\mathbf{m} \cdot \mathbf{d})^2 < (\mathbf{m} \cdot \mathbf{d})$, for $(\mathbf{m} \cdot \mathbf{d}) < 1$, and $(\mathbf{m} \cdot \mathbf{d})^2 > (\mathbf{m} \cdot \mathbf{d})$,

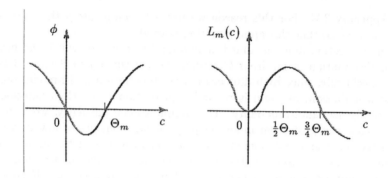

Figure 3.1: The function ϕ and the loss functions for a fixed m and θ_M.

for $(\mathbf{m} \cdot \mathbf{d}) > 1$.

The risk (expected value of the loss) is given by:

$$R_m = -\mu E\{\frac{1}{3}(\mathbf{m} \cdot \mathbf{d})^3 - \frac{1}{4}E[(\mathbf{m} \cdot \mathbf{d})^2](\mathbf{m} \cdot \mathbf{d})^2\}$$
$$= -\mu\{\frac{1}{3}E[(\mathbf{m} \cdot \mathbf{d})^3] - \frac{1}{4}E^2[(\mathbf{m} \cdot \mathbf{d})^2]\}. \qquad (3.2)$$

Since the risk is continuously differentiable, its minimization can be achieved via a gradient descent method with respect to m, namely:

$$\frac{dm_i}{dt} = -\frac{\partial}{\partial m_i}R_m = \mu\ \{E[(\mathbf{m} \cdot \mathbf{d})^2 d_i] - E[(\mathbf{m} \cdot \mathbf{d})^2]E[(\mathbf{m} \cdot \mathbf{d})_i]\}$$
$$= \mu\ E[\phi((\mathbf{m} \cdot \mathbf{d}), \theta_M)d_i]. \qquad (3.3)$$

A more general form according to the objective function formulation has the form:

$$\theta_M = E[(\mathbf{m} \cdot \mathbf{d})^p],$$

and

$$R_m = -\mu\frac{1}{2p-1}E[(\mathbf{m} \cdot \mathbf{d})^{2p-1} + \frac{1}{2p}E^2[(\mathbf{m} \cdot \mathbf{d})^p].$$

The implied stochastic synaptic modification equation has the form:

$$\dot{m} = \mu(\mathbf{m} \cdot \mathbf{d})^{p-1}\{(\mathbf{m} \cdot \mathbf{d})^{p-1} - \theta_M\}\mathbf{d}. \qquad p > 1 \qquad (3.4)$$

The resulting differential equations give a somewhat different version of the law governing synaptic weight modification of the BCM theory (1982). The difference lies in the way the threshold θ_M is defined. In the original form this threshold was $\theta_M = E^p(c)$ for $p > 1$, while in the current form $\theta_M = E(c^p)$ for $p > 1$. The latter takes into account the variance of the activity (for $p = 2$) and therefore is always positive, this ensures stability even when the average of the inputs is zero. It should be noted here, that the original theory (1982) assumed that the inputs were positive, whereas the present threshold relaxes this assumption and yields stability for a larger class of bounded inputs. In the special case of $p = 2$, we obtain a quadratic form of the modified BCM learning rule, which we term QBCM.

Either form seems consistent with presently available experimental results as has been shown in [Clothiaux et al., 1991; Blais et al., 1996] but imply quite different underlying physiological mechanisms. The original BCM form requires that a history of activity (likely cell depolarization) be stored and then via a non-linear process produce the modification threshold. The present form of θ_M requires that the non-linear process occurs first.

3.2.2 *Extension to a Nonlinear Neuron*

The fact that the distribution has part of its mass on both sides of θ_M makes it plausible as a projection index that seeks multi- modalities. However, this projection index will be more general if, in addition, the sensitivity to outliers can be regulated and if we allow any projected distribution to be shifted so that the part of the distribution that satisfies $c < \theta_M$ will have its mode at zero. The over-sensitivity to outliers is addressed by considering a nonlinear neuron in which the neuron's activity is defined to be $c = \sigma(\mathbf{m} \cdot \mathbf{d})$, where σ usually represents a smooth sigmoidal function. The ability to shift the projected distribution so that one of its modes is at zero is achieved by introducing a threshold β so that the projection is defined to be $c = \sigma((\mathbf{m} \cdot \mathbf{d}) + \beta)$. From the biological viewpoint, β can be related to spontaneous activity. The modification equations for finding the optimal threshold β are easily obtained by observing that this threshold effectively adds one dimension to the input vector and vector of synaptic weights so that $\mathbf{d} = (d_1 \ldots, d_n, 1)$, $\mathbf{m} = (m_1, \ldots, m_n, \beta)$, and therefore, β can be found by using the same synaptic modification equations. For the rest of the chapter we shall assume that this threshold is added to the projection, without specifically writing it.

For the nonlinear neuron, θ_M is defined to be $\theta_M = E[\sigma^2(\mathbf{m} \cdot \mathbf{d})]$. The loss function is given by:

$$
\begin{aligned}
L_m(\mathbf{d}) &= -\mu \int_0^{\sigma(\mathbf{m} \cdot \mathbf{d})} \hat{\phi}(s, \theta_M) ds \\
&= -\mu \left\{ \frac{1}{3}\sigma^3(\mathbf{m} \cdot \mathbf{d}) - \frac{1}{4}E[\sigma^2(\mathbf{m} \cdot \mathbf{d})]\sigma^2(\mathbf{m} \cdot \mathbf{d}) \right\}
\end{aligned}
\tag{3.5}
$$

The gradient of the risk becomes:

$$\begin{aligned}
-\nabla_m R_m &= \mu \left\{ E[\sigma^2(\mathbf{m} \cdot \mathbf{d})\sigma'\mathbf{d}] \right. \\
&\quad \left. -E[\sigma^2(\mathbf{m} \cdot \mathbf{d})]E[\sigma(\mathbf{m} \cdot \mathbf{d})\sigma'\mathbf{d}] \right\} \\
&= \mu\, E[\phi\big(\sigma(\mathbf{m} \cdot \mathbf{d}), \theta_M\big)\sigma'\mathbf{d}],
\end{aligned} \tag{3.6}$$

where σ' represents the derivative of σ at the point $(\mathbf{m} \cdot \mathbf{d})$. Note that the multiplication by σ' reduces sensitivity to outliers of the differential equation since for outliers σ' is close to zero.

3.2.3 *Extension to a Network with Feed-Forward Inhibition*

We now define a network with feed-forward inhibition. The activity of neuron k in the network is $c_k = (\mathbf{m} \cdot \mathbf{d})_k$, where m_k is the synaptic weight vector of neuron k. The *inhibited* activity and threshold of the k'th neuron is given by

$$\tilde{c}_k = c_k - \eta \sum_{j \neq k} c_j, \qquad \tilde{\Theta}_M^k = E[\tilde{c}_k^2]. \tag{3.7}$$

This feed-forward network should be contrasted with a lateral inhibition network (used for example by Cooper and Scofield, 1988) in which the inhibited activity is given by $c_k = c_k(0) + \sum L_{ij}c_j$. The relation between these two networks is discussed in the next section and in Chapter 4.

For the feed-forward network the loss function is similar to the one defined in a single feature extraction with the exception that the activity $c = (\mathbf{m} \cdot \mathbf{d})$ is replaced by $\tilde{c}$. Therefore the risk for node k is given by:

$$R_k = -\mu\{\frac{1}{3}E[\tilde{c}_k^3] - \frac{1}{4}E^2[\tilde{c}_k^2]\}, \tag{3.8}$$

and the total risk is given by

$$R = \sum_{k=1}^{N} R_k. \tag{3.9}$$

To find the gradient of R we write:

$$\frac{\partial \tilde{c}_k}{\partial \mathbf{m}_j} = -\eta \mathbf{d}, \quad \frac{\partial \tilde{c}_k}{\partial \mathbf{m}_k} = \mathbf{d},$$

$$\frac{\partial R_k}{\partial \mathbf{m}_k} = \frac{\partial R_k}{\partial \tilde{c}_k} \frac{\partial \tilde{c}_k}{\partial \mathbf{m}_k} = -\mu\{E[\tilde{c}_k^2 \mathbf{d}] - E[\tilde{c}_k^2]E[\tilde{c}_k \mathbf{d}]\},$$

$$\frac{\partial R_j}{\partial \mathbf{m}_k} = \frac{\partial R_j}{\partial \tilde{c}_j} \frac{\partial \tilde{c}_j}{\partial \mathbf{m}_k} = -\eta \frac{\partial R_j}{\partial \mathbf{m}_j},$$

$$\Rightarrow \quad \frac{\partial R}{\partial \mathbf{m}_k} = \frac{\partial R_k}{\partial \mathbf{m}_k} - \eta \sum_{j \neq k} \frac{\partial R_j}{\partial \mathbf{m}_j}$$

$$= \mu \left[E[\phi(\tilde{c}_k, \tilde{\Theta}_M^k)\mathbf{d}] - \eta \sum_{j \neq k} E[\phi(\tilde{c}_j, \tilde{\Theta}_m^j)\mathbf{d}] \right]. \quad (3.10)$$

The coupling given by Equation 3.7 suggests that maximization of activity and consequently of the objective function can occur if each neuron is mostly active when other neurons are quiet. Since the solution of single neuron dynamics is such that its weight vector becomes orthogonal to most of the inputs, this leaves a large space to which the other neurons may become selective. The dynamics does not require any matrix inversion and demonstrates the ability of the network to perform exploratory projection pursuit in parallel, since the minimization of the risk involves minimization of nodes $1, \ldots, N$, which are loosely coupled.

When the non-linearity of the neuron is included, the inhibited activity is defined (as in the single neuron case) as $\tilde{c}_k = \sigma(c_k - \eta \sum_{l \neq k} c_l)$. $\tilde{\Theta}_M^k$, and R_k are defined as before. However, in this case

$$\frac{\partial \tilde{c}_k}{\partial m_j} = -\eta \sigma'(\tilde{c}_k)x, \qquad \frac{\partial \tilde{c}_k}{\partial m_k} = \sigma'(\tilde{c}_k)x. \quad (3.11)$$

Therefore the total gradient becomes:

$$\dot{m}_k = \frac{\partial R}{\partial m_k} = \mu\{E[\phi(\tilde{c}_k, \tilde{\Theta}_M^k)\sigma'(\tilde{c}_k)\mathbf{d}] - \eta \sum_{j \neq k} E[\phi(\tilde{c}_j, \tilde{\Theta}_m^j)\sigma'(\tilde{c}_j)\mathbf{d}]\}(3.12)$$

The lateral inhibition network performs a search of k-dimensional projections together; thus it may find a richer structure that a step-wise approach might miss. An illustration of such structure is given in Figure 3.2 (See also example 14.1, Huber, 1985). It shows a two dimensional struc-

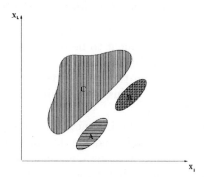

Figure 3.2: Concurrent projection of Structure in one direction can not be found without knowing the structure in the other direction.

ture that contains a bi-modal structure that might be missed due to the "shadow" from the other cluster.

3.3 The BCM Feature Extraction and Coding

The main mathematical results concerning the type of features detected by a BCM neuron and coding of these features [Intrator and Cooper, 1992] roughly says: with n clusters in an n-dimensional space, the only stable solutions are projections which are orthogonal to all but one of the clusters. There are at most n such solutions and each such solution occurs with probability p_i (the probability of cluster i). Moreover, the neuronal activity of a neuron that becomes tuned to cluster i (in the linear case) is $1/p_i$.

This fundamental result of the quadratic version of the BCM rule (QBCM) suggests an efficient coding of the extracted features. It indicates that features which appear with high probability are coded with smaller neuronal activity, while features which occur with a small probability, are coded with higher neuronal activity. By adding a monotone truncated log function on top of the neuronal activity, we get a close to optimal coding of the features which is given by $\log 1/p_i$ where p_i is the probability of occurrence of the feature. For this result to hold, only non-negative neuronal activity should be considered, thus, we require a truncated log function (a thresholded monotone function that is biologically plausible.)

In practice, while the activity of a neuron becomes close to the inverse of the probability of the feature, this is not always the case. If the feature is only partially detected, namely, the probability that the feature appears in the input at a certain time is not close to one, then the activity of the neuron is degraded accordingly. A model for the separation of these two probabilities would be desirable but currently not available.

3.3.1 *BCM and suspicious coincidence detection*

So far, we have been concerned with the type of features that can be extracted from the input environment to be relayed to higher cortical areas. The assumption was that if the information is carried in the data, then it can somehow be decoded from the data. However, we have ignored *optimal coding* issues. Below, we discuss some coding considerations and their relevance to the BCM theory.

Barlow argues that a basic brain function is to adjust expectations according to past context. Examples include the ability to understand speech in a noisy environment, understanding under contextual constraints, or to drive a car. He further claims that while it is largely assumed that when sensory neurons detect features in their input representation, they should transmit the probability of occurrence of the features they learn to detect; such coding is not optimal and in fact neurons can and should transmit additional information. Following his seminal work on minimal entropy codes and unsupervised learning [Barlow, 1989; Barlow et al., 1989], we attempt to address some fundamental problems concerning neuronal coding, neuronal goals for learning, feature detection and information transmission. In particular, the need to transmit the probability of events is put into a practical neuronal framework for detecting suspicious events. We derive these assertions from basic principles of information theory, from energy conservation considerations, and from some assumptions about neuronal goals.

Several other researchers have been interested in these questions. Atick (1992) compared information coding patterns in flies and mammalians retinal coding and supports the notion of redundancy reduction through effective information coding. Field et al. [Field, 1994; Olshausen and Field, 1996c] inferred the goal of visual sensory coding from properties of the statistics of natural images. Their main conclusions are the need to extract higher order statistics (i.e., more than linear and pairwise) and the need for sparse coding as a mean to achieve efficient information relay.

Barlow has been arguing for the last four decades that *suspicious coincidences* is the basic type of event to which the cerebral cortex must attune itself [Barlow, 1961; Barlow, 1985; Barlow, 1990; Barlow, 1994]. Assuming that a major task of the brain is to form a statistical model of the world, Barlow asked what kind of events would be worth noting and keeping a record of. Clearly, neither isolated events (the falling of an individual stone) nor repeated occurrences of events (the ticking of a clock) deserve too much attention. In contrast, a co-occurrence of two events may call for investigation or may justify remembering, but only if this co-occurrence is *surprising* (i.e., unlikely), given prior knowledge regarding the occurrence of the individual events. Coincidence detection is also a key idea in the *Compositional Machine* framework presented by Geman and Bienenstock [Geman and Bienenstock, 1995]. Barlow has presented a *Probabilistic Pandemonium* which is constructed so that the response strength of a feature-detector demon is proportional to $-\log P$, where P is the *posterior probability* of occurrence of the feature the demon detects. The feature-detector signals are then propagated to an association network which receives *unconditional* inputs as well – inputs that follow and are assumed to be related to the *conditional* input. The main innovation in this setup, is the argument that each demon (feature detector) propagates information inversely proportional to the likelihood of the feature that is detected. This is very different from conventional feature detectors. In conventional feature detectors such as Principal Components, the output is proportional to the degree of similarity between the input and the feature (when extracting PC from the correlation of inputs matrix), or the amount of variance explained by that feature (when extracting PC from the covariance matrix).

Following the result described in Section 3.3 (See the appendix and [Intrator and Cooper, 1992] for full details), it is clear that the BCM rule relays the prior probability of features that are detected and is thus different than conventional feature detectors and is suitable for coincidence detection.

3.4   Information Theoretic Considerations

In order to get a better perspective of the relation between different high order learning rules (rules that depend on higher order correlations between inputs) we have to address some fundamental questions concerning the nature of projections from high dimensional spaces as well as the nature of information that can be conveyed between neuronal layers. We motivate the need for higher order correlation rules and distinguish between, second order statistics rules and present a mathematical technique which, we believe, can lead to a clearer distinction between the large family of rules based on higher order correlations, and give a more accurate definition for such synaptic plasticity rules. For further discussion of second order statistics rules, the reader is referred to Chapter 5.

We note that our main interest is in studying the theoretical concepts that suggest a distinction between learning rules on the basis of their information theoretic properties. Only after such distinction between neuronal learning goals, can one continue further and distinguish between learning rules aimed at achieving the same objective on the basis of their detailed mathematical or computational properties.

We start with a motivation for the search for non-Gaussian distribution using information theoretic considerations.

3.4.1   *Information theory and synaptic modification rules*

A general class of learning rules follows from the information theoretic idea of maximizing the mutual information between the net output and input, or as it is sometimes called: minimizing the information loss across the network[Barlow, 1961]. This idea has been suggested as a general principle for cortical and artificial network models [Linsker, 1986b; Bichsel and Seitz, 1989; Atick and Redlich, 1992].

Information theory was developed about 50 years ago for the study of communication channels [Shannon, 1948]. Shannon considers information as a loss of *uncertainty*. The information is a function of the probability distribution of the variables. If, for example, the probability distribution $P(X)$ is concentrated on a single value, then the information we can transmit when choosing values from this distribution is zero since we always transmit the same value. Thus, it is a measure of the variability of the distribution that determines the amount of information of a random variable. This quantity that we denote by $H(X)$ should satisfy an additivity constraint that states that when two random variables are independent, the information contained in both of them should be the sum of the information contained in each of them, namely

$$P(X_1, X_2) = P_1(X_1)P_2(X_2) \Rightarrow H(X_1, X_2) = H(X_1) + H(X_2). \quad (3.13)$$

Shannon has shown that the only function that is consistent with this condition and with some other simple constraints is the Boltzmann entropy of statistical mechanics.[†] The entropy[‡] in the continuous and discrete cases respectively is given by:

$$H(X) = -\int P(x) \log P(x) dx, \quad H(X) = -\sum_{i=1}^{K} p(x_i) \log p(x_i), \quad (3.14)$$

where $p(x_i)$ is the probability of observing the value x_i out of a possible K discrete values of the random variable X. An intuitive way to look at this function is by considering the average number of bits that is needed to produce an efficient code; it is desirable to use a small number of bits for sending those words that appear with high probability, and use larger number of bits for sending words that appear with lower probability. In the special case of n words arriving at the same probability, the number of bits that are required for each word is $\log_2 n$.

Shannon formulated this idea for the problem of information flow through a bottleneck, in order to optimize the code so as to send the smallest number of bits on average. This led to questions such as how does the receiver, given the transmitted information only, maximize his knowledge about the data available at the sender side. We formulate the mutual information idea in terms of a neural network of a single layer. Let $\mathbf{d}^i \in R^n$ be an input vector to the network occurring with the probability distribution P_d, and let $\mathbf{c}^i \in R^k$ be the corresponding k-dimensional network activity with its probability distribution P_c. The *relative entropy* or the *Kullback Leibler distance* between the two probability distributions is defined as[§]

$$D(P_d \parallel P_c) = \sum_{\mathbf{d}_i} P_d(\mathbf{d}_i) \log \frac{P_d(\mathbf{d}_i)}{P_c(\mathbf{c}_i)} = E_{P_d}[\log(P_d) - \log(P_c)]. \quad (3.15)$$

[†] E. T. Jaynes has demonstrated the connection between information theory, statistics and statistical mechanics in two papers[Jaynes, 1957a; Jaynes, 1957b]. They are also in his book [Jaynes, 1982] and in a forthcoming book about his work (http://bayes.wustl.edu).

[‡] In information theory, it is customary to neglect the Boltzmann constant that sets up the units correctly, and to use the logarithm of base 2 so that the information is measured in bits.

[§] Note that this is not symmetric and does not satisfy the triangle inequality.

Consider now the joint probability distribution of the input and output random variables $P(\mathbf{d}, \mathbf{c})$ such that $P_{\mathbf{d}}$ and $P_{\mathbf{c}}$ are the corresponding marginal distributions. The *mutual information* $I(\mathbf{d}, \mathbf{c})$ is the relative entropy between the joint distribution and the product distribution, namely,

$$
\begin{aligned}
I(\mathbf{d}, \mathbf{c}) &= D(P(\mathbf{d}, \mathbf{c}) \parallel P(\mathbf{d})P(\mathbf{c})) \\
&= \sum_{\mathbf{d}^i} \sum_{\mathbf{c}^j} P(\mathbf{d}^i, \mathbf{c}^j) \log \frac{P(\mathbf{d}^i, \mathbf{c}^j)}{P(\mathbf{d}^i)P(\mathbf{c}^j)} \\
&= \sum_{\mathbf{d}^i} \sum_{\mathbf{c}^j} P(\mathbf{d}^i, \mathbf{c}^j) \log \frac{P(\mathbf{d}^i|\mathbf{c}^j)}{P(\mathbf{d}^i)} \\
&= H(\mathbf{d}) - H(\mathbf{d}|\mathbf{c}). \tag{3.16}
\end{aligned}
$$

Note that by symmetry $I(\mathbf{d}, \mathbf{c}) = H(\mathbf{c}) - H(\mathbf{c}|\mathbf{d})$, and $I(\mathbf{d}, \mathbf{c}) = H(\mathbf{c}) + H(\mathbf{d}) - H(\mathbf{d}, \mathbf{c})$. Additional properties of mutual information can be found in [Cover and Thomas, 1991].

By maximizing the mutual information we effectively minimize $H(\mathbf{d}|\mathbf{c})$ namely, we reduce the uncertainty about the input $\mathbf{d}$ by knowing the output $\mathbf{c}$. Synaptic modification rules can be derived from solving the mutual information maximization problem under different assumptions about the probability distribution of input words. The solution to such learning rules is based on gradient ascent or a more sophisticated optimization algorithm, such as conjugate gradient. Mathematical properties of this information criterion are worked out for simple distributions, although the general solution is not given in a closed form.

Maximization of entropy is often done under some constraints. For example, the Gibbs distribution maximizes the entropy for the class of positive valued distributions that has a bounded second order statistics (variance) and the Gaussian distribution maximizes the entropy for the class of unbounded distributions with bounded variance. Random projections of high dimensional data carry no information, therefore the uncertainty (entropy) is high. It is therefore clear that in order to find projections which carry some information and therefore reduce the uncertainty about their output, one is looking for projections of lower entropy. This makes the clear connection between projection pursuit and entropy minimization algorithms and demonstrates that the task of searching for non-Gaussian distributions is a specific case of entropy minimization algorithms.

3.4.2   *Information theory and early visual processing*

A coding scheme that generates a probability distribution that is different from the one that maximizes entropy under the appropriate coding constraints is said to be *redundant*. It is thus natural to study the signal distribution at various information junctions in the brain and determine the rate of redundancy of code at those locations. The first place to start in the visual pathway is of course the images themselves. It was demonstrated recently [Ruderman, 1994] that the single log intensity of pixel distribution of a small collection of natural images is not Gaussian. This indicates that the multi-dimensional distribution of pixel images is not Gaussian, since otherwise, every (linear) projection (including single pixel projections) should have been Gaussian. Ruderman suggests a transformation of the pixel intensity, based on its local variance, which makes the new distribution Gaussian. While the optimality of such a transformation is demonstrated from information theory considerations, the biological basis of such transformation has yet to be found.

Atick and Redlich (1992) hypothesis that the main goal of retinal transformations is to eliminate redundancy in input signals, particularly that due to pairwise correlations among pixels (second order correlation). Their discussion of the optimal response of Ganglion cells is motivated by information maximization.

Field (1987) suggests an interesting match between the spectrum of natural images, and the log polar mapping from retina to cortex. Based on a small number of images, he observes that the power spectrum goes down like $1/f^2$ where f is the frequency of the changes of grey level in the image. Assuming that the coding is done similarly in each of the frequency bands, this implies that different frequency bands do not carry the same amount of information, thus, leading to sub-optimal coding of the information. He suggests that log polar retinotopic mapping, in which, the bandwidth of each frequency band is a fraction of the central frequency, causes each frequency band to carry the same amount of information, and is thus, optimal from information theory view point. More recently Field suggested that the redundancy can be utilized to produce a more constant response from highly varying spectra that is frequency dependent [Field and Brady, 1997].

The above examples hypothesize that the goal of neuronal learning and data relay maybe to reduce redundancy and transfer a non-Gaussian distribution into a Gaussian one or to utilize the redundancy to gain other desired properties such as sensitivity to varying spatial frequency. So far, we have not seen a reduction in the amount of information relay, but merely a recoding that makes the code more efficient. We now turn to methods that actually attempt to *reduce* the amount of relayed-information by extracting *important* information (based on some criteria to be discussed) and ignoring the rest. These methods actually emphasize the parts of the data that are not Gaussian in a manner that is described below.

3.4.3   *Information properties of Principal Components*

In the late 90's there was a surge in the flow of work about neural networks performing principal components extraction. See for example [Sejnowski, 1977; Oja, 1982; Linsker, 1986b; Miller et al., 1989; Sanger, 1989]. Analysis of principal components is given in Chapter 5. Here we briefly review some properties that are needed for the comparison with other methods.

The Linsker model [Linsker, 1986b] which is based on mutual information maximization, could generate receptive fields that resemble simple and complex cells. However, this required a Gaussian arbor function (a function that controls the initial synaptic strengths as a function of spatial location) and a particular set of parameters related to the width of the arbor function, and to the constraints on the weights. A simplified form of these equations which ignores saturation constraints on the weights leads to principal components extraction in each layer.

Principal components are optimal solutions of the maximum information preservation (mutual information maximization) *under Gaussian data distribution*. They are also optimal when the goal is to linearly reconstruct the inputs. They are not optimal when the goal is classification, as can be seen by the simple example in Figure 3.3 (see also p. 212, Duda and Hart, 1973). Two clusters each belonging to a different class are presented.

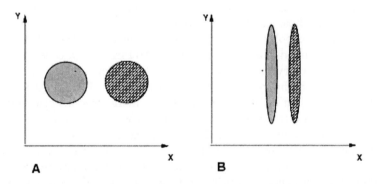

Figure 3.3: Principal components finding useful structure in data (A) and fail when the variance of each cluster is different in each direction (B).

As before, the goal is to simplify the representation with minimal loss in information, and in this case it amounts to finding a single dimensional projection that will capture the structure that is exhibited in the data. In Figure 1B clusters have different variance in either direction, whereas in Figure 1A the variance in both directions is equal. Clearly, the structure in the data is conveyed in the x projection and is not related to the direction that maximizes the variance of the projection. The projection onto the y direction, which maximizes the variance also minimizes the mean squared error (MSE) of the reconstructed image, and is the direction of the principal component of the data. We therefore have a simple example in which the goal of maximum information preservation conflicts with the goal of finding the principal component of the data. Further, the example also demonstrates the superiority of the goal of maximum information preservation over the goal of extracting principal components.

One can then ask, why is it that the principal component misses the important structure in the data, while another projection does not. The answer, as we have already stated, lies in the fact that principal components are concerned with first and second order moments of the data; when there is important information in higher order moments, it is not revealed by principal components.

Another way to view what principal components do to the data is by observing that they define a new system of coordinates in which the covariance matrix is diagonal, namely, they eliminate the second order correlation in the data i.e., correlation between pairs of pixels. Contrary to independent components analysis, this procedure, however, does not eliminate higher order correlations in the data.

3.5   Extraction of Optimal Unsupervised Features

The issue of neuronal data representation is highly linked with the presentation of very high dimensional data. For example a small image patch of 25x25 pixels can be represented as a point in a 625-dimensional vector space; thus the properties of such high dimensional spaces play an important role in understanding neuronal goals. When detection and classification of high dimensional vectors is sought, the *curse of dimensionality* [Bellman, 1961] becomes the main factor affecting the classification performance. The curse of dimensionality is due to the inherent sparseness of high dimensional spaces; thus, the amount of training data needed in order to get reasonably low variance estimators¶, becomes ridiculously high. Much work in recent years is aimed at constructing methods that specifically avoid this problem. For example, when important structure in the data actually lies in a much smaller dimensional space, it becomes reasonable to try and reduce the dimensionality before attempting the classification. This approach can be successful if the dimensionality reduction/feature extraction method loses as little significant information as possible during the dimensionality reduction.

At a first glance, it seems that a supervised feature extraction method,

---

¶The Variance portion of the error has a stronger effect than the Bias; for a review see [Geman et al., 1992].

Demonstration of the Curse of Dimensionality

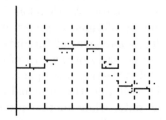

Figure 3.4: In a one dimensional situation, $k * n$ observations are needed for robust density estimation which is done by splitting the range into n segments and estimating the mean of the function from k observations in each segment. In a two-dimensional case, when splitting each dimension into n segments, we get n^2 such volumes so that the number of samples needed for estimation is $n^2 * k$. Thus, the number of required points to train a network grows exponentially with the dimensionality.

such as multiple discriminant analysis [Bryan, 1951; Sebestyen, 1962, for reference] is superior to an unsupervised one, because it uses more information about the problem. However, the supervision imposes constraints which do not easily direct a gradient descent method to a good solution as they are not smooth. Thus, the error surface of a supervised scheme tends to be rough, so that a network can often get stuck in a local minimum which is far from an optimal solution. Unsupervised methods however, often use constraints on some smooth function of the moments of the distribution, such as variance or skewness, leading to a smoother error surface, and therefore are less sensitive to the number of estimated parameters. This has been suggested as a potential way to avoid the curse of dimensionality [Barron and Barron, 1988].

3.5.1 *Projection Pursuit and Deviation from Gaussian Distributions*

We see that information preservation may be very different from extraction of principal components, and that principal components may not be useful in the case of non-Gaussian distribution. Now it becomes relevant to ask, what constitutes an interesting structure (important information) in high dimensional non-Gaussian distribution.

A general class of unsupervised dimensionality reduction methods, called exploratory projection pursuit is based on seeking *interesting* projections of high dimensional data points [Kruskal, 1969; Switzer, 1970;

Kruskal, 1972; Friedman and Tukey, 1974; Friedman, 1987; Huber, 1985, for review]. The notion of interesting projections is motivated by an observation made by Diaconis and Freedman (1984), that for most high-dimensional clouds, most low-dimensional projections are approximately normal. This finding suggests that the important information in the data is conveyed in those directions whose single dimensional projected distribution is far from Gaussian. Various projection indices differ on the assumptions about the nature of deviation from normality, and in their computational efficiency. Friedman (1987) argues that the most computationally efficient measures are based on polynomial moments. However although many synaptic plasticity models are based on second order statistics and lead to extraction of the principal components [Sejnowski, 1977; von der Malsburg, 1973; Oja, 1982; Linsker, 88; Miller et al., 1989], second order polynomials are not sufficient to characterize the important features of a distribution (see examples in Duda and Hart (1973) p. 212, and the example in Figure 3.3). This suggests that in order to use polynomials for measuring deviation from normality, higher order polynomials are required, and care should be taken in order to avoid their over-sensitivity to outliers. From our earlier discussion it follows that these polynomial moments should be of higher order than two. In some special cases where the data is known in advance to be bi-modal, it is relatively straightforward to define a good projection index [Hinton and Nowlan, 1990], however, when the structure is not known in advance, it is still valid to seek multi-modality in the projected data.

Despite the computational attractiveness, projection indices based on polynomial moments are not directly applicable, since they very heavily emphasize departure from normality in the tails of the distribution (Huber, 1985). Friedman (1987) addresses this issue by applying an inverse cumulative normal distribution function that compresses the projected data from R to $[-1, 1]$. This transformation takes a Gaussian distribution to a uniform one. We address the problem by applying a sigmoidal function to the projections, and then applying an objective function based on polynomial moments.

The following should be viewed as different measures that seek non-Gaussian projections. Since we are not sure what exact properties of non-Gaussian distributions one should be looking for, it is not possible to decide a-priori which measures would prove more useful. Below, we describe the learning rules that are based on the skewness and kurtosis of the distribution. Note that the BCM algorithm attempts to find (at least) two disjoint distributions in the projection (one around zero and one away from zero).

The quadratic form of BCM was already viewed as a method for finding projections that produce an activity profile that strongly deviates from Gaussian. As mentioned in Section 3.5.1, this can be approached more generally by the projection pursuit formalism, which aims at studying interesting projections in the form of deviation from Gaussian distribution. Below we describe a few specific index measures that are commonly used in the context of neuronal learning, and use them to derive a family of learning rules. We then show what types of receptive fields they produce in a natural image environment.

Each of the indices used is defined to be zero for a Gaussian distribution, and has two forms: one which is *multiplicative* and one which is *subtractive*. Although they are dependent on the same moments, and have the same value for a Gaussian distribution, the multiplicative and subtractive forms have different biological implications.

3.5.2 *Skewness*

The first standard measure of deviation from the Gaussian distribution is skewness. It measures the degree to which the distribution symmetry is broken using the third moment of the distribution normalized by the variance [Stuart et al., 1987].

Neural activity is assumed to be a positive quantity, so for biological plausibility, we denote by c the rectified activity $\sigma(\mathbf{d} \cdot \mathbf{m})$ and assume that the sigmoid is a smooth monotone function with a positive output (a slight negative output is also allowed). The derivative $\sigma' > 0$ as σ is strongly monotonic. The rectification is required for all rules that depend on odd moments because these vanish in a symmetric distribution such as natural scenes. We also demonstrate later that the rectification makes little difference on learning rules that depend on even moments.

(a) Skewness 1
This measures the deviation from symmetry [Kendall and Stuart, 1977, for review] and is of the form:

$$S_1 = E[c^3]/E^{1.5}[c^2]. \tag{3.17}$$

A maximization of this measure via gradient ascent gives

$$\nabla S_1 = \frac{1}{\theta_M{}^{1.5}} E\left[c\left(c - E[c^3]/E[c^2]\right)\sigma'\mathbf{d}\right]$$

$$= \frac{1}{\theta_M{}^{1.5}} E\left[c\left(c - E[c^3]/\theta_M\right)\sigma'\mathbf{d}\right] \tag{3.18}$$

where Θ_m is defined as $E[c^2]$.

(b)   Skewness 2

A subtractive skewness measure is given by

$$S_2 = E[c^3] - E^{1.5}[c^2]. \tag{3.19}$$

This measure requires a stabilization mechanism, because it is not invariant under constant multiples of the activity c or $\mathbf{m}$. We stabilize the rule by requiring that the vector of weights, which we denote by $\mathbf{m}$, has a fixed norm, say $\parallel \mathbf{m} \parallel = 1$. The gradient of this measure is

$$\nabla S_2 = 3E\left[c^2 - c\sqrt{E[c^2]}\right] = 3E\left[c\left(c - \sqrt{\theta_M}\right)\sigma'\mathbf{d}\right], \tag{3.20}$$

subject to the constraint $\parallel \mathbf{m} \parallel = 1$.

3.5.3   *Kurtosis*

Kurtosis measures deviation from Gaussian distribution mainly in the tails of the distribution. It depends primarily on the fourth moment of the distribution.

(a)   Kurtosis 1

This version of kurtosis has the form

$$K_1 = E[c^4]/E^2[c^2] - 3. \tag{3.21}$$

so that

$$\begin{aligned}\nabla K_1 &= \frac{1}{\theta_M{}^2}E\left[c\left(c^2 - E[c^4]/E[c^2]\right)\sigma'\mathbf{d}\right] \\ &= \frac{1}{\theta_M{}^2}E\left[c\left(c^2 - E[c^4]/\theta_M\right)\sigma'\mathbf{d}\right].\end{aligned} \tag{3.22}$$

(b)   Kurtosis 2

The subtractive version that requires some stabilization is given by:

$$K_2 = E[c^4] - 3E^2[c^2]. \tag{3.23}$$

and has a gradient of the form

$$\nabla K_2 = 4E\left[c^3 - cE[c^2]\right] = 3E\left[c(c^2 - \theta_M)]\sigma'\mathbf{d}\right]. \tag{3.24}$$

In all the above, the maximization of the measure can be used as a goal for projection seeking, so the variable c can be thought of as a (nonlinear) projection of the input distribution onto a certain vector of weights, and the maximization then defines a learning rule for this vector of weights. The multiplicative forms of both kurtosis and skewness do not require an extra stabilization constraint, due to the normalizing factor $1/\theta_M{}^p$ in each rule.

Kurtotic distributions are special deviation from Gaussian in the sense that tail of the distribution is thicker. This means that events with high neuronal activity (few standard deviations above the mean) are much more likely than in Gaussian distribution. The higher tail implies narrower center of the distribution, namely a higher probability of very small random values (or neuronal activity). This could be viewed as a way to produce a sparse coding where a cell is mostly quiet but produces quiet large activity with a non-significant probability. It has been suggested that natural images have a sparse structure [Mumford, 1995; Olshausen and Field, 1996c; Olshausen and Field, 1996a] and so forming an internal representation which is sparse as well is a natural neuronal learning goal [Field, 1994; Fyfe and Baddeley, 1995].

3.5.4   *Quadratic BCM*

The Quadratic form of BCM (QBCM), first presented in [Intrator and Cooper, 1992], is described in Section 3.2;

$$\text{QBCM} = \frac{1}{3}E[c^3] - \frac{1}{4}E^2[c^2]. \tag{3.25}$$

Maximizing this form using gradient ascent gives the learning rule:

$$\text{QBCM} = E\left[c^2 - cE[c^2]\right] = E[c(c - \theta_M)\sigma'\mathbf{d}]. \tag{3.26}$$

Unlike the measures S_2 and K_2 above, the Quadratic BCM rule does not require any additional stabilization. This turns out to be an important property [Intrator, 1996, Section 3.3], since additional information can then be transmitted using the resulting norm of the weight vector $\mathbf{m}$.

The Quadratic BCM rule is one of several possible forms for BCM modification. In fact, Skewness 1 and Kurtosis 1, which do not require additional constraints to converge, have the general properties proposed by BCM: the gradient is zero when the activity $c = 0$, there is a negative Hebbian region followed by a positive Hebbian region and the shift from negative to positive occurs at a threshold level which is a nonlinear function of the past (expected) activity. The other two measures share those properties but use a different form of stabilization and so that they are less like BCM.

3.5.5   *Constrained BCM measure*

For the purpose of comparison with other projection indices it is useful to look at a special case of the QBCM form – a constrained gradient maximization version of the BCM projection index that we call *length free*.

Since the weight modification attempts to maximize the following objective:

$$\mathcal{E}(\mathbf{m}) = \frac{1}{3}E[(\mathbf{m}\cdot\mathbf{d})^3] - \frac{1}{4}E^2[(\mathbf{m}\cdot\mathbf{d})^2], \tag{3.27}$$

we extract a non-zero λ and study instead:

$$\begin{aligned}
\mathcal{E}_\lambda(\mathbf{m}) &= \frac{1}{3}\lambda^3 E[(\mathbf{m}\cdot\mathbf{d})^3] - \frac{1}{4}\lambda^4 E^2[(\mathbf{m}\cdot\mathbf{d})^2] \\
&= \lambda^3\Big(\frac{1}{3}E[(\mathbf{m}\cdot\mathbf{d})^3] - \frac{\lambda}{4}E^2[(\mathbf{m}\cdot\mathbf{d})^2]\Big).
\end{aligned} \tag{3.28}$$

In this version we split the search for an optimal direction from the search for an optimal norm of the weight vector $\mathbf{m}$. We further restrict the search for an optimal direction to the restricted path in which the vector length is already optimized for each direction. Let us therefore first attempt to maximize $\mathcal{E}_\lambda$ with respect to λ only, so as to achieve an optimal length for a fixed direction. We therefore write

$$\begin{aligned}
0 = \frac{\partial}{\partial\lambda}\mathcal{E}_\lambda(\mathbf{m}) &= 3\lambda^2\Big(\frac{1}{3}\lambda^3 E[(\mathbf{m}\cdot\mathbf{d})^3] - \frac{\lambda}{4}E^2[(\mathbf{m}\cdot\mathbf{d})^2]\Big) - \lambda^3\frac{1}{4}E^2[(\mathbf{m}\cdot\mathbf{d})^2] \\
&= \lambda^2 E[(\mathbf{m}\cdot\mathbf{d})^3] - \lambda^3 E^2[(\mathbf{m}\cdot\mathbf{d})^2].
\end{aligned} \tag{3.29}$$

Assuming $\lambda \neq 0$, it follows that the optimal λ (denoted by λ^*) has the form

$$\lambda^* = \frac{E[(\mathbf{m}\cdot\mathbf{d})^3]}{E^2[(\mathbf{m}\cdot\mathbf{d})^2]}, \tag{3.30}$$

therefore

$$\begin{aligned}
\mathcal{E}_{\lambda^*}(\mathbf{m}) &= \Big(\frac{E(\mathbf{m}\cdot\mathbf{d})^3}{E^2(\mathbf{m}\cdot\mathbf{d})^2}\Big)^3\Big(\frac{1}{3}E[(\mathbf{m}\cdot\mathbf{d})^3] - \frac{1}{4}E[(\mathbf{m}\cdot\mathbf{d})^3]\Big) \\
&= \frac{1}{12}\Big(\frac{E^2(\mathbf{m}\cdot\mathbf{d})^3}{E^3(\mathbf{m}\cdot\mathbf{d})^2}\Big)^2,
\end{aligned} \tag{3.31}$$

which gives skewness to the fourth power.

We can therefore, regard skewness as a special case of the QBCM measure restricted to be scale invariant.

3.5.6 *Independent Components and Receptive Fields*

Independent components [Comon, 1994] are those directions that maximize the independence between projections. In comparison, *principal components* are those orthogonal directions that maximize the second order correlation between direction projections. Jutten and Herault have introduced an adaptive algorithm in a network-like architecture that can separate several unknown independent sources.

Recently it has been claimed that the independent components of natural scenes are the edges found in simple cells[Bell and Sejnowski, 1997]. This was achieved through the maximization of the mutual entropy of a set of mixed signals. Others[Hyvarinen and Oja, 1997] have claimed that maximizing kurtosis, with the proper constraints, can also lead to the separation of mixed signals into independent components. This alternate connection between kurtosis and receptive fields leads us into a discussion of ICA. We start with a brief review of ICA and explore the single cell implementations of ICA in the natural scene environment.

Independent Component Analysis (ICA) is a statistical signal processing technique whose goal is to express a set of random variables as linear combinations of statistically independent component variables. We observe k scalar variables $(d_1, d_2, \ldots, d_k)^{\mathrm{T}} \equiv \mathbf{d}$ that are assumed to be linear combinations of n unknown *statistically independent* variables $(s_1, s_2, \ldots, s_n)^{\mathrm{T}}$. We can express this mixing of the sources $\mathbf{s}$ as

$$\mathbf{d} = \mathbf{As} \qquad (3.32)$$

where $\mathbf{A}$ is an unknown $k \times n$ mixing matrix. The problem for ICA is then to estimate both the mixing matrix $\mathbf{A}$ and the sources $\mathbf{s}$ using only the observation of the mixtures d_i. Using the feature extraction properties of ICA, the columns of $\mathbf{A}$ represent features, and s_i represent the amplitude of each feature in the observed mixtures $\mathbf{d}$. These are the features in which we are interested.

In order to perform ICA, we first make a linear transformation of the observed mixtures

$$\mathbf{c} = \mathbf{Md} \qquad (3.33)$$

These linearly transformed variables would be the outputs of the neurons, in a neural network implementation and $\mathbf{M}$, the de-mixing matrix or matrix of features, would be the weights. Two well known methods for performing ICA involve maximizing the entropy of the transformed mixtures, $\mathbf{c}$, and minimizing the mutual information of c with respect to the transformation matrix, $\mathbf{M}$, so that the components of $\mathbf{c}$ are independent. These methods are, by their definition, multi-neuron algorithms. We continue now with a single cell implementation, based on maximizing kurtosis.

3.5.7 *Kurtosis and ICA*

We start with kurtosis defined as $K_2(c) = E\left[c^4\right] - 3E^2\left[c^2\right]$. Using a property of this kurtosis measure [Kendall and Stuart, 1977], $K_2(x_1+x_2) = K_2(x_1) + K_2(x_2)$ for independent variables, and defining $\mathbf{z} = \mathbf{A}^T\mathbf{m}$, we get [Hyvarinen and Oja, 1996]

$$K_2(\mathbf{m} \cdot \mathbf{d}) \equiv K_2(\mathbf{m}^T\mathbf{d}) = K_2(\mathbf{m}^T\mathbf{As})$$

$$= K_2(\mathbf{z}^T\mathbf{s}) = \sum_{j=1}^{n} z_j^4 K_2(s_j) \qquad (3.34)$$

The extremal points of Equation 3.34 with respect to $\mathbf{z}$ under the constraint $E\left[(\mathbf{m} \cdot \mathbf{d})^2\right] = $ constant occur when one component, z_j, of $\mathbf{z}$ is ± 1 and all the rest are zero[Delfosse and Loubaton, 1995]. In other words, finding the extremal points of kurtosis leads to projections where $\mathbf{m} \cdot \mathbf{d} \equiv \mathbf{m}^T\mathbf{d} = \mathbf{z}^T\mathbf{s}$ equals (up to a sign) a single component, s_j, of $\mathbf{s}$. Thus, finding the extrema of kurtosis of the projections enables the estimation of the independent components *individually*, rather than all at once, as is done by the previous ICA rules.

Maximizing K_2 under the constraint $E\left[(\mathbf{m} \cdot \mathbf{d})^2\right]$, and defining the co-variance matrix of the inputs $\mathbf{C} = E\left[\mathbf{dd}^T\right]$, yields the following learning rule

$$\mathbf{m} = \frac{2}{\lambda}\left(\mathbf{C}^{-1}E\left[\mathbf{d}(\mathbf{m} \cdot \mathbf{d})^3\right] - 3\mathbf{m}\right) \qquad (3.35)$$

This equation leads to an iterative "fixed-point algorithm", which converges very quickly and works both for single cell and network implementations.

3.5.8 *Friedman's distance from uniform measure*

Friedman [Friedman, 1987] used Legendre polynomial expansion for measuring deviation from Gaussian distributions:

$$R_k = \sum_{j=1}^{J}\left(\frac{2j+1}{2}\right)E^2(P_j(R)) \quad J = 2, \dots, 6$$

where:

$$R = 2\Phi(C_k) - 1$$

Φ is a standard normal cumulative distribution function (CDF) given by:

$$\Phi(a|\eta, \sigma) = 1/\sqrt{2\pi}\int_{-\infty}^{a} \exp^{-\frac{t-\eta^2}{2\sigma^2}} dt$$

The polynomials P_i are given by the recursive relation: $P_0(R) = 1$; $P_1(R) = R$; $P_j(R) = \frac{(2j-1)}{j}RP_{j-1}(R) - \frac{(j-1)}{j}P_{j-2}(R)$ The gradient of this index is given by:

$$\frac{\partial R_k}{\partial w_k} = \sum_{j=1}^{J} E(P_j(R))E[P_j'(R)\exp^{\frac{-C_k{}^2}{2}}(X_k - w_kC_k)]$$

where: $P_1'(R) = 1$; $P_j' = RP_{j-1}'(R) + jP_{j-1}(R)$

The distance can be found by measuring directly the deviation (of the transformed distribution) from a uniform distribution using mean squared error.

3.5.9 *Entropy*

There are several information theoretic ways to measure deviation from Gaussian distributions and few more statistically motivated methods. The above methods measured features in the data which are particular deviations of the more general entropy measure. One can either measure a general deviation from the normal distribution via some approximation (for computational efficiency), or concentrate on specific departures from normal distribution and measure them specifically. General deviations are often measured via the relative entropy between the unknown distribution and a normal distribution with similar variance. The measure relies on an approximation to the entropy, so as to avoid the integration over the distribution space. As the general information-theoretic measure of deviation from Gaussian distribution – negative entropy – can be approximated by skewness and kurtosis [Jones and Sibson, 1987] it becomes relevant to study the ability of these two measures to extract relevant information from high-dimensional data, in particular from natural scenes. A difference between various measures would appear when the original signals are not independent as is likely in the case of natural scenes. We thus, base our review on the Gram-Charlier expansion of the probability density function [Stuart and Ord, 1994] as it is based on the third and fourth moments of the distribution.

Since Gaussian distribution maximizes entropy it is possible to test deviation from Gaussians as a difference between the entropy of a Gaussian (with similar variance) and the given distribution. This measure (sometimes called *negative entropy* is non-negative and provides a measure of the information content of the distribution relative to the maximal content of a Gaussian with the same variance. The index is given by

$$J_I(p) = H(p_G) - H(p)$$

$$= \frac{1}{2}\log(2\pi) + \log(\sigma) + \int p(x)\log p(x)dx, \tag{3.36}$$

where p is the distribution-density and σ is the standard deviation of the distribution. It turns out that this index also leads to redundancy reduction and independent component analysis [Girolami and Fyfe, 1996] (discussed in Section 3.5.10.)

As the density $p(x)$ is unknown, it has to be estimated from the data. This is computationally expensive and not very robust. While it is possible to estimate non-parametrically the density from the observed data, e.g, via kernel estimation [Wand, 1994; Viola and Wells, 1995], such methods are sensitive to the curse of the dimensionality and data sparseness [Bellman, 1961] and it is, thus, usually preferable to estimate the desired integral by some moment approximation to the density. Often the third and fourth cumulants:

$$\kappa_3 = \frac{E[(x - \bar{x})^3]}{\sigma^3},$$

$$\kappa_4 = \frac{E[(x - \bar{x})^4]}{\sigma^4} - 3, \tag{3.37}$$

are used. The *Edgeworth expansion* [Stuart and Ord, 1994] has been proposed for the estimation of the entropy [Comon, 1994] and more recently, the *Gram-Charlier expansion* [Stuart and Ord, 1994] has been proposed [Amari et al., 1996] as it explicitly depends on the third and fourth cumulant of the distribution. This Gram-Charlier approximation has the form:

$$p(x) \simeq \alpha(x)\{1 + \frac{\kappa_3}{3!}H_3(x) + \frac{\kappa_4}{4!}H_4(x)\}, \tag{3.38}$$

where $\alpha(x) = \frac{1}{\sqrt{2\pi}}\exp(-x^2/2)$ and $H_k(x)$ are Chebyshev-Hermite polynomials defined by the identity

$$(-1)^k \frac{d^k\alpha(x)}{dx^k} = H_k(x)\alpha(x) \tag{3.39}$$

and given in our case by:

$$H_3(x) = 4x^3 - 3x,$$
$$H_4(x) = 8x^4 - 8x^2 + 1. \tag{3.40}$$

The exact measure of deviation from Gaussian distribution is clearly presented in this approximation (3.38) as some measure of the skewness and kurtosis of the distribution. If we plug this approximation into the calculation of the neg-entropy index (3.36) we get

$$\hat{J}_I(p) = \sigma - \frac{(\kappa_3)^2}{2 \cdot 3!} - \frac{(\kappa_4)^2}{2 \cdot 4!} + \frac{5}{8}(\kappa_3)^2\kappa_4 + \frac{1}{16}(\kappa_4)^3. \tag{3.41}$$

This calculation [Jones and Sibson, 1987; Amari et al., 1996] uses results about moments of a Gaussian distribution:

$$\int x^{2k+1}\alpha(x)dx = 0, \quad \int x^{2k}\alpha(x)dx = 1 \cdot 3 \cdot \cdot (2k-1). \qquad (3.42)$$

This measure is dependent on a polynomial of a high degree and thus may sensitive to outliers.

3.5.10 *The concept of minimum mutual information between neurons*

A concept that has gained much attention in recent years is *minimum mutual information* between neurons.[||] This concept was termed *redundancy reduction* [Barlow, 1961] who proposed it as a main goal for neuronal learning. It has been adopted as a learning goal for information transfer from retina to cortex [Atick and Redlich, 1992]. More recently, this concept has been called *independent component analysis (ICA)* [Comon, 1994; Bell and Sejnowski, 1995; Amari et al., 1996; Cardoso and Laheld, 1996] – a method which attempts to decompose a set of signals into their most independent components. Formally, ICA attempts to make the joint probability of neuronal activity be as close as possible to the product of the marginal distribution of each neuron. Conditions on cumulants were given to characterize a large class of learning rules that performs redundancy reduction and ICA [d'Alché Buc and Nadal, 1996].

The different flavors of this algorithm are attributed to different measures of the distance between distributions and different approximations to the probability density function and consequently to the distance between distributions.

Let M be a matrix of neuronal weights which together with the input distribution, define a set of neuronal activities

$$\mathbf{c}(t) = (c_1(t), c_2(t), \ldots, c_N(t)),$$

with a joint probability distribution $p(\mathbf{c}; M)$. Let

$$p_i(c_i; M) = \int p(\mathbf{c}; M)dc_1 \cdots \check{d}c_i \cdots dc_N, \qquad (3.43)$$

be the marginal distribution of c_i, where $\check{d}c_i$ means that the dc_i is omitted in the integration. Then when the neuronal activities are independent, the joint probability is equal to the product of the marginal distributions

$$\tilde{p}(\mathbf{c}; M) = \Pi_{i=1}^{N}p_i(c_i; M). \qquad (3.44)$$

[||]This concept is different from the maximum mutual information between input and output [Linsker, 1986b] (see discussion in Section 3.4.3).

If we measure the distance between these probabilities using the Kullback-Leibler divergence [Kullback, 1959], we are led to minimize (with respect to M):

$$D(p; \tilde{p}) = \int p(\mathbf{c}; M) \log \frac{p(\mathbf{c}; M)}{\tilde{p}(\mathbf{c}; M)} d\mathbf{c}. \qquad (3.45)$$

Unfortunately, this minimization is nontrivial as the calculation of the entropy requires the integration over the distribution which is unknown.

As discussed before, when the third and fourth cumulants of the distribution are known, it is possible to estimate the integrals using some approximation to the probability density function resulting in a similar learning rule to the Entropy measure (Equation 3.41) [Amari et al., 1996].

3.5.11 *Some Related Statistical and Computational Issues in BCM*

The proposed method uses low order polynomial moments which are computational efficient and its sensitivity to outliers can be regulated by the saturating limit of the sigmoidal (see Section 3.3). It naturally extends to multi-dimensional projection pursuit using the feed-forward inhibition network. The number of calculations of the gradient grows linearly with the dimensionality and *linearly* with the number of projections sought. The projection index contains a single dimensional scaling which actually allows the transmission additional information in the cell's activity (this has been elaborated on in Section 3.3.) This also removes the need for sphering the data, but if one is interested in scale invariant projection, sphering can still be useful[**]. The projection index has a natural stochastic gradient descent version which further speeds the calculation by eliminating the need to calculate the empirical expected value of the gradient. All the above lead to a fully parallel algorithm that may be implemented on a multi-processor machine, and produce a practical feature extractor for very high dimensional problems.

Although, the projection index is motivated by the desire to search for clusters in the high dimensional data, the resulting feature extraction method is quite different from other pattern recognition methods that search for clusters. Since the class labels are not used in the search, the projection pursuit is not biased to the class labels. This is in contrast with classical methods such as discriminant analysis [Fisher, 1936; Sebestyen, 1962]. The issue of using an unsupervised method vs. supervised for revealing structure in the data has been discussed extensively elsewhere. We would only like to add that it is striking that in various low-dimensional

---

[**]This will result in a type III projection index (see Huber, 1985).

examples [Friedman and Tukey, 1974; Jones, 1983; Friedman, 1987] the exploratory capabilities of PP were not worse than those of supervised method such as discriminant analysis and factor analysis in discovering structure, thus suggesting that in high dimensions where supervised methods may fail, still PP can find useful structure.

The resulting method concentrates on projections that allow discrimination between clusters and not faithful representation of the data, namely reconstruction ability of the features. This is in contrast to principal components analysis (as demonstrated in Figure 3.3 and discussed in Section 3.4.3), or factor analysis which tend to combine features that have high correlation (see review in Harman, 1967).

The method differs from cluster analysis by the fact that it searches for clusters in the low dimensional projection space, thus avoiding the inherent sparsity of the high dimensional space. The search for multi-modality is further constrained by the desire to seek those projections that are orthogonal to all but one of the clusters (or have a mode at zero). This constraint simplifies the search, since it implies that under the assumption of K linearly independent clusters, there may be at most K optimal projections as opposed to at most $\binom{K}{2}$ separating hyper-planes.

3.6   Analysis of the Fixed Points of BCM in High Dimensional Space

In Appendix 3A we show using a general result on random differential equations [Intrator, 1990a] that the solution of the random differential equations remains as close as we like, in the L^2 sense, to the solution of the deterministic equations. We have shown in Section 3.2 that the deterministic equation converges to a local minimum of the risk. This implies that the solution of the random differential equation converges to a local minimum of the risk in L^2. Based on the statistical formulation, we can say that the local minima of the risk are *interesting features* extracted from the data, which correspond to directions in which the single dimensional distribution of the projections is far from a Gaussian distribution, by means of penalized skewness measure.

In the following, we attempt to analyze the shape of the high dimensional risk function, with specific inputs, namely, we look for the location of the critical points of the risk, and locate those that have a local minima given a specific training set. This completely characterizes the solution of the synaptic modification equations, and sheds some more light on the power of the risk functional in finding interesting directions in the data. In doing so we gain some detailed information on the behavior of the solution of the random differential equations, as a model for learning in visual cortex, under various rearing conditions.

Since the introduction of the threshold β does not pose any mathematical difficulty as was described before, we omit it in the analysis.

First, we analyze the limiting behavior of the solution in the case where we have n linearly independent inputs (not necessarily orthogonal). The introduction of noise into the system will be done in the next sections.

3.6.1 n linearly independent inputs

The random differential equation is given by

$$\dot{\mathbf{m}}_\epsilon = \epsilon \, \mu(t)\phi((\mathbf{m} \cdot \mathbf{d}), \Theta_m)\mathbf{d}, \quad \mathbf{m}_\epsilon(0) = \mathbf{m}_0, \tag{3.46}$$

the averaged (batch) version of the gradient descent is given by:

$$\dot{\overline{\mathbf{m}}}_\epsilon = \epsilon \, \mu(t)E\big[\phi((\overline{\mathbf{m}} \cdot \mathbf{d}), \Theta_m)\mathbf{d}\big] \quad \overline{\mathbf{m}}_\epsilon(0) = \mathbf{m}_0. \tag{3.47}$$

The main tool in establishing the following results is the connection between the solution to the deterministic differential equation 3.47 and the solution of the random differential equation 3.46. A general result which yields this connection is given in [Intrator, 1990a] and will be discussed in the appendix. When applied to this specific differential equation, the result says that

$$\sup_{t>T} E|\mathbf{m}_\epsilon - \overline{\mathbf{m}}_\epsilon|^2 \xrightarrow[\epsilon \to 0]{} 0. \tag{3.48}$$

Proposition 3.1 *Let* $\mathbf{d}^{(1)}, \ldots, \mathbf{d}^{(n)}$ *be* n *linearly independent bounded vectors in* R^n. *Let* D *be the random process so that* $P[D = \mathbf{d}^{(i)}] = p_i, \quad p_i > 0, \; i = 1, \ldots, n, \; \sum p_i = 1$.

Then the critical points of Equation 3.46 are the 2^n *weight vectors* $\mathbf{m}^{(i)} \in R^n$, *each a solution to one of the equations:* $A\mathbf{m}^{(i)} = v^{(i)}$, $i = 0, \ldots, 2^n - 1$, *where* A *is the matrix whose* i*'th row is the input vector* $\mathbf{d}^{(i)}$, *and* $\{v^{(i)}, \quad i = 0, \ldots, 2^n - 1\}$, *is the* n *dimensional set of vectors of the form:*

$$
\begin{aligned}
v^{(0)} &= (0, \ldots, 0), \\
v^{(1)} &= (\frac{1}{p_1}, 0, \ldots, 0), \\
v^{(2)} &= (0, \frac{1}{p_2}, 0, \ldots, 0), \\
v^{(3)} &= (\frac{1}{p_1 + p_2}, \frac{1}{p_1 + p_2}, 0, \ldots, 0), \\
v^{(4)} &= (0, 0, \frac{1}{p_3}, 0, \ldots, 0), \\
& , \ldots,
\end{aligned}
$$

$$v^{(2^n-1)} = (1, \ldots, 1).$$

Proof: Rewrite Equation 3.46 in the form

$$\dot{\mathbf{m}}_\epsilon = \epsilon\mu(t)((\mathbf{m} \cdot \mathbf{d})_\epsilon)[(\mathbf{m} \cdot \mathbf{d})_\epsilon - \theta_M]\mathbf{d}, \qquad (3.49)$$

where $\theta_M = E[((\mathbf{m} \cdot \mathbf{d})_\epsilon)^2]$. Since $\epsilon\mu(t) > 0$, then $\mathbf{m}_\epsilon$ is a critical point if either $\mathbf{d}^{(i)} \cdot \mathbf{m}_\epsilon = 0$, or $\mathbf{d}^{(i)} \cdot \mathbf{m}_\epsilon = \theta_M \neq 0$, $i = 1, \ldots, n$.

There are exactly 2^n possibilities for the set of n numbers $\mathbf{d}^{(i)} \cdot \mathbf{m}_\epsilon$ to be either 0, or nonzero. Therefore there are only 2^n possible solutions.

Let $\mathbf{m}_\epsilon^{(1)}$ be such that $\mathbf{m}_\epsilon^{(1)} \cdot \mathbf{d}^{(1)} \neq 0$, and $\mathbf{m}_\epsilon^{(1)} \cdot \mathbf{d}^{(i)} = 0$, $i > 1$. Then for $\mathbf{m}_\epsilon^{(1)}$,

$$\theta_M = E[((\mathbf{m} \cdot \mathbf{d})_\epsilon)^2] = \sum_{i=1}^{N} p_i(\mathbf{d}^{(i)} \cdot \mathbf{m}_\epsilon^{(1)})^2 = p_1(\mathbf{d}^{(1)} \cdot \mathbf{m}_\epsilon^{(1)})^2. \quad (3.50)$$

When we combine the condition $\theta_M = \mathbf{d}^{(1)} \cdot \mathbf{m}_\epsilon^{(1)}$, we get $\mathbf{d}^{(1)} \cdot \mathbf{m}_\epsilon^{(1)} = \frac{1}{p_1}$.

Now suppose $m = \mathbf{m}_\epsilon^{(3)}$, is such that $\mathbf{d}^{(1)} \cdot \mathbf{m}_\epsilon^{(3)} = \mathbf{d}^2 \cdot \mathbf{m}_\epsilon^{(3)} = \theta_M$, and $\mathbf{d}^{(i)} \cdot \mathbf{m}_\epsilon^{(3)} = 0$, $i > 2$. In this case $\theta_M = p_1(\mathbf{d}^{(1)} \cdot \mathbf{m}_\epsilon^{(3)})^2 + p_2(\mathbf{d}^2 \cdot \mathbf{m}_\epsilon^{(3)})^2$, which yields, $\mathbf{d}^j \cdot \mathbf{m}_\epsilon^{(3)} = \frac{1}{p_1+p_2}$, $j = 1, 2$.

The other cases are treated similarly. $\diamond$

Stability of the solution

Let $m(t)$ be a solution of a random differential equation, then $\mathbf{m}_0$ is said to be a stable point if for any $\delta > 0$ there is a $\tau(\delta)$ such that for any $K > 0$, $t \geq \tau$

$$P\{|m(t) - \mathbf{m}_0|^2 > K\} \leq \frac{\delta}{K}. \qquad (3.51)$$

This roughly says that the $\mathbf{m}_0$ is a stable point, then the probability of finding the solution *far* from this point is *small*.

Lemma 3.1 *Let m be a critical point for the random differential equation. Then m is a stable (unstable) critical point, if it is a stable (unstable) critical point for the averaged deterministic version. The stability of the stochastic equation is in the L^2 sense.*

Proof: From Equation 3.48 follows that if $\mathbf{m}_\epsilon$ is a critical point of the random version, then it is a critical point of the averaged deterministic equation. If this point is a stable (unstable) point of the deterministic equation, then perturbing both equations (i.e. starting from an initial condition that is close to $\mathbf{m}_\epsilon$), will yield that the deterministic equation will converge back to (diverge from) the original critical point. This is independent of ϵ and with probability one since it is a deterministic equation. Consequently, the random solution must stay close to the deterministic solution which in this case, implies the stability (instability) of the random solution. ◇

Theorem 3.1 *Under the conditions of proposition 3.1, the critical points $m_e^{(i)}$ that are stable are only those in which the corresponding vector v^i, has one and only one nonzero element in it.*

Proof: From the above two lemmas it follows that it is enough to check the stability on the deterministic version of the equations, at the critical points of the random version.

The gradient is then given by:

$$-\nabla_m R_m = E[(\mathbf{m} \cdot \mathbf{d})^2 \mathbf{d}] - E[(\mathbf{m} \cdot \mathbf{d})^2] E[(\mathbf{m} \cdot \mathbf{d})\mathbf{d}], \qquad (3.52)$$

and the second order derivative is given by:

$$-\nabla_m^2 R_m = 2E[(\mathbf{m} \cdot \mathbf{d})\mathbf{d} \times \mathbf{d}] - E[(\mathbf{m} \cdot \mathbf{d})^2] E[\mathbf{d} \times \mathbf{d}]$$
$$-2E[(\mathbf{m} \cdot \mathbf{d})\mathbf{d}] \times E[(\mathbf{m} \cdot \mathbf{d})\mathbf{d}]. \qquad (3.53)$$

The critical point $m = 0$ is clearly unstable, since the second derivative matrix is zero, and changes sign around $m = 0$. For selective solution, we can choose without loss of generality, $\mathbf{m}^{(1)}$ which is the solution for $v^{(1)}$. Putting $\mathbf{m}^{(1)}$ into the gradient equation gives:

$$-\nabla_m R \big|_{m=m^{(1)}} = p_1(\mathbf{d}^{(1)} \cdot \mathbf{m}^{(1)})^2 \mathbf{d}^{(1)} - p_1(\mathbf{d}^{(1)} \cdot \mathbf{m}^{(1)})^2 p_1(\mathbf{d}^{(1)} \cdot \mathbf{m}^{(1)})\mathbf{d}^{(1)}$$
$$= p_1(\mathbf{d}^{(1)} \cdot \mathbf{m}^{(1)})^2 [1 - p_1](\mathbf{d}^{(1)} \cdot \mathbf{m}^{(1)})\mathbf{d}^{(1)}. \qquad (3.54)$$

Since $\mathbf{m}^{(1)}$ is a critical point and $\mathbf{d}^{(1)}$ is the preferred input, we get from the fact that the gradient is equal to zero at $\mathbf{m}^{(1)}$: $(\mathbf{d}^{(1)} \cdot \mathbf{m}^{(1)}) = \frac{1}{p_1}$, $E(\mathbf{m} \cdot \mathbf{d})^2 = \frac{1}{p_1}$.

Define the matrix B to be

$$B = E[\mathbf{d} \times \mathbf{d}] = \sum_{i=1}^{N} p_i \mathbf{d}^{(i)} \times \mathbf{d}^{(i)}, \qquad (3.55)$$

since the inputs are independent and span the whole space, it follows that B is positive definite. Putting $(\mathbf{d}^{(1)} \cdot \mathbf{m}^{(1)})$ into Equation 3.53 gives:

$$-\nabla_m^2 R \big|_{m=m^{(1)}} = p_1(\mathbf{d}^{(1)} \cdot \mathbf{m}^{(1)})$$
$$\times \left(2\mathbf{d}^{(1)} \times \mathbf{d}^{(1)} - \frac{1}{p_1} B - 2\mathbf{d}^{(1)} \times \mathbf{d}^{(1)} \right), \qquad (3.56)$$

which is negative definite, thus leading to a stable critical point.

Now, assume, without loss of generality, that $m = \mathbf{m}^{(3)}$, then

$$-\nabla_m R \big|_{m=m^{(3)}} = [p_1(\mathbf{d}^{(1)} \cdot \mathbf{m}^{(3)})^2 \mathbf{d}^{(1)} + p_2(\mathbf{d}^{(2)} \cdot \mathbf{m}^{(3)})^2 \mathbf{d}^{(2)}]$$

$$-[p_1(\mathbf{d}^{(1)} \cdot \mathbf{m}^{(3)})^2 + p_2(\mathbf{d}^{(2)} \cdot \mathbf{m}^{(3)})^2]$$
$$[p_1(\mathbf{d}^{(1)} \cdot \mathbf{m}^{(3)})\mathbf{d}^{(1)} + p_2(\mathbf{d}^{(2)} \cdot \mathbf{m}^{(3)})\mathbf{d}^{(2)}]. \quad (3.57)$$

Since $\mathbf{m}^{(3)}$ is a critical point, we have from proposition 3.1 that $(\mathbf{d}^{(1)} \cdot \mathbf{m}^{(3)}) = (\mathbf{d}^{(2)} \cdot \mathbf{m}^{(3)}) = \frac{1}{p_1+p_2}$, and $E(\mathbf{m} \cdot \mathbf{d})^2 = \frac{1}{p_1+p_2}$.

Putting this into Equation 3.53 gives:

$$-\nabla_{\mathbf{m}}^{(3)} R\big|_{m=m^{(3)}} = 2p_1(\mathbf{d}^{(1)} \cdot \mathbf{m}^{(3)})\mathbf{d}^{(1)} \times \mathbf{d}^{(1)} + 2p_2(\mathbf{d}^{(2)} \cdot \mathbf{m}^{(3)})\mathbf{d}^{(2)} \times \mathbf{d}^{(2)}$$

$$- \frac{1}{p_1+p_2} B$$

$$-2\Big([p_1(\mathbf{d}^{(1)} \cdot \mathbf{m}^{(3)})\mathbf{d}^{(1)} + p_2(\mathbf{d}^{(2)} \cdot \mathbf{m}^{(3)})\mathbf{d}^{(2)}]$$

$$\times [p_1(\mathbf{d}^{(1)} \cdot \mathbf{m}^{(3)})\mathbf{d}^{(1)} + p_2(\mathbf{d}^{(2)} \cdot \mathbf{m}^{(3)})\mathbf{d}^{(2)}]\Big)$$

$$= \Big(\frac{2p_1}{p_1+p_2} - \frac{2p_1^2}{(p_1+p_2)^2}\Big)\mathbf{d}^{(1)} \times \mathbf{d}^{(1)}$$

$$+ \Big(\frac{2p_2}{p_1+p_2} - \frac{2p_2^2}{(p_1+p_2)^2}\Big)\mathbf{d}^{(2)} \times \mathbf{d}^{(2)}$$

$$- \frac{1}{p_1+p_2} B$$

$$- \frac{2p_1 p_2}{(p_1+p_2)^2}(\mathbf{d}^{(1)} \times \mathbf{d}^{(2)} + \mathbf{d}^{(2)} \times \mathbf{d}^{(1)}). \quad (3.58)$$

Denote the above gradient matrix by G. Without loss of generality we may assume that $p_1 \geq p_2$. Then consider a vector, y which is orthogonal to all but $\mathbf{d}^{(2)}$. Then

$$y^T G y = y^T \mathbf{d}^{(2)} \times \mathbf{d}^{(2)} y \frac{p_2}{p_1+p_2}\Big(6 - \frac{6p_2}{p_1+p_2} - 3\Big) \geq 0, \quad (3.59)$$

since $\frac{p_2}{p_1+p_2} \leq \frac{1}{2}$. It is easy to see, by replacing $\mathbf{m}^{(3)}$ with $\lambda\mathbf{m}^{(3)}$, that the second derivative along $\mathbf{m}^{(3)}$ changes sign at $\lambda = 1$, which implies instability.

The proof for the other critical points follows in the exactly same way.
◇

3.6.2   *Noise with no Patterned Input*

This is a special case, which is related to the binocular deprivation environment discussed earlier and hence is analyzed separately. In general, we consider input as being composed of pattern and noise. The patterned input represents a highly correlated set of patterns that appear at random, and are supposed to mimic key features in visual environment such as edges with different orientation, etc. The noise is an uncorrelated type of input, which is assumed to exist in large network of neurons receiving inputs from several parts of cortex. Patterned input is associated with open eyes, pure noise with closed eyes.

When the input contains only noise, the averaged deterministic solution has a stable critical point, and the random solution stays close to the deterministic one as is shown in the appendix. When the input is composed of noise with zero mean only, we find that the averaged version has a stable zero solution (as opposed to the case with patterned input). This implies that the solution of the random version wanders about the origin but stays close to zero in L^2 norm.

Noise with Zero Mean

The crucial property of white noise x is the fact that it is symmetric around zero, thus, when $\mathbf{d} = (x_1, x_2, \ldots, x_n)^T$, this implies that $E[(\mathbf{m} \cdot \mathbf{d})^3] = 0$, and the risk,

$$R_m = -\{E[(\mathbf{m} \cdot \mathbf{d})^3] - E^2[(\mathbf{m} \cdot \mathbf{d})^2]\} = E^2[(\mathbf{m} \cdot \mathbf{d})^2] \geq 0. \quad (3.60)$$

It is easy to see that only for $\mathbf{m} = 0$, $R_m = 0$, and this is the only critical point in this case. Since this result is related to binocular deprivation experiments, it should be emphasized again that the solution to the stochastic version of the differential equations will wander around zero in a random manner but with a small magnitude controlled by the learning rate μ.

In view of the properties of the risk, we can say that when the distribution of x has zero skewness in every direction, the only stable minima of the risk is $\mathbf{m} = 0$. This is not true when the noise has a positive or a negative average as analyzed in the next section.

Noise with Positive Mean

We assume that x is now bounded random noise, with $\overline{x} > 0$, and with the same single dimensional distribution in all directions, which implies that for $\mathbf{d} = (x_1, x_2, \ldots, x_n)^T$, $x = \overline{d_i} = \overline{d_1} > 0$, $i \geq 0$. Let $\mathbf{d} = \overline{\mathbf{d}} + \mathbf{y}$, where $\mathbf{y}$ is vector of random noise with zero average. Denote $\text{Var}(y_1) = \lambda$. The following identities can easily be verified:

$$E(\mathbf{m} \cdot \mathbf{d})^2 = (\overline{\mathbf{m} \cdot \mathbf{d}})^2 + \text{Var}(\mathbf{m} \cdot \mathbf{y}),$$
$$E(\mathbf{m} \cdot \mathbf{y})\mathbf{y} = \lambda m,$$
$$E(\mathbf{m} \cdot \mathbf{y})^2 \mathbf{y} = 0. \quad (3.61)$$

Putting these identities in the first and second gradient (Equations 3.52 and 3.53) we get:

$$-\nabla_m R_m = [(\overline{\mathbf{m} \cdot \mathbf{d}})^2 + \text{Var}(\mathbf{m} \cdot \mathbf{y})]\overline{x}$$
$$-[(\overline{\mathbf{m} \cdot \mathbf{d}})^2 + \text{Var}(\mathbf{m} \cdot \mathbf{y})][(\overline{\mathbf{m} \cdot \mathbf{d}})\overline{x} + \lambda m]. \quad (3.62)$$

We are looking for critical points of the gradient,

$$\nabla_m R_m = 0 \Rightarrow \quad m_i = [\frac{1}{\lambda} - \frac{\overline{(\mathbf{m} \cdot \mathbf{d})}}{\lambda}]\overline{d}_i. \tag{3.63}$$

Equation 3.63 suggests a consistency condition that has to be filled, namely, if we multiply both sides of this equation by $\overline{d}_i$ and sum over all $i's$ we get:

$$\overline{(\mathbf{m} \cdot \mathbf{d})} = [\frac{1}{\lambda} - \frac{\overline{(\mathbf{m} \cdot \mathbf{d})}}{\lambda}] \parallel \overline{\mathbf{d}} \parallel^2, \tag{3.64}$$

therefore,

$$\overline{(\mathbf{m} \cdot \mathbf{d})} = \frac{\parallel \overline{\mathbf{d}} \parallel^2}{\lambda + \parallel \overline{\mathbf{d}} \parallel^2}. \tag{3.65}$$

When substituting Equation 3.65 into Equation 3.63 we get the explicit ratio between m_i and $\overline{d}_i$, namely,

$$m_i = [\frac{1}{\lambda + \parallel \overline{\mathbf{d}} \parallel^2}]\overline{d}_i. \tag{3.66}$$

This is a displaced critical point for the case of non-zero mean noise.

The second derivative is given by:

$$\begin{aligned}
-\nabla_m^2 R_m = &\ [2\overline{(\mathbf{m} \cdot \mathbf{d})}^2 \overline{(\mathbf{m} \cdot \mathbf{d})}^2 - \text{Var}(\mathbf{m} \cdot \mathbf{y})](\overline{\mathbf{d}} \times \overline{\mathbf{d}}) \\
&+ E[\{2(\mathbf{m} \cdot \mathbf{y}) - 2(\mathbf{m} \cdot \mathbf{y})\overline{(\mathbf{m} \cdot \mathbf{d})}\}(\mathbf{y} \times \overline{\mathbf{d}})] \\
&- 2\lambda \overline{(\mathbf{m} \cdot \mathbf{d})}(\overline{\mathbf{d}} \times m) \\
&- 2\lambda (\mathbf{m} \cdot \mathbf{y})(\mathbf{y} \times m) \\
&- \lambda[\overline{(\mathbf{m} \cdot \mathbf{d})}^2 + \text{Var}(\mathbf{m} \cdot \mathbf{y})]I.
\end{aligned} \tag{3.67}$$

Using relations 3.61 and 3.65 of the critical points, we get to a gradient in terms of $\overline{\mathbf{d}} \times \overline{\mathbf{d}}$, and λ – the variance of the noise. Let $\tau = \frac{1}{\lambda + \|\overline{d}\|^2}$, then

$$\begin{aligned}
-\nabla_m^2 R_m = &\ \tau^2(\overline{\mathbf{d}} \times \overline{\mathbf{d}})[(2 - 4) \\
&- \lambda \parallel \overline{\mathbf{d}} \parallel^2 + 2\lambda^2\tau \\
&- 2\lambda^2 \parallel \overline{\mathbf{d}} \parallel^2 - 2\lambda^2].
\end{aligned} \tag{3.68}$$

It follows that the gradient is positive definite for any noise with variance $\lambda > 0$. This implies stability of the averaged version, and stability in the L^2 sense of the random version.

3.6.3   *Patterned Input with Noise*

We now explore the change in the position of critical points under small noise. The result relies on the smoothness of the projection index, and on the fact that noise can be presented as a small perturbation.

Let the input $\mathbf{d} = \hat{\mathbf{d}} + \mathbf{x}$, where $\hat{\mathbf{d}}$ is the patterned input and $\mathbf{x}$ is a vector of small random noise with zero mean. (If the mean of the noise is non-zero it can always be absorbed in the patterned input and the resulting noise will have a zero mean.) Let $\lambda = \text{Var}(\mathbf{m} \cdot \mathbf{x})$ which is small as well. Consider the projection index

$$
\begin{aligned}
R_m &= -\mu\{\frac{1}{3}E[(\mathbf{m}\cdot\mathbf{d})^3] - \frac{1}{4}E^2[(\mathbf{m}\cdot\mathbf{d})^2]\} \\
&= -\mu\{\frac{1}{3}E[\mathbf{m}\cdot\hat{\mathbf{d}}^3] - \frac{1}{4}E^2[\mathbf{m}\cdot\hat{\mathbf{d}}^2] \\
&\quad + \lambda\{E\mathbf{m}\cdot\hat{\mathbf{d}} - \frac{\lambda}{4}[1 + E\mathbf{m}\cdot\hat{\mathbf{d}}^2]\}\}.
\end{aligned}
\tag{3.69}
$$

Thus $R_m(\hat{\mathbf{d}} + \mathbf{x}) = R_m(\hat{\mathbf{d}}) + O(\lambda)$. Therefore our results are robust to the addition of small noise.

3.7 Application to Various Rearing Conditions

In the following section, we apply the analysis described above to some visual cortical plasticity experiments.

3.7.1 *Normal Rearing(NR)*

This case has been covered by the Theorem 3.1 from which it follows that a neuron will become selective to one of the inputs. Note that it also follows that the synaptic weights of both eyes become selective to the same orientation.

3.7.2 *Monocular Deprivation (MD)*

From Theorem 3.1 we can get an explicit expression to θ_M in the case of n linearly independent inputs. Recall that the only stable points in such case are those in which the synaptic weight m is orthogonal to all but one of the inputs. Assuming that all the K inputs have the same probability $\frac{1}{K}$, we get: $\theta_M = E(\mathbf{m}\cdot\mathbf{d})^2 = \frac{1}{K}\sum_{i=1}^{K}(\mathbf{m}\cdot\mathbf{d}_i)^2 = \frac{1}{K}(\mathbf{m}\cdot\mathbf{d}_{i_0})^2$ where $\mathbf{d}_{i_0}$ is the input which is not orthogonal to $\mathbf{m}$. Putting that into the deterministic version of the gradient descent it follows immediately that $\mathbf{m}\cdot\mathbf{d}_{i_0} = K$, which implies that $\theta_M = \frac{1}{K}(d_{i_0}\cdot m)^2 = K$, and $E(\mathbf{m}\cdot\mathbf{d}) = \frac{1}{K}(\mathbf{m}\cdot\mathbf{d}_{i_0}) = 1$. This result will be used in the following MD analysis.

The assumptions in the monocular deprivation case are that the input to the left (right) eye is composed of noise only, namely $\mathbf{d}^r$ represents patterned input plus noise, and $\mathbf{d}^l = x$. We also assume that the noise has zero average and has a symmetric distribution uniform in all directions.

We relax the assumption that $\mathbf{d}^r$ has zero mean, and instead assume that $E(\mathbf{m}^r \cdot \mathbf{d}^r) < \frac{1}{2}E(\mathbf{m}^r \cdot \mathbf{d}^r)^2$, this is easily achieved when the dimensionality is larger than 2 (following from the calculation at the beginning of this section). We have:

$$
\begin{aligned}
R &= -\{\frac{1}{3}E(\mathbf{m} \cdot \mathbf{d})^3 - \frac{1}{4}E^2(\mathbf{m} \cdot \mathbf{d})^2\} \\
&= -\{\frac{1}{3}E[(\mathbf{m}^r \cdot \mathbf{d}^r + \mathbf{m}^l \cdot \mathbf{x})^3] - \frac{1}{4}E^2[(\mathbf{m}^r \cdot \mathbf{d}^r + \mathbf{m}^l \cdot \mathbf{x})^2]\} \\
&= -\{\frac{1}{3}E[(\mathbf{m}^r \cdot \mathbf{d}^r)^3] + \frac{1}{3}E[(\mathbf{m}^l \cdot \mathbf{x})^3] \qquad\qquad (3.70) \\
&\quad + E[(\mathbf{m}^r \cdot \mathbf{d}^r)^2(\mathbf{m}^l \cdot \mathbf{x})] + E[(\mathbf{m}^r \cdot \mathbf{d}^r)(\mathbf{m}^l \cdot \mathbf{x})^2] \\
&\quad - \frac{1}{4}[E^2[(\mathbf{m}^r \cdot \mathbf{d}^r)^2] + E^2[(\mathbf{m}^l \cdot \mathbf{x})^2] + 2E[(\mathbf{m}^r \cdot \mathbf{d}^r)^2]E[(\mathbf{m}^l \cdot \mathbf{x})^2] \\
&\quad + 4E[\mathbf{m}^r \cdot \mathbf{d}^r]E[\mathbf{m}^l \cdot \mathbf{x}]\left(E[(\mathbf{m}^r \cdot \mathbf{d}^r)^2] + E[(\mathbf{m}^l \cdot \mathbf{x})^2]\right. \\
&\quad \left. + E[\mathbf{m}^r \cdot \mathbf{d}^r]E[\mathbf{m}^l \cdot \mathbf{x}])]\} \\
&= -\{\frac{1}{3}E[(\mathbf{m}^r \cdot \mathbf{d}^r)^3] - \frac{1}{4}E^2[(\mathbf{m}^r \cdot \mathbf{d}^r)^2]\} \\
&\quad + \frac{1}{4}\mathrm{Var}(\mathbf{m}^l \cdot \mathbf{x})\left(\mathrm{Var}(\mathbf{m}^l \cdot \mathbf{x}) + 2E[(\mathbf{m}^r \cdot \mathbf{d}^r)^2] - 4E[\mathbf{m}^r \cdot \mathbf{d}^r]\right).
\end{aligned}
$$

The first term of the risk is due to the open eye and is therefore minimized when the neuron becomes selective as in the regular normal rearing case. The second term is non-negative due to the previous assumption, and therefore can be minimized only if $\mathbf{m}^l = 0$. It can be seen that when the right eye becomes selective (implying that the term $2E[(\mathbf{m}^r \cdot \mathbf{d}^r)^2] - 4E[\mathbf{m}^r \cdot \mathbf{d}^r]$ becomes larger), then the driving force for $\mathrm{Var}(\mathbf{m}^l \cdot \mathbf{x})$ to go to zero becomes larger. This is consistent with the experimental observation which suggests that the synapses of the closed eye do not go down until the open eye becomes selective.

3.7.3　*Binocular Deprivation (BD)*

This case has been analyzed in Section 3.6.2. During BD we assume that the input is noise; the conclusion was that either synaptic weights perform a random walk around zero, or in case of positive average noise, a random walk about a positive weight that is a function of the average of the noise and its variance.

3.7.4　*Reverse Suture (RS)*

The limiting behavior of RS is similar to that of MD, described above. Computer simulations show that it is possible to achieve a disconnection of the newly closed eye before the newly open eye becomes selective [Clothiaux et al., 1991; Blais et al., 1996].

3.7.5 *Strabismus*

From Theorem 3.1 we infer that a stable fixed point is such that its projection to one of the inputs is positive, and it is orthogonal to all the other inputs. Under strabismus we assume that the input to both eyes is uncorrelated, therefore this situation is possible only if the vector of synaptic weights of one eye is orthogonal to all but one of the inputs; thus the vector of synaptic weights of the other eye is orthogonal to all the inputs. Since the inputs span the whole space this vector must be zero.

3.8 Discussion

We have presented an objective function formulation of the BCM theory of visual cortical plasticity. This permits us to demonstrate the connection between the unsupervised BCM learning procedure and the statistical method of projection pursuit and provides a general method for stability analysis of the fixed points. Relating this unsupervised learning to statistical theory enables comparison with various other statistical and unsupervised methods for feature extraction.

Analysis of the behavior and the evolution of the network under various visual rearing conditions is in agreement with experimental results. An experimental question of great interest is posed: how does the modification threshold depend on the average activity of the cell; $\theta_M \simeq \bar{c}^2$ as in the original BCM, $\theta_M \simeq \overline{c^2}$ as presented here, or some more general non-linear form? Extensive simulation, comparing theory and experiments on visual cortical plasticity, have shown that the modified version of θ_M is consistent with the experimental results. We thus have the result that a biological neuron may be performing a sophisticated statistical procedure.

Appendix 3A

Convergence of the Solution of the Random Differential Equations

To show the explicit dependence on the learning rate, we rewrite the random modification equations in the form:

$$\dot{\mathbf{m}}_\epsilon = \epsilon \, \mu(t)\phi((\mathbf{m} \cdot \mathbf{d})_\epsilon, \theta_M)\mathbf{d}, \quad \mathbf{m}_\epsilon(0) = \mathbf{m}_0, \tag{3A.1}$$

and the deterministic differential equations,

$$\dot{\overline{\mathbf{m}}}_\epsilon = \epsilon \, \mu(t)E[\phi(\overline{\mathbf{m}_\epsilon} \cdot \mathbf{d}, \theta_M)\mathbf{d}], \quad \overline{\mathbf{m}}_\epsilon(0) = \mathbf{m}_0, \tag{3A.2}$$

The convergence of the solution will be shown in two steps; First we show that the solution of the averaged deterministic equation converges, and then we use theorem 3A.1 to show the convergence of the solution of the random differential equation to the solution of its averaged deterministic equation.

3A.1 Convergence of the Deterministic Equation

The deterministic differential equations represent a negative gradient of the risk. Therefore, in order to show convergence of the solution, we only need to show that the risk is bounded from below. This will assure that the solution converges to a local minimum of the risk.

We can assume that $\mathbf{m}$ the synaptic weight vector lies in the space spanned by the random variable $\mathbf{d}$. When we replace the random variable $\mathbf{d}$ with a training set $\mathbf{d}^1, \ldots, \mathbf{d}^n$, this assumption says that $\mathbf{m} \in$ Span$\{\mathbf{d}^1, \ldots, \mathbf{d}^n\}$. This implies that there is a $\lambda > 0$, so that $\forall \mathbf{m}$ Var$(\mathbf{m} \cdot \mathbf{d}) \geq \lambda \| m \|^2 > 0$.

To show that the vector $\overline{\mathbf{m}}_\epsilon$ is bounded we assume that none of its components is zero (since zero is definitely bounded), and multiply both sides of the above equation by $\overline{\mathbf{m}}_\epsilon$, this implies:

$$\frac{1}{2}\frac{d}{dt} \| \overline{\mathbf{m}}_\epsilon \|_{l^2}^2 = E[\overline{\mathbf{m}}_\epsilon^3 \cdot \mathbf{d}] - E^2[\overline{\mathbf{m}}_\epsilon^2 \cdot \mathbf{d}]$$

$$\leq \| \, \overline{\mathbf{m}}_\epsilon \, \|^3 - \mathrm{Var}^2(\overline{\mathbf{m}}_\epsilon \cdot \mathbf{d})$$
$$\leq \| \, \overline{\mathbf{m}}_\epsilon \, \|^3 - \lambda^2 \| \, \overline{\mathbf{m}}_\epsilon \, \|^4$$
$$= \| \, \overline{\mathbf{m}}_\epsilon \, \|^3 \, \{1 - \lambda^2 \| \, \overline{\mathbf{m}}_\epsilon \, \|\}, \tag{3A.3}$$

which implies that $\| \, \overline{\mathbf{m}}_\epsilon \, \| \leq \frac{1}{\lambda^2}$.

Using this fact we can now show the convergence of $\overline{\mathbf{m}}_\epsilon$. We observe that $\overline{\mathbf{m}}_\epsilon = -\nabla R$, where $R(\overline{\mathbf{m}}_\epsilon) = -\mu\{\frac{1}{3}E[(\overline{\mathbf{m}}_\epsilon \cdot \mathbf{d})^3] - \frac{1}{4}E^2[(\overline{\mathbf{m}}_\epsilon \cdot \mathbf{d})^2]\}$ is the risk. R is bounded from below since $\| \, \overline{\mathbf{m}}_\epsilon \, \|$ is bounded, therefore $\overline{\mathbf{m}}_\epsilon$ converges to a local minimum of R as a solution to the gradient descent.

3A.2   Convergence of the Random Equation

Using the fact that the averaged deterministic version converges we shall now show the convergence of the random version. For this we need a general result on random differential equations [Intrator, 1990a] which is cited below. This result is an extension of a result by Geman (1977) and roughly says that under some smoothness conditions on the second order derivatives of the differential equations, the solution of the random differential equation remains close (in the L^2 sense) to the deterministic solution *for all times*.

We start with some preliminary notation. let $H(x, \omega, t)$ be a continuous and mixing R^m valued random process for any fixed x and t, where ω is a sample point in a probability space. Define $G(x, t) = E[H(x, \omega, t)]$, the expected value with respect to ω. Let $\mu(t)$ be a continuous monotone function decreasing to zero, and let $\epsilon > 0$ be arbitrary. Consider the following random differential equation together with its associated averaged version,

$$\dot{x}_\epsilon(t, \omega) = \epsilon \, \mu(t) H(x_\epsilon(t, \omega), \omega, t), \; x_\epsilon(0, \omega) = x_0 \in R^n.$$
$$\dot{y}_\epsilon(t) = \epsilon \, \mu(t) G(y_\epsilon(t), t), \qquad y_\epsilon(0) = x_0 \in R^n. \tag{3A.4}$$

ϵ generates a family of solutions x_ϵ, and y_ϵ.

Theorem 3A.1   *Given the above system of random differential equations, assume:*

1 $H \in R^n$ is jointly measurable with respect to its three arguments, and is of Type II φ mixing.
2 $G(x, t) = E[H(x(s, \omega), t)]$, and for all i and j

$$\frac{\partial}{\partial x_j} G_i(x, t) \text{ exists, and is continuous in } (x, t).$$

3(a) There exists a unique solution, $x(t, \omega)$, on $[0, \infty)$ for almost all ω; and

(b) A solution to

$$\frac{\partial}{\partial t}g(t,s,x) = G(g(t,s,x),t), \quad g(s,s,x) = x,$$

exists on $[0,\infty) \times [0,\infty) \times R^n$.

4 *There exist continuous functions $B_1(r), B_2(r)$, and $B_3(r)$, such that for all $i,j,k,\tau \geq 0$, and ω:*

(a) $| H_i(x,\omega,t) | \leq B_1(| x |)$;
(b) $| (\partial/\partial x_j)H_i(x,\omega,t) | \leq B_2(| x |)$;
(c) $| (\partial^2/\partial x_j \partial x_k)H_i(x,\omega,t) | \leq B_3(| x |)$.

5 $\sup_{\epsilon>0,t} | y_\epsilon(t) | \leq B_4$ *for some B_4.*

6 $\exists \, \gamma > 0, \, c > 0, \,$ *such that $\varphi(\delta) \leq \delta^{-\gamma}$, and $\mu(t) \leq t^{-(\frac{1}{\gamma}+1+c)}$, for a monotone decreasing μ.*

Then under conditions 1-6:

$$\limsup_{\epsilon \to 0 \atop t \geq 0} E \mid x_\epsilon - y_\epsilon \mid^2 = 0, \tag{3A.5}$$

To use this result, we need only to show that the deterministic and the random solutions are bounded, which will ensure conditions 2-5. Then under the mixing conditions 1 and 6 on the input x, we get the desired result.

Verifying that the random solution is bounded for every ω can be done by multiplying both sides of the random differential equations by $\mathbf{m}_\epsilon$, assuming its components are not zero, and applying the assumptions made above on $\text{Var}((\mathbf{m} \cdot \mathbf{d})_\epsilon)$, we get

$$\begin{aligned}
\frac{1}{2}\frac{d}{dt}\| \, m_\epsilon \, \|^2 &= (\mathbf{m}_\epsilon \cdot \mathbf{d})^3 - (\mathbf{m}_\epsilon \cdot \mathbf{d})^2 E[(\mathbf{m}_\epsilon \cdot \mathbf{d})^2] \\
&= (\mathbf{m}_\epsilon \cdot \mathbf{d})^2\{(\mathbf{m}_\epsilon \cdot \mathbf{d}) - E[(\mathbf{m}_\epsilon \cdot \mathbf{d})^2]\} \\
&\leq (\mathbf{m}_\epsilon \cdot \mathbf{d})^2\{(\mathbf{m}_\epsilon \cdot \mathbf{d}) - \text{Var}(\mathbf{m}_\epsilon \cdot \mathbf{d})\} \\
&\leq (\mathbf{m}_\epsilon \cdot \mathbf{d})^2\{(\mathbf{m}_\epsilon \cdot \mathbf{d}) - \lambda\| \, m_\epsilon \, \|^2\} \\
&\leq (\mathbf{m}_\epsilon \cdot \mathbf{d})^2\{\| \, m_\epsilon \, \| - \lambda\| \, m_\epsilon \, \|^2\}, \tag{3A.6}
\end{aligned}$$

which implies that the derivative of the norm will become negative whenever $\| \, m_\epsilon \, \| > \lambda$, therefore $\| \, m_\epsilon \, \| \leq \frac{1}{\lambda}$.

Finally, since the random solution remains close to a converging deterministic solution, it remains close (in the L^2 sense) to its limit for large enough t.

δ is arbitrary, which implies that

$$E|\mathbf{m}_\epsilon(t) - \tilde{\mathbf{m}} \mid^2 \xrightarrow[\epsilon \to 0]{} 0 \tag{3A.7}$$

Appendix 3B

Analysis and Comparison of BCM and Kurtosis in Extended Distributions

Most of the analysis presented above assumes an environment of linearly independent vectors. When we introduce natural images we will see that this environment cannot be approximated with linearly independent vectors. In this appendix we use the objective function formulation explored in Chapter 3 to analyze some specific low-dimensional extended distributions in order to compare two forms of learning algorithms: BCM and Kurtosis. We demonstrate that many of the results from the linearly independent cases still hold.

As an example, we take a one dimensional neuron (a neuron with one synapse), and assume that the input distribution is a Laplace (or double exponential) distribution. The distributions presented here represent the distributions of projections in a higher dimensional space.

$$f_d(d) = \frac{1}{2\lambda} e^{-|d|/\lambda} \qquad (3B.1)$$

The output of the neuron is simply

$$c = d \cdot m \text{ (note: no sigmoid)}$$

$$\tilde{c} \equiv \sigma(c) \equiv \begin{cases} c \text{ if } c \geq 0 \\ 0 \text{ otherwise} \end{cases}$$

where we have introduced the notation c for the *pre-sigmoid* output, and $\tilde{c}$ as the *post-sigmoid* output. The sigmoid we are using here has a lower value of 0 and no upper limit. This choice makes the analysis tractable, and becomes inappropriate in some cases (see Section 3B.3), but does lead to a significantly better understanding of the deprivation results.

To calculate the distribution of the outputs, c and $\tilde{c}$, we use some statistical theorems (see Appendix 3B.5.2).

$$f_c(c) = \frac{1}{2\lambda|m|}e^{-|c/m|/\lambda}$$

$$f_{\tilde{c}}(\tilde{c}) = \begin{cases} f_c(\tilde{c}) & \text{if } \tilde{c} > 0 \\ \frac{1}{2}\delta(\tilde{c}) & \text{if } \tilde{c} = 0 \\ 0 & \text{if } \tilde{c} < 0 \end{cases}$$

We will assume that m is positive, so we don't have to carry the absolute value through the calculations. Note that any solution we find, say $m = m_o$, *must* be positive, because it represents $|m| = m_o$, but that the solution will really be $m = \pm m_o$.

To calculate the values of, say, R_{QBCM} and K_2, we calculate the moments of the distribution $f_{\tilde{c}}(\tilde{c})$.

$$E\left[\tilde{c}^2\right] = \int_{-\infty}^{\infty} \tilde{c}^2 f_{\tilde{c}}(\tilde{c})d\tilde{c}$$
$$= \frac{1}{2\lambda m}\int_0^{\infty} \tilde{c}^2 e^{-\tilde{c}/m\lambda}d\tilde{c}$$
$$= m^2\lambda^2$$
$$E\left[\tilde{c}^3\right] = \int_{-\infty}^{\infty} \tilde{c}^3 f_{\tilde{c}}(\tilde{c})d\tilde{c}$$
$$= \frac{1}{2\lambda m}\int_0^{\infty} \tilde{c}^3 e^{-\tilde{c}/m\lambda}d\tilde{c}$$
$$= 3m^3\lambda^3$$
$$E\left[\tilde{c}^4\right] = \int_{-\infty}^{\infty} \tilde{c}^4 f_{\tilde{c}}(\tilde{c})d\tilde{c}$$
$$= \frac{1}{2\lambda m}\int_0^{\infty} \tilde{c}^4 e^{-\tilde{c}/m\lambda}d\tilde{c}$$
$$= 12m^4\lambda^4$$

which gives us

$$R_{QBCM} = \frac{1}{3}E\left[\tilde{c}^3\right] - \frac{1}{4}E^2\left[\tilde{c}^2\right]$$
$$= m^3\lambda^3 - \frac{1}{4}m^4\lambda^4 \qquad (3B.2)$$
$$K_2 = E\left[\tilde{c}^4\right] - 3E\left[\tilde{c}^2\right]$$
$$= 9m^4\lambda^4 \qquad (3B.3)$$

Clearly, K_2 is unstable (its maximum is with $m = \infty$) so we have to add the constraint that $|m|^2 = 1$. With this constraint, the one dimensional solution if trivially $m = 1$.

The equation for R_{QBCM} can be maximized with respect to the weights,

$$\frac{\partial R_{\text{QBCM}}}{\partial m} = 3m^2\lambda^3 - m^3\lambda^4$$

$$= m^2\lambda^3(3 - m\lambda) = 0 \tag{3B.4}$$

$$\Rightarrow m = 0, \frac{3}{\lambda} \tag{3B.5}$$

and we can evaluate the stability of any fixed points found.

$$\frac{\partial^2 R_{\text{QBCM}}}{\partial m^2} = 6m\lambda^3 - 3m^2\lambda^4$$

$$= 3m\lambda^3(2 - m\lambda)$$

$$= \begin{cases} \frac{\partial^2 R_{\text{QBCM}}}{\partial m^2}\big|_{m=0} = 0 & \text{unstable} \\ \frac{\partial^2 R_{\text{QBCM}}}{\partial m^2}\big|_{m=3/\lambda} < 0 & \text{stable} \end{cases}$$

Notice that the length of the weight vector also gives extra information about the distribution, namely the inverse of the environmental parameter λ. We can also get some dynamics by setting dm/dt equal to the gradient of the cost function.

$$\frac{dm}{dt} = \frac{\partial R_{\text{QBCM}}}{\partial m}$$

$$= 3m^2\lambda^3 - m^3\lambda^4 \tag{3B.6}$$

$$\Rightarrow \frac{1}{9\lambda^3 m} - \frac{1}{9\lambda^2}\log\left(\frac{\lambda m - 3}{m}\right) = t + \text{const} \tag{3B.7}$$

3B.1 Two Dimensions

We introduce a low dimensional, two-eye model, by having one dimension for each eye. For two eyes we have the following

$$c = m_1 d^l + m_2 d^r$$

If the eyes see the same thing, this becomes

$$c = (m_1 + m_2)d$$
$$= m^{\text{eff}} d$$

We notice that we can use our solutions for the 1D case to find m^{eff}, but that the solution is not uniquely defined. *Any* solution satisfying $m_1 + m_2 =$

m^{eff} would work, so we have a continuum of solutions. If we look at the change in the *difference* between the left and right eye weights

$$\frac{dm_1}{dt} - \frac{dm_2}{dt} = E\left[\phi(c)(d^l - d^r)\right]$$
$$= 0$$

it is clear that the difference in the weights does not change, so if our initial weights are small, $|\mathbf{m}_o| \ll 1$, the final weights for left and right eye will be approximately the same.

Thus, for normal rearing using BCM in the Laplace environment, we have

$$m_{\text{eff}} \equiv m_1 + m_2 \tag{3B.8}$$
$$= \pm 3/\lambda \tag{3B.9}$$

$$\mathbf{m} \equiv \begin{pmatrix} m_1 \\ m_2 \end{pmatrix}$$
$$= \begin{pmatrix} \pm 3/2\lambda - \frac{\delta}{2} \\ \pm 3/2\lambda + \frac{\delta}{2} \end{pmatrix} \tag{3B.10}$$

where $\delta \equiv (m_2)_o - (m_1)_o$ is the difference between the initial conditions. This is shown in Figure 3B.1A.

For K_2, with the normalization condition, the normal rearing fixed point is simply

$$\mathbf{m} \equiv \begin{pmatrix} m_1 \\ m_2 \end{pmatrix}$$
$$= \begin{pmatrix} \pm \frac{\sqrt{2}}{2} - \frac{\delta}{2} \\ \pm \frac{\sqrt{2}}{2} + \frac{\delta}{2} \end{pmatrix} \tag{3B.11}$$

In order to model monocular deprivation we start from the fixed point of normal rearing and alter the distribution, presenting uniform (or Gaussian) noise to one of the eyes, as shown in Figure 3B.1B. We will see that the neuron comes to respond to that eye which has structure, or in our case the one with the highly kurtotic input distribution.

The basic idea is that deprivation effects occur because of a competition between the input distributions. When presented with two different distributions, the neuron responds more strongly to the more kurtotic distribution and responds more weakly to the less kurtotic distribution (see Figure 3B.1).

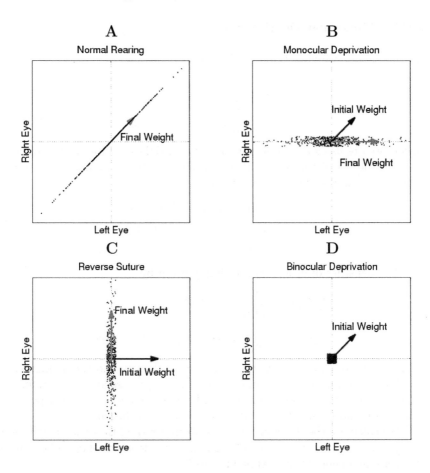

Figure 3B.1: 2D Rearing Conditions. Normal rearing (A) is modeled with numbers chosen from a Laplace distribution presented to each eye. The eyes see identical inputs, so the input distribution (samples shown with dots) lies along the 45° line. The initial weights are small, and the final weights are equal for each eye (Equation 3B.10 for BCM and Equation 3B.11 for kurtosis). Monocular deprivation (B) is modeled with Laplace numbers to one eye, representing the structure from the natural environment, and uniform (or Gaussian) numbers to the other eye, representing the noise of activity from the closed eye. The initial weight is from normal rearing, and the final weight is in the direction of the open eye: the cell comes to respond only to the open eye. Reverse suture (C) is modeled with Laplace numbers to one eye and uniform (or Gaussian) numbers to the other eye, following monocular deprivation. Binocular deprivation (D) is modeled using uniform (or Gaussian) noise presented to both eyes, following normal rearing.

3B.2   Monocular Deprivation

In this model, we have the following input densities

$$f_{d_1}(d_1) = \frac{1}{2\lambda} e^{-|d_1|/\lambda} \qquad\qquad (3B.12)$$

$$f_{d_2}(d_2) = \frac{1}{2a} \text{ in the range } [-a..a] \qquad\qquad (3B.13)$$

where we are using d_1 and d_2 for the left and right eye inputs, respectively.

The output of the cell is broken up into a sum of two one dimensional outputs, each of which we know the distribution.

$$c = \mathbf{d} \cdot \mathbf{m} = d_1 m_1 + d_2 m_2$$
$$\equiv c_1 + c_2 \text{ (note: no sigmoid)}$$
$$\tilde{c} \equiv \sigma(c)$$

The densities of c_1 and c_2 are simply given by

$$f_{c_1}(c_1) = \frac{1}{2\lambda m_1} e^{-|c_1|/m_1\lambda}$$

$$f_{c_2}(c_2) = \frac{1}{2m_2 a} \text{ in the range } [-m_2 a .. m_2 a]$$

from which we can calculate the total output density and the moments.

We are still using the assumption that $m_i = |m_i|$, so any solution for m_i that we find must be positive. We also have to remember that any positive solution found for m_i, the negative of it is also a solution.

We calculate the distribution of the output c (and thus the distribution of $\tilde{c}$) by taking the convolution of the individual densities of c_1 and c_2, since they are independent (see Appendix 3B.5.2).

$$f_c(c) = \int_{-\infty}^{\infty} f_{c_1}(c - c_2) f_{c_2}(c_2) dc_2$$

$$= \frac{1}{4\lambda a m_1 m_2} \int_{-am_2}^{am_2} e^{-|c-c_2|/m_1\lambda} dc_2$$

$$\equiv \frac{1}{4\lambda a m_1 m_2} \int_{-am_2-c}^{am_2-c} e^{-|u|/m_1\lambda} du$$

assume, for now, that $c > 0$.

if $c < am_2$: $f_c(c) = \frac{1}{4\lambda a m_1 m_2} \left(\int_{-am_2-c}^{0} e^{u/m_1\lambda} du + \int_{0}^{am_2-c} e^{-u/m_1\lambda} du \right)$

$$= \frac{2\lambda m_1 - \lambda m_1 e^{(-am_2-c)/\lambda m_1} - \lambda m_1 e^{(-am_2+c)/\lambda m_1}}{4\lambda a m_1 m_2}$$

$$\text{if } c > am_2: \; f_c(c) = \frac{1}{4\lambda a m_1 m_2} \int_{-am_2-c}^{am_2-c} e^{u/m_1\lambda} du$$

$$= \frac{\lambda m_1 e^{(am_2-c)/\lambda m_1} - \lambda m_1 e^{-(am_2+c)/\lambda m_1}}{4\lambda a m_1 m_2}$$

which generalizes for the $c < 0$ case in the following

$$\text{if } |c| < am_2: \; f_c(c) = \frac{1}{4am_2} \left(2 - e^{(-am_2+|c|)/\lambda m_1} - e^{(-am_2-|c|)/\lambda m_1} \right)$$

$$\text{if } |c| > am_2: \; f_c(c) = \frac{1}{4am_2} \left(e^{(am_2-|c|)/\lambda m_1} - e^{-(am_2+|c|)/\lambda m_1} \right)$$

$$f_{\tilde{c}}(\tilde{c}) = \begin{cases} f_c(\tilde{c}) & \text{if } \tilde{c} > 0 \\ \frac{1}{2}\delta(\tilde{c}) & \text{if } \tilde{c} = 0 \\ 0 & \text{if } \tilde{c} < 0 \end{cases}$$

With moments

$$E[\tilde{c}^2] = \frac{1}{6}a^2 m_2^2 + \lambda^2 m_1^2$$

$$E[\tilde{c}^3] = \frac{1}{8am_2} \left(12\lambda^2 m_1^2 a^2 m_2^2 + a^4 m_2^4 + 24\lambda^4 m_1^4 (1 - e^{-am_2/\lambda m_1}) \right)$$

$$E[\tilde{c}^4] = \frac{1}{10}a^4 m_2^4 + 12\lambda^4 m_1^4 + 2\lambda^2 a^2 m_1^2 m_1^2$$

We present two forms of learning, Kurtosis and BCM. These forms have been defined in Chapter 3 under the names of Subtractive Kurtosis (Section 3.5.3) and Quadratic BCM (Section 3.5.4).

3B.2.1 *Kurtosis*

Kurtosis is calculated from the moments, as defined and explored earlier in Section 3.5.3, and converted to polar coordinates (due to the simplifying contraint, $|m|^2 = 1$)

$$K_2 = \frac{1}{60}a^4 m_2^4 + 9\lambda^4 m_1^4 + \lambda^2 a^2 m_1^2 m_2^2 \qquad (3B.14)$$

$$= \frac{1}{60}a^4 R^4 + R^4 \cos^4(\theta) \left(9\lambda^4 - \lambda^2 a^2 + \frac{1}{60}a^4 \right) +$$

$$R^4 \cos^2(\theta) \left(-\frac{1}{30}a^4 + a^2 \lambda^2 \right)$$

We then take derivatives with respect to θ, evaluate at $R = 1$, and look a the fixed points.

$$\frac{\partial K_2}{\partial \theta} = \left(-36\lambda^4 + 4\lambda^2 a^2 - \frac{1}{15}a^4\right)\sin(\theta)\cos^3(\theta) +$$

$$\left(\frac{1}{15}a^4 - 2\lambda^2 a^2\right)\sin(\theta)\cos(\theta) \qquad (3B.15)$$

This has fixed points at $\theta = 0$ and $\theta = \pi/2$. The $\theta = 0$ fixed point corresponds to the weight equal to zero for the input receiving uniform noise (m_2, or the closed eye), or in other words, the cell losing responsiveness to the closed eye. This fixed point is stable for $a < \lambda 3\sqrt{2}$, or small noise compared to the structure in the environment, which makes physiological sense. We are using "structure" here as synonymous with "high λ", because the structure in the natural scenes arises from directions of high kurtosis. The $\theta = \pi/2$ is unstable in this noise regime, so the neuron will lose responsiveness to the closed eye starting from the initial conditions from normal rearing, $\mathbf{m} = \left(\sqrt{2}/2 \ \sqrt{2}/2\right)$, or in polar coordinates, $\theta = \pi/4$.

How *quickly* does the cell lose responsiveness, and how does it depend on the *noise level*. To do this we set, as before, Equation 3B.15 equal to $d\theta/dt$ to get the dynamics. We expand $\cos(\theta)$ and $\sin(\theta)$ in the resulting equation about the initial point $\theta = \pi/4$, drop high order terms in the expansion, and introduce a low noise approximation.

$$\cos(\pi/4 + x) \approx \frac{\sqrt{2}}{2} - \frac{\sqrt{2}}{2}x$$

$$\sin(\pi/4 + x) \approx \frac{\sqrt{2}}{2} + \frac{\sqrt{2}}{2}x$$

$$\frac{dx}{dt} \approx \left(\frac{1}{30}a^4 + 18\lambda^4 - 2\lambda^2 a^2\right)x + \left(-9\lambda^4 + \frac{1}{60}a^4\right)(3B.16)$$

$$\equiv \xi_1 x + \xi_2 \qquad (3B.17)$$

which has an exponential solution. Putting in $x(0) = 0$, we get

$$x(t) = \frac{\xi_2}{\xi_1}\left(\exp(\xi_1 t) - 1\right) \qquad (3B.18)$$

The rate of the cutoff from the closed eye is determined by the value of ξ_1. The larger the value of ξ_1, the *faster* the cutoff of response to the closed eye. Since the noise to the closed eye is an experimentally controllable parameter, we want to know how the rate depends on the noise level, a. This is simply done by looking at the sign of the change in ξ_1 with respect to a.

$$\frac{\partial \xi_1}{\partial a} = \frac{2a}{15}(a^2 - 30\lambda^2)$$

$$< 0 \text{ if } a^2 < 30\lambda^2 \tag{3B.19}$$

which is certainly true if $a < \lambda 3\sqrt{2}$, which was the requirement for stability of the biologically reasonable solution. This means that for kurtosis, the noise tends to *slow down* the decay of response to the closed eye, as we have seen in the simulations.

3B.2.2 BCM

The BCM equations depend not only on the *direction* but the *magnitude* of the weights. We can't simply convert to polar coordinates, and reduce the dimensionality of the problem. The cost function is calculated from the moments of the Laplace-Uniform environment.

$$R_{QBCM} = \frac{1}{2}\lambda^2 m_1^2 a m_2 \tag{3B.20}$$

$$+ \frac{1}{24}a^3 m_2^3 + \lambda^4 m_1^4 \left(1 - e^{-am_2/\lambda m_1}\right)/am_2$$

$$- \frac{1}{144}a^4 m_2^4 - \frac{1}{12}a^2 m_2^2 \lambda^2 m_1^2 - \frac{1}{4}\lambda^4 m_1^4$$

If $a \ll \lambda$, (and we assume that the weights themselves are not particularly large), then we can expand the exponential in the risk function (Equation 3B.20) to powers of $(a/\lambda)^2$.

$$R_{QBCM} = \frac{1}{2}\lambda^2 m_1^2 a m_2 + \frac{1}{24}a^3 m_2^3$$

$$+ \frac{\lambda^4 m_1^4}{am_2} - \lambda^4 m_1^4 \left(1 - \frac{am_2}{\lambda m_1} + \frac{a^2 m_2^2}{2\lambda^2 m_1^2}\right)/am_2$$

$$- \frac{1}{144}a^4 m_2^4 - \frac{1}{12}a^2 m_2^2 \lambda^2 m_1^2 - \frac{1}{4}\lambda^4 m_1^4$$

$$= \frac{1}{24}a^3 m_2^3 + \lambda^3 m_1^3 - \frac{1}{144}a^4 m_2^4 - \frac{1}{12}a^2 m_2^2 \lambda^2 m_1^2 - \frac{1}{4}\lambda^4 m_1^4$$

The modification equations are then

$$\frac{dm_1}{dt} \equiv \frac{\partial R_{QBCM}}{\partial m_1} = 3\lambda^3 m_1^2 - \frac{1}{6}a^2\lambda^2 m_1 m_2^2 - \lambda^4 m_1^3 \tag{3B.21}$$

$$\frac{dm_2}{dt} \equiv \frac{\partial R_{QBCM}}{\partial m_2} = \frac{1}{8}a^3 m_2^2 - \frac{1}{111}a^4 m_2^3 - \frac{1}{6}a^2\lambda^2 m_2 m_1^2 \tag{3B.22}$$

which have a single stable fixed point at $m_1 = 3/\lambda, m_2 = 0$, much like the case with kurtosis.

In the small noise approximation, the second term in Equation 3B.21 is small, and we end up with an equation identical to the weight modification in the one dimensional Laplace environment (Equation 3B.4). In other words, in small noise, the input with structure (the open eye) develops normally to the fixed point for the lower dimensional environment.

For the closed eye (m_2) the dynamics are quite different. If we keep only the last term in Equation 3B.22, which is clearly larger than the others, and we assume that the other weight has converged quickly and is at the fixed point ($m_1 = 3/\lambda$), then we obtain a simple exponential decay of m_2 with $(3/2)a^2$ as the exponent of decay, where a is related to the variance of the noise with $\frac{3}{2}\sigma^2 = a^3$. Keeping further terms yields qualitatively similar forms. For BCM, then, more noise into the closed eye during MD yields a *faster* cutoff of response to the closed eye. This is consistent with experiment[Rittenhouse et al., 1999].

3B.3   Binocular Deprivation

3B.3.1   *Gaussian Noise*

In this model, we have the following input densities

$$f_{d_i}(d_i) = \frac{1}{\sqrt{2\pi\sigma^2}}e^{-d_i^2/2\sigma^2} \tag{3B.23}$$

and the outputs are defined as before.

$$c = \mathbf{d}\cdot\mathbf{m} = d_1 m_1 + d_2 m_2$$
$$\equiv c_1 + c_2 \text{ (note: no sigmoid)}$$
$$\tilde{c} \equiv \sigma(c)$$

The densities of c_i are simply given by

$$f_{c_i}(c_i) = \frac{1}{m_i\sqrt{2\pi\sigma^2}}e^{-c_i^2/2\sigma^2 m_i^2} \tag{3B.24}$$

from which we can calculate the total output density and the moments.

$$
\begin{aligned}
f_c(c) &= \int_{-\infty}^{\infty} f_{c_1}(c - c_2)f_{c_2}(c_2)dc_2 \\
&= \frac{1}{m_1 m_2}\frac{1}{2\pi\sigma^2}\int_{-\infty}^{\infty} e^{-(c-c_2)^2/2\sigma^2 m_1^2}e^{-c_2^2/2\sigma^2 m_2^2} \\
&= \sqrt{\frac{1}{m_1^2 + m_2^2}}\sqrt{\frac{1}{2\pi\sigma^2}}e^{-c^2/2\sigma^2(m_1^2 + m_2^2)}
\end{aligned}
\tag{3B.25}
$$

With moments

$$E[\tilde{c}^2] = \frac{\sigma^2}{2}\left(m_1^2 + m_2^2\right) \tag{3B.26}$$

$$E[\tilde{c}^3] = \sqrt{\frac{2}{\pi}}\sigma^3 \left(m_1^2 + m_2^2\right)^{3/2} \tag{3B.27}$$

$$E[\tilde{c}^4] = \frac{3\sigma^4}{2}\left(m_1^2 + m_2^2\right)^2 \tag{3B.28}$$

3B.3.2 *Kurtosis*

Kurtosis is calculated from the moments, and converted to polar coordinates.

$$K_2 = \frac{3\sigma^4}{4}\left(m_1^2 + m_2^2\right)^2 \tag{3B.29}$$

$$= \frac{3\sigma^4}{4}R^4 \tag{3B.30}$$

which doesn't depend on the angle at all. Since we are starting from the $R = 1$ point, the weights do a random walk in the $R = 1$ circle. A picture of this is in Figure 3B.2.

3B.3.3 *BCM*

In this case, the BCM cost function can also be converted to polar coordinates, because it doesn't depend on the length of the weights.

$$R_{\text{QBCM}} = \frac{1}{3}\sqrt{\frac{2}{\pi}}\sigma^3 \left(m_1^2 + m_2^2\right)^{3/2} - \frac{\sigma^4}{16}\left(m_1^2 + m_2^2\right)^2 \tag{3B.31}$$

$$= \frac{1}{3}\sqrt{\frac{2}{\pi}}\sigma^3 R^3 - \frac{\sigma^4}{16}R^4 \tag{3B.32}$$

which has a fixed point at

$$\left(m_1^2 + m_2^2\right) \equiv R$$

$$= \pm 4\sqrt{\frac{2}{\pi\sigma^2}} \tag{3B.33}$$

Once the weights reach this circle, they do a random walk around the circle (Figure 3B.2).

One conclusion we make from these calculations, is that the cells remain binocular. Selectivity could be lost (if the weights decrease), but the cells remain, on average, binocular. The uniform distribution actually contains enough structure to have stable fixed points, so weights actually converge to the fixed point, and do not wander.

One peculiar consequence of the BCM fixed point Equation 3B.33 is that, because the noise variance, σ^2, is in the denominator, for small noise the weights increase! Analytically this makes sense when we think of the behavior of BCM in the one dimensional case, because the lower the input, the larger the weight fixed point is in order to keep the output constant (both Equations 2.27 and 3B.4).

Gaussian Noise

Uniform Noise

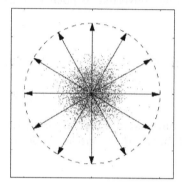
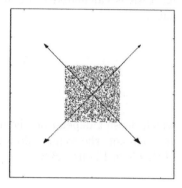

Figure 3B.2: Binocular Deprivation Fixed Points in a low dimensional environment. For the Gaussian case (left), the fixed points for both K_2 and R_{BCM} fall on a circle. For the uniform case (right), they point in the direction of the corners of the distribution.

The reason we have this behavior in these examples, and not in the simulations, is that the sigmoid in this simple analysis has a lower cutoff of zero. This sigmoid defines what we mean by spontaneous activity. This is the first time where the definition of spontaneous activity becomes crucial to the model. We can see where this comes from by looking at two extremes, low and high noise, rectified by a sigmoid with non-zero minimum.

Figure 3B.3 shows the unrectified and rectified Gaussian distributions, for both a high and a low noise case. In the low noise case the sigmoid doesn't change the distribution much, so we would only have a fixed point at $\mathbf{m} = 0$. In the high noise case the sigmoid introduces a significant skew, so our fixed point would have a non-zero value, but because it is the large noise case, the value would be small. Therefore, if the sigmoid has a minimum far enough from zero, we can keep the weights from growing in binocular deprivation. This point requires further examination. As the cellular and molecular interpretations of the variables c and d become clear it should be possible to refine the equations near zero and to clarify these points.

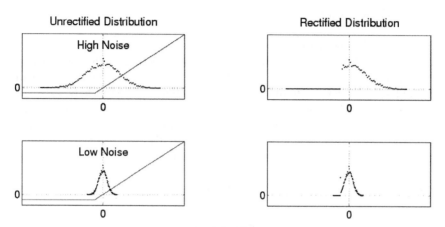

Figure 3B.3: Shown are the unrectified (left) and rectified (right) Gaussian distributions, along with the rectifying sigmoid. In the high noise case (above) the sigmoid introduces a significant skew, whereas in the low noise case (below) the sigmoid doesn't change the distribution much.

3B.4 Reverse Suture

The environment for reverse suture is identical to that for monocular deprivation (Figure 3B.1C), so all of the results we derived for MD apply here as well. The only difference is the initial conditions. Essentially, if there is some component of the closed eye remaining in MD, then reverse suture will eventually lead to the proper fixed point: the direction of the newly open eye. The sigmoid plays a crucial role here, as it does with binocular deprivation. At the start of reverse suture, conditions are similar to binocular deprivation. We have small responses from each eye, because we have noise coming in from one eye, and a small weight (initially) for the other eye. If the responses are too small, and the sigmoid has a non-zero lower value, then reverse suture will not work for the same reasons that binocular deprivation *requires* such a sigmoid: all of the moments will vanish.

This apparent inconsistency can be resolved by making sure that there is some, somewhat significant, residual left from monocular deprivation and that the bottom value of the sigmoid is not so large (in magnitude) to make all of the moments equal to zero. The particular timing of the reverse suture depends, then, on the residual left from monocular deprivation and the lower level of the sigmoid.

3B.5   Strabismus

Strabismus is the procedure where the eyes of the kitten were artificially misaligned. Simulations that demonstrate the resulting change from binocular to monocular cells are shown in Shouval et. al. (1995). This result can be understood very easily in this simple environment. Essentially, each eye is presented with structured input (numbers taken from a Laplace distribution), but the eyes are uncorrelated. The distribution does not lie on the 45° line, as it does for normal rearing (Figure 3B.1A), but the two input directions are independent, as shown in Figure 3B.4.

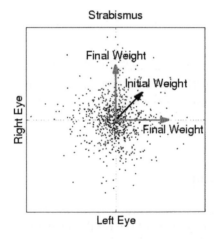

Figure 3B.4: 2D Strabismus. Strabismus is modeled with numbers chosen from a Laplace distribution presented to each eye. The eyes have *independent* inputs (samples shown with dots). The initial weight is from normal rearing, and the final weight is in the direction of one of the eyes alone: the cell comes to respond only to only one eye.

In this case we have an input vector **d** whose elements are chosen independently from a Laplace distribution.

$$f_{d_i}(d_i) = \frac{1}{2\lambda} e^{-|d_i|/\lambda} \tag{3B.34}$$

We can see from Figure 3B.4 that the tails of the distribution extend out in the $\hat{d}_1$ and $\hat{d}_2$ directions, which are the directions of highest kurtosis.

Again we have

$$c = \mathbf{d} \cdot \mathbf{m} = d_1 m_1 + d_2 m_2 \tag{3B.35}$$

$$\equiv c_1 + c_2 \text{ (note: no sigmoid)} \tag{3B.36}$$

$$\tilde{c} \equiv \sigma(c) \tag{3B.37}$$

$$f_{c_i}(c_i) = \frac{1}{2\lambda m_i} e^{-|c_i|/m_i\lambda} \tag{3B.38}$$

and we calculate the distribution of the output c (and thus the distribution of $\tilde{c}$) by taking the convolution of the individual densities of c_1 and c_2.

$$f_c(c) = \int_{-\infty}^{-\infty} f_{c_1}(c - c_2) f_{c_2}(c_2) dc_2$$

$$= \frac{1}{4\lambda^2 m_1 m_2} \int_{-\infty}^{-\infty} e^{-\left|\frac{c-c_2}{m_1}\right|/\lambda} e^{-|c_2/m_2|/\lambda} dc_2 \tag{3B.39}$$

$$= \frac{1}{2\lambda(m_1 - m_2)(m_1 + m_2)}$$
$$\times \left(m_1 e^{-|c|/m_1\lambda} - m_2 e^{-|c|/m_2\lambda} \right) \tag{3B.40}$$

$$f_{\tilde{c}}(\tilde{c}) = \begin{cases} f_c(\tilde{c}) & \text{if } \tilde{c} > 0 \\ \frac{1}{2}\delta(\tilde{c}) & \text{if } \tilde{c} = 0 \\ 0 & \text{if } \tilde{c} < 0 \end{cases} \tag{3B.41}$$

The moments are calculated in a straightforward fashion.

$$E\left[\tilde{c}^2\right] = \frac{1}{2\lambda(m_1 - m_2)(m_1 + m_2)} \left(m_1 2\lambda^3 m_1^3 - m_2 2\lambda^3 m_2^3 \right)$$
$$= \lambda^2 \left(m_1^2 + m_2^2 \right) \tag{3B.42}$$

$$E\left[\tilde{c}^3\right] = \frac{1}{2\lambda(m_1 - m_2)(m_1 + m_2)} \left(6m_1^5\lambda^4 - 6m_2^5\lambda^4 \right)$$
$$= 3\lambda^3 \frac{m_1^5 - m_2^5}{m_1^2 - m_2^2} \tag{3B.43}$$

$$E\left[\tilde{c}^4\right] = \frac{1}{2\lambda(m_1 - m_2)(m_1 + m_2)} \left(24\lambda^5 m_1^6 - 24\lambda^5 m_2^6 \right)$$
$$= 12\lambda^4 (m_1^4 + m_1^2 m_2^2 + m_2^4) \tag{3B.44}$$

3B.5.1 *Kurtosis*

The value of K_2 is then simply

$$K_2 = E\left[\tilde{c}^4\right] - 3E\left[\tilde{c}^2\right]$$
$$= 9\lambda^4 m_1^4 + 6\lambda^4 m_1^2 m_2^2 + 9\lambda^4 m_2^4 \tag{3B.45}$$

$$K_2(R, \theta) = \lambda^4 R^4 \left(12 \cos^4(\theta) - 12 \cos^2(\theta) + 9 \right) \qquad (3\text{B}.46)$$

where we have converted K_2 to polar coordinates, as before.

This function has stable maxima at $\theta = 0$ and $\theta = \pi/2$, which are the monocular solutions.

3B.5.2 BCM

The cost function is calculated from the moments, as before.

$$
\begin{aligned}
R_{\text{QBCM}} &= \frac{1}{3} E \left[\tilde{c}^3 \right] - \frac{1}{4} E^2 \left[\tilde{c}^2 \right] \\
&= \lambda^3 \frac{m_1^5 - m_2^5}{m_1^2 - m_2^2} - \frac{\lambda^2}{4} \left(m_1^2 + m_2^2 \right)^2 \qquad (3\text{B}.47)
\end{aligned}
$$

which has stable maxima

$$\mathbf{m} = \begin{pmatrix} 0 \\ 3/\lambda \end{pmatrix}, \begin{pmatrix} 3/\lambda \\ 0 \end{pmatrix} \qquad (3\text{B}.48)$$

which are also monocular solutions.

Appendix 3C

Statistical Theorems

The following are some theorems from [Papoulis, 1984], useful in the analysis of extended probability distributions.

$$y = g(x) \tag{3C.1}$$

$$\text{(all possible solutions) } x_i \equiv g^{-1}(y) \tag{3C.2}$$

$$f_y(y) = \frac{1}{|g'(x_1)|} f_x(x_1)$$

$$+ \frac{1}{|g'(x_2)|} f_x(x_2) + \cdots \tag{3C.3}$$

$$y = ax + b \tag{3C.4}$$

$$f_y(y) = \frac{1}{|a|} f_x \left(\frac{y - b}{a} \right) \tag{3C.5}$$

$$z = x + y \tag{3C.6}$$

$$f_z(z) = \int_{-\infty}^{-\infty} f(z - y, y) dy \tag{3C.7}$$

$$\text{if independent: } f(x, y) = f_x(x) f_y(y) \tag{3C.8}$$

$$f_z(z) = \int_{-\infty}^{-\infty} f_x(z - y) f_y(y) dy \tag{3C.9}$$

Chapter 4

Cortical Network Theory

4.1 Introduction

In previous chapters we analyzed a simplified single cell theory of synaptic plasticity. The actual cortical network is very complex. It includes different cell types, intra-cortical interactions, and recurrent collaterals. Most of the input, both excitatory and inhibitory, to cortical cells in visual cortex arises from other cortical cells and not from thalamo-cortical projections. Therefore, theories of synaptic plasticity must address the effect of network dynamics. Networks of many interacting neurons are simulated in detail in Chapter 8. In this chapter we present two complementary forms of analysis that can help elucidate some of the effects of the cortical network, without resorting to complex simulations.

The cells of visual cortex form a network in which inhibitory and excitatory cells receive input from the lateral geniculate nucleus (LGN), from each other and feedback from higher cortical levels. Such a network is a highly complex, non-linear, system. Some of the key questions concern the necessary levels of connectivity, the importance of instantaneous signaling, stochastic behavior as well as the approach to equilibrium. For example, the amount of connectivity is of significance both from a theoretical point of view as well as for the possible embodiment of neural networks in electronic circuitry.

Interacting cortical networks can have two distinct effects on the outcome of synaptic plasticity. Such networks can: (1) alter the development of single cell properties. (2) effect the organization of single cell properties across the cortical map. Our analysis concentrates on addressing the former issue. Analysis in the previous sections has concentrated on single BCM neurons, in an environment composed of linearly independent inputs (for a linear algebra review, see the Appendix to [Dayan and Abbott, 2001]). In some descriptions of cortical plasticity, network interactions are essential for obtaining selective receptive fields [Kohonen, 1984; Olshausen and

111

Field, 1996c]. In contrast, we have shown that BCM obtains selective receptive fields for single cells. However, the effect of lateral connectivity and neuronal non-linearity might have a large impact on the form of selectivity and receptive fields obtained with BCM neurons. Using two complementary techniques we will examine this issue. As in previous sections our analysis typically assumes a simplified environment composed of linearly separable input vectors. Further, this analysis is restricted to cases in which the lateral connectivity itself in non-plastic.

In section 4.2 we describe a mean field approximation of the cortical network. We show that there exists a mapping between single cell and network results. In addition, we show that if inhibition is strong enough, fully selective fixed points can be reached even if thalamo-cortical synapses are solely excitatory.

In section 4.3 a more complex matrix based analysis of networks of interacting BCM neurons [Castellani et al., 1999] is reviewed. This analysis extends our previous analytical single cell results to networks of non-linear neurons, without using the approximations of the mean-field theory. However, as in the mean field approximation we assume there is no plasticity in the cortico-cortical connections. Although this analysis is complex it reveals quite simple and surprising results. We find that both non-linearities and network interactions do not fundamentally alter the nature of the fixed points of BCM neurons. In terms of the output responses, the same fixed points exist for single cells and for networks of interacting non-linear neurons. What is altered is the structure of the synaptic weights and the basins of attraction of the different stable fixed points.

4.2 Mean Field Theory

In what follows we present a mean field analysis of this complex system. The first step is to divide the inputs to any cell into those from LGN and those from other sources. In a network generalization of Equation 2.1, we may therefore write

$$c_i = \mathbf{m}_i \cdot \mathbf{d} + \sum_j L_{ij} c_j, \qquad (4.1)$$

where c_i is the activity of cortical neuron i, $\mathbf{m}_i$ is the synaptic weight vector between thalamus and cortical neuron i, and L_{ij} are the cortico-cortical synapses between neurons with activity level c_j to neuron with activity level c_i. In this approximation we exclude feedback from cells that are not directly linked to LGN. We can also break up the input to cortical cells into left and right eye inputs, and weights thus $\mathbf{m}_i = (\mathbf{m}_i^l, \mathbf{m}_i^r)$ and

$\mathbf{d}_i = (\mathbf{d}_i^l, \mathbf{d}_i^r)$. Our description is based on the theory discussed in Scofield and Cooper (1985) and Cooper and Scofield (1988). Inhibition is more likely to contribute to sharpening RF's and for making them diverse. Therefore we concentrate on $(L_{ij} < 0)$.

Given a matrix of cortical synaptic weights M, the output of the cells of the full network can be written as

$$\mathbf{c} = \sigma(M\mathbf{d} + L\mathbf{c}) \tag{4.2}$$

where $\mathbf{c} = (c_1, \ldots, c_N)^T$, and c_i is the output activity of the ith cortical cell and $L = (L_{ij})$ is the matrix of cortical-cortical connections so that L_{ij} is the synapse from the jth cell to the ith cell. $M = (M_{ik}^l, M_{ik}^r)$ where M_{ik}^l and M_{ik}^r are the kth LGN synapses from the left and right eye to the ith cortical cell. $\mathbf{d} = (\mathbf{d}^l, \mathbf{d}^r)^T$, where $\mathbf{d}^{l(r)} = (d_1^{l(r)}, \ldots, d_n^{l(r)})^T$.

The learning rule is as for the single cell

$$\dot{M} = \mathbf{d} \times \phi(\mathbf{c}, \boldsymbol{\theta}_M).$$

except that, in this equation, $\mathbf{c}$ is a vector of outputs with the corresponding vector of thresholds, $\boldsymbol{\theta}_M$, and the product is an *outer* product between the input vector, $\mathbf{d}$, and the vector of modification values, $\phi(\mathbf{c}, \boldsymbol{\theta}_M) \equiv (\phi(c_1, (\boldsymbol{\theta}_M)_1), \phi(c_2, (\boldsymbol{\theta}_M)_2), \cdots)$.

Further, in what follows, we assume for maximum simplicity that there is no modification of cortico-cortical synapses although what experimental results there are suggest only that modification of inhibitory cortico-cortical synapses is slow. Thus

$$\dot{L}_{ij} = 0.$$

In the linear region of the sigmoidal activity function the output of a cell is given by the weighted sum of the LGN inputs and the cortical inputs. Thus the activity is given by:

$$\mathbf{c} = M\mathbf{d} + L\mathbf{c}. \tag{4.3}$$

We consider a region of cortex for which the neural mapping of the input from the visual field is constant (all of the cells, in effect, look at a given region of the visual field). Under these conditions, for an input $\mathbf{d}$ constant in time, the equilibrium state of this network would be

$$\mathbf{c} = (I - L)^{-1} M\mathbf{d}. \tag{4.4}$$

It is interesting to note that if we expand $(1 - L)^{-1}$, we obtain an expansion in mono, di, tri ... synaptic events:

$$(1 - L)^{-1} = 1 + L + L^2 + \ldots.$$

How many synaptic events one includes depends on the time interval of importance. For synaptic modification we assume that time intervals of the order of a half second are appropriate. Thus c represents the average over about one-half second of the number of spikes that are the result of an external presentation. The post stimulus time histogram can be broken into much smaller time intervals thus separating mono, di, tri synaptic events and excitatory and inhibitory inputs.

Recall from Equation 4.1, that for a given LGN-cortical vector of synapses, $\mathbf{m}_i$, and for a given input from both eyes, $\mathbf{d}$, the activity of the ith cortical cell is given by

$$c_i = \mathbf{m}_i \cdot \mathbf{d} + \sum_j L_{ij} c_j, \tag{4.5}$$

where the first term is the input from LGN and the second represents intra-cortical input to the cell. We define c_{mf} as the average activity of all of the cortical cells under *the conditions above:*

$$c_{mf} = \frac{1}{N} \sum_i c_i. \tag{4.6}$$

The mean field approximation is obtained by replacing c_j in the sum in Equation 4.5 by its average value so that c_i becomes

$$c_i = \mathbf{m}_i \cdot \mathbf{d} + c_{mf} L(i), \tag{4.7}$$

where

$$L(i) = \sum_j L_{ij}.$$

Here, in a manner similar to that in the theory of magnetism, we have replaced the effect of individual cortical cells by their average effect (as though all other cortical cells can be replaced by an 'effective' cell with activity c_{mf} and synaptic connection to cell i denoted by $L(i)$).

From Equations 4.6 and 4.7 we obtain the solution (consistency condition)

$$c_{mf} = \frac{1}{N} \sum_i c_i = \overline{\mathbf{m}} \cdot \mathbf{d} + c_{mf} L_0, \tag{4.8}$$

where

$$L_0 = \frac{1}{N} \sum_i L(i),$$

is the average inhibition constant

$$\overline{\mathbf{m}} = \frac{1}{N} \sum_i \mathbf{m}_i.$$

is the average of all the input weight vectors to the different neurons. Using this we obtain

$$c_{mf} = (1 - L_0)^{-1} \overline{\mathbf{m}} \cdot \mathbf{d}.$$

Note that the average magnitude of cortico-cortical inhibition, (L_0), must be smaller than one. Otherwise c_{mf} would be smaller than zero, and there would be so much inhibition that on average no cells would fire.

This analysis yields

$$c_i = \left(\mathbf{m}_i + \frac{L(i)}{1 - L_0} \overline{\mathbf{m}} \right) \cdot \mathbf{d}. \tag{4.9}$$

If we assume that the lateral connection strengths are a function only of $i-j$ (not dependent on the absolute position of a cell in the network, therefore dependent only on the distance of two cells from one another), L_{ij} becomes a circular matrix so that

$$\sum_i L_{ij} = \sum_j L_{ij} = L(i) = L_0, \tag{4.10}$$

independent of the cortical cell, i.

We then obtain

$$c_i = \left(\mathbf{m}_i + \frac{L_0}{1 - L_0} \overline{\mathbf{m}} \right) \cdot \mathbf{d}. \tag{4.11}$$

In the mean field approximation we can therefore write that the output of the cell is the combined effect of the feed-forward inputs, $\mathbf{m}_i \cdot \mathbf{d}$, and a background inhibition, $-\boldsymbol{\alpha} \cdot \mathbf{d}$, giving

$$c_i = (\mathbf{m}_i - \boldsymbol{\alpha}) \cdot \mathbf{d}, \tag{4.12}$$

where

$$\boldsymbol{\alpha} = -\frac{L_0}{1 - L_0} \overline{\mathbf{m}} \tag{4.13}$$

is the mean background inhibition. Note that $\boldsymbol{\alpha}$ is a vector, proportional to the $\overline{\mathbf{m}}$ vector.

For two eyes, this can be written as

$$c_j(\boldsymbol{\alpha}) = (\mathbf{m}_i - \boldsymbol{\alpha}) \cdot \mathbf{d} = (\mathbf{m}_i^l - \boldsymbol{\alpha}^l) \cdot \mathbf{d}^l + (\mathbf{m}_i^r - \boldsymbol{\alpha}^r) \cdot \mathbf{d}^r, \tag{4.14}$$

where the mean field

$$\alpha = (\alpha^l, \alpha^r) = -a(\overline{\mathbf{m}}^l, \overline{\mathbf{m}}^r)$$

with

$$a = |L_0|(1 + |(L_0|)^{-1},$$

and we assume that $L_0 < 0$ (the network is, on average, inhibitory).

For BCM neurons it is often the case that the selective fixed points occur in a region of space where at least some components of $\mathbf{m}_i$ are less then zero, or inhibitory. For BCM to reach these fixed points it must be able to freely alter the sign of these synaptic connections; this is unlikely to be biologically plausible.

We note that even if m_i the LGN-cortical synapses are excitatory ($m_i \geq 0$), if there is average inhibition ($\alpha > 0$), then $m_i - \alpha$ may be negative.

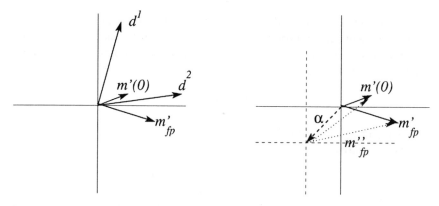

Figure 4.1: Fixed points of BCM in a mean field network. (Left) Input vectors d_1, d_2, the initial weight vector $m'(0)$ and the final weight vector m'_{fp}, in the absence of cortical interactions and restrictions on synaptic weights, in a simple 2D example. The axes represent both input magnitude (for the $\mathbf{d}$ vectors) and weight magnitude (for the $\mathbf{m}$ vectors). It is conceptually simpler to view the inputs and the weights on the same plot, even though in reality these quantities would be measured in different units. A selective fixed point is reached but some synaptic weights must be negative. (Right) Cortical interactions between different neurons in a network result in an effective mean field inhibition, α. Thus in this network an analogous fixed point m''_{fp}, is reached which is fully excitatory. The fixed point in the cortical network is the fixed point of $\alpha = 0$ network but is measured with respect to a new coordinate system shifted by α.

If α is large enough, the selective fixed points lying in the $\mathbf{m}_i < 0$ region may be reached (see Figure 4.1). However, it is not obvious that it will indeed be reached using the same BCM synaptic dynamics. This is addressed in the following section.

4.2.1 Position and Stability of Fixed Points of LGN-Cortical Synapses in the Mean Field Network

We now generalize the arguments given in BCM for the position and stability of the fixed points of the stochastic non-linear synaptic modification equations. In the mean field network

$$\dot{m}_i(\alpha) = \phi(c_i(\alpha), \theta_M(\alpha))d = \phi[m_i(\alpha) - \alpha]d \qquad (4.15)$$

The mean field inhibition, $\alpha^{l(r)}$ as given by Equation 4.13, has a time dependent component $\bar{m}^{l(r)}$. This varies as the average over all of the network modifiable synapses and, in most environmental situations, should change slowly compared to the change of the modifiable synapses to a single cell:

$$|\dot{\bar{m}}| << |\dot{m}_i|. \qquad (4.16)$$

We, therefore, define an approximation in which we assume that α is slowly varying and determine the trajectory of m_i for fixed α. (We imagine that m_i reaches its fixed point before α varies*. In the adiabatic approximation we can write

$$\frac{d}{dt}(m_i(\alpha) - \alpha) = \phi[m_i(\alpha) - \alpha]d. \qquad (4.17)$$

We see that there is a mapping

$$m_i' \leftrightarrow m_i(\alpha) - \alpha \qquad (4.18)$$

such that for every $m_i(\alpha)$ there exists a corresponding (mapped) point m_i' which satisfies

$$\dot{m}_i' = \phi[m_i']d, \qquad (4.19)$$

the original equation for the mean field zero theory. Therefore, if we start from the corresponding initial point

---

*The non-adiabatic situation is analyzed in Appendix 4A, where it is shown that, in any case, the position and stability of the fixed points is unaltered.

$$m_i'(t_o) = m_i(\alpha, t_o) - \alpha, \tag{4.20}$$

the m_i' trajectory viewed from the m_i coordinate system is the trajectory of $m_i(\alpha = 0)$. Thus, we can compute $m_i(\alpha)$ from the $\alpha = 0$ trajectory using

$$m_i(\alpha) = m_i' + \alpha = m_i(\alpha = 0) + \alpha. \tag{4.21}$$

The transformation

$$m_i'' = m_i + \alpha \tag{4.22}$$

gives the weight vector in a new coordinate system, whose origin is displaced from the zero mean-field coordinates by α (Figure 4.1). The trajectory of a solution of the $\alpha = 0$ theory measured from this coordinate system gives a solution of the $\alpha \neq 0$ theory for the corresponding point:

$$m_i''(\alpha) = m_i'(\alpha) + \alpha = m_i(0) + \alpha = m_i(\alpha). \tag{4.23}$$

It follows that at corresponding points

$$c_i(\alpha) = c_i(0) \tag{4.24}$$

for every input, and thus

$$\theta_m(\alpha) = \theta_m(0) \tag{4.25}$$

Applied to the fixed points we conclude that for every fixed point of $m_i(\alpha = 0)$ there exists a corresponding fixed point for $m_i(\alpha)$ with the same selectivity and stability properties. Therefore, just as for the $\alpha = 0$ theory, for arbitrary α only selective fixed points are stable. Further, at corresponding fixed points we obtain the same cell output.

From this we see that if the background inhibition is changed (e.g. by long term application of bicuculline or a GABA agonist) and the LGN-cortical synapses are allowed to evolve to the new fixed points in the same visual environment, the outputs of the cortical cells will evolve to what they were before the background inhibition was altered. [It is presumed that a cortical cell does not jump from one stable fixed point to another in this process.]

The above is limited as follows:

(1) The LGN-cortical synapses are restricted to be positive (excitatory). Therefore, if α is too small (insufficient background inhibition), $m_i(\alpha)$ will not be able to reach its fixed points with only positive components.

(2) The LGN-cortical synapses cannot increase beyond some physiological and/or molecular limit. Therefore, if α is too large, the cell will never fire thus restricting the evolution of $m_i(\alpha)$.

In Scofield and Cooper (1988) this work was extended to cases in which not all thalamo-cortical neurons are plastic and to different rearing conditions.

4.2.2 *Comparison of Linear Feed-Forward with Lateral Inhibition Network: Mean Field Approximation*

For the linear case, using the notation of Cooper and Scofield, (1988), neuron activity in the lateral inhibition network is given by

$$c = Md + Lc. \tag{4.26}$$

In the mean field approximation this becomes

$$c = Md + L\bar{c}, \tag{4.27}$$

where M is the synaptic matrix for N neurons, $c = (c_1, \ldots, c_N)^T$, L is the inhibitory connection matrix with norm less than 1 and $\bar{c}$ is the averaged activity over all neurons in the network. In the context of visual cortex, the first term is due to the input from LGN and the second due to input from other cortical cells. If we define $c(0) = Md$, then the averaged inhibited activity can be written as

$$\bar{c} = \bar{c}(0) + L\bar{c}, \tag{4.28}$$

or

$$\bar{c} = (I - L)^{-1}\bar{c}(0) = (I + L + L^2 + L^3 + \ldots)\,\bar{c}(0). \tag{4.29}$$

Using this notation, the activity of a neuron in the feed-forward network as defined in Section 3.2.3 can be written

$$\tilde{c} = c(1) = c(0) + Lc(0), \tag{4.30}$$

which leads to an averaged activity of the form

$$\bar{c}(1) = (I + L)\bar{c}(0), \tag{4.31}$$

which is a first order approximation of Equation 4.28; it is useful primarily because it removes the need to invert a matrix or in the non-linear case, have relaxation dynamics. In addition, successive approximations

$$\begin{aligned} \bar{c}(1) &= \bar{c}(0) + L\bar{c}(0) = (I + L)\bar{c}(0), \\ \bar{c}(2) &= \bar{c}(0) + L\bar{c}(1) = (I + L + L^2)\bar{c}(0), \end{aligned} \tag{4.32}$$

$$\vdots$$

can be thought of as including mono-synaptic, bi-synaptic, tri-synaptic etc. events and thus follow the time course of the post-synaptic potentiation. It follows that $\bar{c}(k) \to \bar{c}$, as $k \to \infty$, thus converging to the lateral inhibition network described in Equation 4.29. Within a scaling factor, the first order feed-forward network, as will be shown below, generates the same synaptic modification equations as the lateral inhibition network in the Cooper and Scofield mean field approximation.

For a feed-forward network with neuron activity given by $\tilde{c}_i = m_i \cdot d + \sum_j L_{ij} c_j$, as in section 3.2,

$$\dot{m}_k = -\frac{\partial R}{\partial m_k} = -\left[\frac{\partial R_k}{\partial m_k} + \sum_j L_{kj} \frac{\partial R_j}{\partial m_j}\right]$$

$$= \mu\left[E[\phi(\tilde{c}_k, \tilde{\Theta}_M^k)\mathbf{d}] + \sum_j L_{kj} E[\phi(\tilde{c}_j, \tilde{\Theta}_m^j)\mathbf{d}]\right]. \quad (4.33)$$

Let $\overline{\mathbf{m}} = \frac{1}{N}\sum_j m_j \; (m_j \in R^n)$. We assume that the inhibitory contributions are a function only of the $i - j$ (not dependent on the absolute position of a cell in the network), so that

$$\sum_i L_{ij} = L_0 = \sum_j L_{ij}, \quad (4.34)$$

and that $\sum_i L_{ij} E[\phi(\tilde{c}_i, \tilde{\Theta}_m^i)\mathbf{d}] = \sum_j L_{ij} E[\phi(\tilde{c}_j, \tilde{\Theta}_m^j)\mathbf{d}]$. Then we get:

$$N\dot{\overline{\mathbf{m}}} = \sum_j \dot{m}_j = \mu\left[\sum_k E[\phi(\tilde{c}_k, \tilde{\Theta}_M^k)\mathbf{d}] + \sum_j L_0 E[\phi(\tilde{c}_j, \tilde{\Theta}_m^j)\mathbf{d}]\right]$$

$$= \frac{(1 + L_0)}{L_0}\mu\sum_k\sum_j L_{kj} E[\phi(\tilde{c}_k, \tilde{\Theta}_M^k)\mathbf{d}]. \quad (4.35)$$

This implies that

$$\frac{L_0}{1 + L_0}\dot{\overline{\mathbf{m}}} = \mu\sum_k L_{jk} E[\phi(\tilde{c}_k, \tilde{\Theta}_M^k)x, \quad (4.36)$$

and hence,

$$\dot{m}_k = \mu\left[E[\phi(\tilde{c}_k, \tilde{\Theta}_M^k)\mathbf{d}] + \frac{L_0}{1 + L_0}\dot{\overline{\mathbf{m}}}\right]. \quad (4.37)$$

Compare this with Cooper and Scofield, (1988) (eq. A3):

$$\dot{m}_k = \mu\left[E[\phi(c_k, \Theta_m^k)\mathbf{d}] + L_0\dot{\overline{\mathbf{m}}}\right], \quad (4.38)$$

Equations 4.37 and 4.38 differ only in the constant of inhibition. Thus, under the uniform lateral inhibition assumption in Equation 4.34, the mean field approximation of the feed-forward network yields the lateral inhibition mean field result merely by scaling the average inhibition.

4.3 Matrix-based Analysis of Networks of Interacting and Non-linear BCM Neurons

A more complex and comprehensive approach based on a matrix formulation of the input environment [Castellani et al., 1999] has allowed us to analytically address networks of interacting non-linear BCM neurons. This analysis is too complex to carry out here. However, we will review here its somewhat surprising results. As in previous analysis we assume an input environment composed of K linearly independent vectors, $D = (\mathbf{d}^1, \mathbf{d}^2, ... \mathbf{d}^K)$, where D is the square matrix composed of the input patterns.

Previously we have shown that the stable fixed points of single linear BCM neurons are such that it is orthogonal to all patterns but one. Therefore, a neuron responds to one input pattern, and this response has the value $c = 1/p_i$ where p_i is the probability of pattern i being chosen randomly. Castellani et. al. (1999) show that this is still the case for a single non-linear neuron, the only difference now is that $\sigma(\mathbf{m}_{fp} \cdot \mathbf{d}^i) = 1/p_i$, where σ is the non-linearity and $\mathbf{m}_{fp}$ is the synaptic weight vector at the fixed point. Formally we have that $\mathbf{m}_{fp} \cdot \mathbf{d}^i = \sigma^{-1}(1/p_i)$. If we choose $\sigma(0) = 0$, the magnitude but not the shape of $\mathbf{m}_{fp}$ is altered, and in all cases the cells output is preserved.

Next Castellani et. al. analyze a network of N output neurons, which interact with each other via a lateral connectivity matrix L. In this analysis the stable fixed points of this network are all possible combinations of the single neuron fixed points. Thus *no novel stable fixed points result from the lateral connectivity.* This is surprising, we could expect that neurons could now have fixed points in which they respond to more than one input pattern if excitation is large enough or to no input patterns for sufficiently strong inhibition. However, our analysis shows that this is not the case. This result is surprising since it is independent of the values of the connectivity matrix L (as long as it is invertible).

What is even more surprising is that all such combinations are stable fixed points. It could be expected that if L is purely excitatory stable fixed points would be such that all neurons respond to the same input pattern, and if it is inhibitory all neurons respond to different input patterns. However, our analysis shows that this is not the case. Thus, the fixed points are the same as for the single cell model in terms of the cells output, but not in terms of the weight vectors. This is similar to what we have found for the non-linear activation function. However, the synaptic weight vectors resulting are different in both magnitude and shape.

While network interactions do not alter the stability of the different fixed points and do not add novel fixed points, they do alter the probability of converging to the different fixed points. We have shown that excitatory connections enhance the probability that the different neurons would become selective to the same input patterns while inhibitory connections enhance the probability of different neurons becoming selective to different input patterns.

In a simple network composed two output neurons, responses can be classified as selective, when the neurons are selective to different input patterns, and associative in which they become selective to the same input pattern. We simulated such networks for different forms of lateral connectivity matrices of the form:

$$L = \begin{pmatrix} 0 & l \\ l & 0 \end{pmatrix}.$$

In Figure 4.2 we show how the value of l effects the fraction of selective states in such a network. As expected, excitatory connections ($l > 0$) favor formation of associative states whereas inhibitory connections ($l < 0$) favor convergence to selective states.

4.4   Discussion

Our analysis in previous chapters has concentrated on single cortical BCM neurons, without lateral interactions with other neurons. Such analysis might be able to account for receptive fields properties of single cortical cells but clearly cannot explain the formation and organization of collective properties of cortical structures, such as organized maps.

Our previous analysis, in simple environments, has shown that the stable fixed points of BCM neurons are maximally selective fixed points. However, this analysis assumed that the feed-forward synaptic weights onto such a neuron can take on both positive and negative values. This does not hold in real synapses that are typically either excitatory or inhibitory. The thalamo-cortical projections, from LGN to a neuron in visual cortex, are purely excitatory. With excitatory weights only, a BCM neuron will be able to achieve only limited selectivity. In this chapter we have shown that a network of cortical neurons, that possesses sufficient inhibition, can attain maximal selectivity even if the thalamo-cortical projections are purely excitatory. Thus lateral inhibition can produce effectively inhibitory thalamo-cortical projections, even if they are physically excitatory. Both the mean

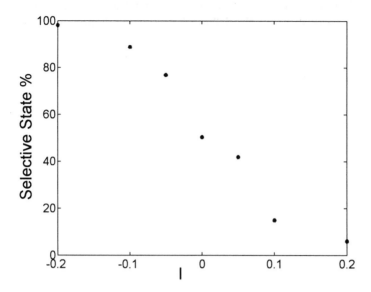

Figure 4.2: Lateral connections effect the probability of converging to selective or associative states. For $l = -0.2, 0.1$ networks usually converge to the selective states. As l increase the chance of converging to a selective state decreases. For $l = 0$ there is an equal probability of converging to selective and associative states, as expected, and for $l = 0.2$, associative states dominate.

field analysis and the matrix based analysis have shown that the lateral connectivity does not alter the identity, selectivity, and stability of the single neuron fixed points. What does change are the synaptic weights at the fixed points.

In a network of laterally connected neurons, the fixed points are combinations of the possible single neuron fixed points. It could be expected that excitatory lateral connections would destabilize combinations of different fixed points, and that inhibitory connections would destabilize combinations where different neurons converge to the same fixed point. Surprisingly, this is not the case. All combinations of stable single neurons fixed points are stable, independent of the lateral connectivity. However, the lateral connectivity does alter the probability of getting different combinations of fixed points. Excitatory connections favor situations in which all neurons converge to the same fixed point, whereas inhibitory connections favor combinations of different fixed points.

This chapter has displayed analytical results concerning networks of laterally connected neurons. With more complex inputs and connectivity schemes, lateral connectivity can be critical for the formation of smooth but diverse cortical maps. We demonstrate this in Chapter 8 with the aid of simulations.

Appendix 4A

Asymptotic Behavior of Mean Field Equations with Time Dependent Mean Field

From Equations 4.18 and 4.19, the trajectory of the corresponding point is

$$\dot{m}'_i = \phi[m'_i]d - \dot{\alpha} \qquad (4A.1)$$

Using Equation 4.2, we have

$$\alpha'_i = a\ \bar{\dot{m}}(\alpha)(1 - a^{-1})\bar{m}', \qquad (4A.2)$$

so that

$$\dot{m}_i = \phi[m'_i]d - a\ (1 - a)^{-1}\bar{\dot{m}}'. \qquad (4A.3)$$

At the fixed points $\dot{m}'_i = 0$. (When all of the cells of the network have reached their respective fixed points $\dot{m}'_i = 0$ for each cell.) Therefore, $\bar{\dot{m}}' = 0$. It follows that at a global fixed point when the network has stabilized at a global fixed point

$$\phi[m'_i]d = 0 \qquad (4A.4)$$

for all inputs. This is the same condition as the $\dot{\alpha} = 0$ (adiabatic) case. Thus the position and stability of the fixed points are the same as those in the adiabatic theory. However, since $0 < (1 - a) < 1$, the absolute value of average movement of the entire network toward the fixed points

$$|\bar{\dot{m}}'| = (1 - a)\phi[\bar{m}'_i]d$$

is slower than in the adiabatic theory.

Appendix 4A

Asymptotic Behavior of Mean Field Equations with Time Dependent Mean Field

Chapter 5

Review and Analysis of Second Order Learning Rules

5.1 Introduction

Many of the qualitative features of the BCM theory depend on its incorporation of statistics beyond the second order. (Other possible learning rules, discussed in the previous chapters, such as kurtosis also incorporate third or higher order statistics). Numerous proposed learning rules that incorporate only second order statistics have been extensively investigated in many complex situations. The simulations used in these investigations employ various initial and final points as well as a variety of parameters so that it is often difficult to tell what features are producing the particular result. To help clarify the connections between assumptions and conclusions for these models, we introduce some new analytic tools. In this chapter, aided by these tools, we analyze the properties of these second order rules as well as their ability to account for the experimental data.

The cornerstone of all unsupervised learning rules is the Hebb rule [Hebb, 1949]. However this rule, in its original form, suffers from two major problems: (1) all modification are positive so that all weights grow (2) it is unstable, i.e., the synaptic weights will all be driven to their maximal value. Numerous learning rules have been proposed to overcome these difficulties. Stability can be attained by normalization of the weights[von der Malsburg, 1973], appropriate decay terms added to the function for the change in the weights [Oja, 1982; Sanger, 1989] or saturation limits on the weights themselves[Linsker, 1986b; Miller et al., 1989]. In addition inputs and outputs can be measured with respect to their mean activity, or to arbitrary reference points. This leads to a family of covariance rules in which weights can decrease as well [Sejnowski, 1977; Linsker, 1986b; Miller et al., 1989]. The outcome of learning in all these models depends only on the first and second order statistics of their inputs. Therefore, to gain understanding of receptive fields extracted by such rules, it is necessary to know what the principal components (eigenvectors) of the inputs are (for a linear algebra review, see the Appendix to Dayan and Abbott, 2001).

Some of these models have been used to model plasticity in the visual system. In order to do this, additional assumptions about the relevant visual environment and the architecture of the network have to be made. We will survey these different assumptions, and try to understand the sources of the differing results: Do they arise from different assumptions about the environment, architecture or the learning rule?

In Section 5.2 we survey the theoretical properties of the Hebbian learning rule as well as of some related learning rules such as Oja's PCA rule [Oja, 1982] and some of the saturated variants of the Hebb rule [Linsker, 1986b; Miller et al., 1989].

In the following sections we describe how known experimental properties of cortical cells can be attained using such learning rules. In Section 5.3 we review the different assumptions that may produce orientation selectivity. We review both simplified correlational models such as those proposed by Linsker [Linsker, 1986b] and models that use actual natural images to drive receptive field development. Section 5.4 reviews models for the development of ocular dominance; again we review both simplified models and more complex models that employ a natural image environment. We also explore the underlying theoretical reasons for the results obtained. Section 5.5 combines results from both previous sections. In it we try to examine conditions under which both orientation selectivity and ocular dominance occur. We show that principal components can not exhibit both ocular dominance and orientation selectivity and examine the conditions under which saturated rules can have both orientation selectivity and ocular dominance. We also show what happens in a mis-aligned natural image environment.

In Section 5.6 we examine both theoretically and using simulations whether such learning rules can produce deprivation results such as Monocular Deprivation, Binocular Deprivation and Reverse Suture.

5.2   Hebb's Rule and Its Derivatives

The original Hebb rule, states how synapse efficacies (or weights) are strengthened [Hebb, 1949]:

> When an axon in cell A is near enough to excite cell B and repeatedly and persistently takes part in firing it, some growth process or metabolic change takes place in one or both cells such that A's efficiency in firing B, is increased.

Later, it was suggested that synaptic strengths may decrease during learning as well. This may happen for two distinct reasons, first strengths change as a function of the correlations between the pre- and post- synaptic neurons, i.e. they increase when the activities of the neurons are correlated, and decrease when they are anti-correlated as was originally suggested by Stent [Stent, 1973] and used subsequently in much of the work on this issue [Oja, 1982; Linsker, 1986b; Miller et al., 1989] . Furthermore, as discussed in the next section, synaptic efficacy decreases may occur in order to stabilize learning [Rochester et al., 1956; von der Malsburg, 1973; Oja, 1982; Linsker, 1986b].

A mathematically simple form, that will nevertheless be general enough for understanding the basic properties of such learning rules, is the linear rule [Linsker, 1986b]

$$\Delta m_i = \eta(d_i - d_o)(c - c_o) \tag{5.1}$$

where d_i are the activities of presynaptic neurons, c is the activity of the postsynaptic neuron, Δm_i is the change in the value of the synaptic efficacy between presynaptic neuron i and the postsynaptic neuron, and η, d_o and c_o are constants. This equation implies that pre- and postsynaptic activity levels are not measured with respect to zero, but with respect to fixed pre- and postsynaptic baselines (d_0, c_0), which could be for example, average pre- and postsynaptic activity levels.

This concept is easiest to analyze in terms of single postsynaptic linear neurons, i.e., when the neuron's activity is given by the following (equivalent to Equation 2.1):

$$c = \sum_j m_j d_j. \tag{5.2}$$

For this case, we can calculate the average of the synaptic efficacies over the input probability distribution. We denote this average by $E[\cdot]$. This average weight change is of interest to us since we define the fixed points as those values of m_i for which the average weight change over the environment is zero.

Using Equations 5.1 and 5.2, averaging the result, and defining the mean input value $\mu = E[d_j] = E[d_i]$, we obtain an equation for the average change in synaptic weight over the entire environment:

$$E[\dot{m}] = \eta(Q - k_2 J)\mathbf{m} + \eta k_1 \hat{\mathbf{e}} \tag{5.3}$$

in which Q is the covariance matrix of the environment, defined as $Q_{ij} = E[(d_i - \mu)(d_j - \mu)]$, J is the matrix of all ones ($J_{ij} = 1$ for all i and j), $k_1 = c_o(d_o - \mu)$, $k_2 = \mu d_o$, and $\hat{\mathbf{e}}$ is the vector of all ones ($e_i = 1$ for all i). We often refer to $Q' = (Q - k_2 J)$ as the pseudo correlation matrix. It does not share some of the mathematical properties of a covariance matrix since it is not necessarily positive definite. It is important to notice that k_1

and k_2 are not free parameters that can be set arbitrarily. For instance, if $d_o = \mu$ then $k_1 = 0$ and if $\mu = 0$ then $k_2 = 0$

This learning rule has no stable fixed points [MacKay and Miller, 1990; Miller and MacKay, 1994] *. The vector $\mathbf{m}$ will asymptotically become parallel to the eigenvector with the largest eigenvalue of the matrix $Q' = Q - k_2 J$ but its magnitude will diverge to infinity.

When $k_1 = 0$ these equations have no fixed points; there is no value of $\mathbf{m}$ for which $E[\dot{\mathbf{m}}] = 0$. The solution of Equation 5.3 with $k_1 = 0$ has the form

$$\mathbf{m}(t) = \sum_j \mathbf{m}_j a_j(0) e^{\lambda_i t}. \tag{5.4}$$

where $\mathbf{m}_i$ is the i'th eigenvector of Q' with eigenvalue λ_i and $a_i(0)$ is a coefficient which accounts for the contribution of this eigenvector to the initial weights $\mathbf{m}(t = 0)$.

When $k_1 \neq 0$ the equation does have a fixed point at $\mathbf{m} = \eta k_1 \hat{e}(Q - k_2 J)^{-1}$, where $\hat{e}$ is a vector all of whose elements are one. However in most interesting cases this fixed point is not stable. This implies that for the deterministic equations any small perturbation from the fixed point would result in the weights diverging; in the stochastic case the weights will diverge even in the absence of a perturbation. It is easy to see this because Equation 5.3 is exactly solvable. The solution has the form:

$$\mathbf{m}(t) = \mathbf{a} e^{Q't} - k_1 \hat{e}(Q')^{-1},$$

where $\mathbf{a}$ is a constant vector determined by the initial conditions such that $\mathbf{a} = \mathbf{m}(t = 0) + k_1 \hat{e}(Q')^{-1}$. Thus if Q' has any eigenvalues that are positive the fixed point is not stable. The true correlation function is positive definite, therefore it has eigenvalues that are all positive. Thus the factor $k_2 J$ has to dominate the correlation function in order for this to happen. Thus the learning rule is stable only if the effect of the environment on the pseudo correlation function Q' is small compared to the constant term $k_2 J$, which is independent of the environment. Furthermore the factor $k_2 J$ can only directly effects eigenvectors that have a non-zero mean value, which we refer to as the DC (direct current) component in analogy with electrical systems.

The instability of the learning rule is not biologically plausible since it implies that the synaptic strengths would grow to arbitrarily large values.

In order to avoid this, one must go beyond the basic Hebb rule by imposing additional constraints. One approach is to assume that there exists a limit which the synapses cannot exceed. This approach, although con-

---

*Unless k_2 is large enough so that all eigenvalues of $(Q - k_2 J)$ are negative, which is not an interesting condition

ceptually simple and easy to implement, does not preserve one of the basic properties of the Hebb rule: the ability to identify the principal component of the data.

Before discussing how this problem can be addressed without a saturation limit, we note that some have avoided this problem by assuming that the neuron learns slowly enough for the receptive field to become approximately parallel to the principal component and that learning stops quickly enough for the synapses to avoid saturation [Linsker, 1986b; Miller et al., 1989; MacKay and Miller, 1990].

The Linsker rule (5.3) supplements the Hebb rule with two additional constraints. The term $\eta k_1 \hat{e}$ subtracts a constant from each synapse. The term $-k_2 J\mathbf{m}$ subtracts from each synapse a term that is proportional to the mean synaptic weight (DC, in analogy with electrical terminology "direct current"). This term discourages the growth of principal components that have a DC term. As we will show below it is sometimes very important to prevent the growth of terms with a DC component. These constraints however do not always totally prevent the growth of these components, they just slow them down. Some use a more stringent constraint in which they subtract at each time-step a term that completely abolishes growth in the DC direction[Miller, 1994; Miller and MacKay, 1994], we call the resulting rule the zero-DC Hebb rule. Although the details of this step do not seem biologically plausible it is sometimes necessary to use it to attain the desired receptive fields.

5.2.1 *Stabilized Hebbian rule*

The absence of a bounded fixed point for the Hebb rule without saturation was first noted by Rochester [Rochester et al., 1956]: Different procedures to stabilize synaptic strengths by supplementing the Hebb rule with additional constraints have been proposed [von der Malsburg, 1973; Kohonen, 1982]. In this section we summarize several of these constraints, including normalization of the weights, threshold levels and saturation limits, and decay terms, evaluating them primarily for their biological plausibility.

The method chosen by von der Malsburg was to renormalize after each Hebbian update by dividing the strength of each synapse by the sum of the synapse strengths of the neuron. Kohonen chose to divide by the sum of the squares of synapse strengths. Dividing by the sum of squares always keeps the weights bounded, whereas dividing by the sum of the weights can fail if the principal component has a sum of weights equal to zero. However, these normalization schemes may be difficult to implement biologically since they are non-local: each synapse has to "know" the weights of all the other synapses terminating on the same neuron, and a mechanism for propagating this non-local information is not known.

Other stabilization procedures terminate learning either when activity levels reach a certain threshold level [Nass and Cooper, 1975] or invoke a bound on synaptic weight strengths [Linsker, 1986b; Miller et al., 1989; Feng et al., 1996], these procedures seem more biologically plausible than the normalization schemes proposed, however they are theoretically less appealing.

Although the above normalization schemes seem biologically implausible a similar form of stabilization can be implemented in another way [Oja, 1982]. Instead of dividing after each Hebbian update, an extra term can be added to the update rule. Setting for simplicity, $\mu = x_0$ which implies that, $k_1 = k_2 = 0$, this rule takes the form

$$\Delta m_i = \eta \left(d_i c - \beta(\mathbf{m}) m_i \right), \tag{5.5}$$

where $\beta(\mathbf{m})$ is a scalar function of the vector $\mathbf{m}$. To determine the fixed point of Equation 5.5, it is convenient to go back to the correlational formulation of the learning rule. In this formulation the fixed points of Equation 5.5 (i.e. the points where we have $E[\Delta \mathbf{m}] = 0$) are given by

$$Q\mathbf{m} = \lambda \mathbf{m} \tag{5.6}$$

where $\lambda = \beta(\mathbf{m})$. Thus the fixed points are the eigenvectors of the correlation matrix Q, and the function $\beta(\mathbf{m})$ sets the normalization of these vectors. If Q is the covariance matrix, its eigenvectors are also called principal components (PC).

Oja chooses $\beta(\mathbf{m}) = y^2$ implying that $E[\beta(\mathbf{m})] = \mathbf{m}^\dagger Q\mathbf{m}$. Therefore the weights will be normalized so that $\mathbf{m}^2 = 1$. In fact, the only stable fixed point is the first principal component. Computationally the importance of the principal component is that it is the projection that maximizes the variance, and in a Gaussian channel carries more information than any other projection. When formulated in this way the stabilized Hebbian learning rule seems more biologically plausible, since the stabilization requires that each synapse have information of its own efficacy, and of the square of the postsynaptic potential.

If instead of using Oja's choice of β we choose $\beta = \hat{\mathbf{e}} \cdot d c = \sum_i d_i c$, this would, when averaged, result in a decay term of the form $\hat{\mathbf{e}} \cdot Q\mathbf{m}$. Thus an eigenvector with eigenvalue λ is normalized such that $\hat{\mathbf{e}} \cdot \mathbf{m} = 1$, equivalent to the normalization proposed by Malsburg [von der Malsburg, 1973]. This type of normalization function β is problematic in the cases where $\hat{\mathbf{e}} \cdot \mathbf{m} = 0$ and normalization is not possible.

There exists an exact solution to Oja's learning rule as was shown by Wyatt and Elfeldel [Wyatt and Elfadel, 1995]. It has the form

$$\mathbf{m}(t) = \frac{e^{Qt}\mathbf{m}_0}{||(e^{Qt}\mathbf{m}_0||^2 + 1 - ||\mathbf{m}_0||)^{\frac{1}{2}}}, \tag{5.7}$$

where $\mathbf{m}_0 = \mathbf{m}(t = 0)$ is the initial state of the weight vector.

5.2.2 *Finding multiple principal components*

Learning rules that extract only the largest principal component generally capture only a fraction of the information in high dimensional data. In order to reduce the dimensionality of the data, yet have a relatively small reconstruction error, it is useful to extract several principal components.

This can be accomplished using a network with lateral inhibition and several different forms for such a network have been proposed [Sanger, 1989; Rubner and Tavan, 1989; Foldia, 1989; Oja, 1992]. Different forms of lateral inhibition may find different features. If we assume that there are k output neurons, where k is smaller than the input dimensionality, then the resulting receptive fields will span the same subspace as the first k principal components but in general will be different from the principal components themselves. However, by adding additional constraints, one can force the features to extract the principal components [Sanger, 1989; Oja, 1992]. A heuristic way of understanding these methods is that the lateral inhibition between the first and second neurons acts effectively to subtract from the input to the second neuron those parts of the input which result from the first neuron's receptive field, and so on for successive neurons.

In this case we have more than one output neuron. We will therefore have a double index on the weights. So m_{ij} now denotes the weight connecting input neuron j to output neurons i. The modified PCA rule proposed by Sanger (1989) has the following form:

$$\Delta m_{ij} = \eta(d_j - \sum_{k=1}^{i} m_{kj}c_k)c_i$$

The second term in the brackets $\sum_{k=1}^{i} m_{kj}c_k$ could be interpreted as a type of inhibition from other neurons in the network, where the self inhibition term $(k = i)$ is identical to the normalization term used in the Oja rule. For the first output neuron $(i = 1)$ this rule is the Oja rule and therefore this neuron would converge to the first principal component. The second neuron has the term $m_{1k}c_1$ subtracted from the input to synapse k. Thus this cell effectively receives a different input than the first neuron, each synapse in the second neuron effectively receives the input pattern $(d_j - m_{1j}c_1)$. If the first neuron has already reached its fixed point (i.e. the first PC) then the second neuron receives an input with all components in the direction of the first PC subtracted. Therefore it will become orthogonal to this direction and will converge to the first PC in the remaining $N - 1$ dimensional subspace. Therefore it will actually converge to the second principal component of the N dimensional space. It can be shown formally

[Sanger, 1989] that this network will find an ordered set of all the principal components of the data.

5.2.3 *Fixed points of saturating Hebb rules*

The fixed points of the Oja and Sanger rules are the eigenvectors of the inputs to the network. A Hebb rule with no decay term and no saturation asymptotically becomes parallel to the eigenvector with the largest eigenvalue. However much of the research in the field concentrates on learning rules that are a saturated variant of the covariance rule (Equation 5.1).

Feng et. al. (1995) have analyzed this situation and have shown which types of receptive field configurations can be stable fixed points of this equation. They use the following method: first they postulate a receptive field shape and then test if it is stable. The advantage of this approach is that it is the only method that truly analyzes the dynamics of the saturated Hebb rule, rather then its linear analog. The disadvantage of this rule is that it does not tell us which RF's would indeed be obtained only which ones are stable. In practice RF's which are stable might be rarely obtained from the dynamics. We will briefly describe a slightly simplified version of their analysis.

The starting point is the averaged synaptic plasticity learning rule, as described by Linsker (Equation 5.3). When the components are explicitly expressed this takes the form:

$$m_i(t+1) = m_i(t) + \eta \sum_j (Q_{ij} - k_2)m_i(t) + k_1,$$

where Q_{ij} is the correlation between inputs i and j and m_i is the i'th component of the input.

This equation is subject to the constraint that m_i can not go above an upper limit m_{max} or below a lower limit m_{min}.

Therefore, this equation can be rewritten as

$$m_i(t+1) = L\left(m_i(t) + \eta \sum_j (Q_{ij} - k_2)m_i + k_1\right).$$

Where L is a limiting function such that

$$L(x) = \begin{cases} m_{max} & \text{if } x \geq m_{max} \\ x & \text{if } m_{min} < x < m_{max} \\ m_{min} & \text{if } x \leq m_{min}. \end{cases}$$

Feng et al. first prove that all fixed points occur when the weights become saturated at either their maximal or their minimal values [†]. Therefore, at fixed points

$$m_i(t) = L\left(m_i(t) + \eta h_i(t)\right),$$

where $h_i(t) = \sum_j (Q_{ij} - k_2)m_j(t) + k_1$. Thus, we see that the sign of h_i at a fixed point has to be the same as m_i. Namely, that $m_i h_i > 0$ for each i, at fixed point.

Assume for simplicity that $m_{max} = 1$ and that $m_{min} = -1$. We can define as sets of weights J^+ and J^-. Where J^+ is the set of all weights that have the value $+1$ and J^- is the set of all weights with value -1. Thus if $m_i \in J^+$ we have

$$k_1 + k_2\left[\sum_{j\in J^+} 1 - \sum_{j\in J^-} 1\right] > \left[\sum_{j\in J^+} Q_{ij} - \sum_{j\in J^-} Q_{ij}\right]$$

This has to hold for all i therefore we have

$$k_1 + k_2\left[\sum_{j\in J^+} 1 - \sum_{j\in J^-} 1\right] > \max_{(i\in J^+)}\left[\sum_{j\in J^+} Q_{ij} - \sum_{j\in J^-} Q_{ij}\right].$$

For $m_i \in J^-$ we get

$$k_1 + k_2\left[\sum_{j\in J^+} 1 - \sum_{j\in J^-} 1\right] < \min_{(i\in J^-)}\left[\sum_{j\in J^+} Q_{ij} - \sum_{j\in J^-} Q_{ij}\right].$$

If we now define

$$S(m) = \left[\sum_{j\in J^+} 1 - \sum_{j\in J^-} 1\right]$$

$$A_1(m) = \max_{(i\in J^+)}\left[\sum_{j\in J^+} Q_{ij} - \sum_{j\in J^-} Q_{ij}\right] \quad \text{if } J^+ = 0 \text{ then } A_1 = -\infty$$

$$A_2(m) = \min_{(i\in J^-)}\left[\sum_{j\in J^+} Q_{ij} - \sum_{j\in J^-} Q_{ij}\right] \quad \text{if } J^- = 0 \text{ then } A_2 = \infty.$$

[†] A fixed point is defined by $m_i(t+1) = m_i(t)$ or $\dot{m}(t) = 0$ in the continuous case.

Then a fixed point is stable if and only if

$$A_2(m) > k_1 + S(m)k_2 > A_1(m).$$

Feng and his co-workers then postulate sets of receptive fields and show for each type of receptive field for which sets of parameters k_1, k_2 these receptive fields can be stable. However this analysis only tells us which types of receptive fields are stable fixed points, not which fixed points are actually reached.

Any initial weight vector can be written as a superposition of the eigen-vectors and therefore initially (before saturation limits are reached) the largest eigenvector would grow the fastest. From simulations it seems that this eigenvector will indeed dominate the shape of the receptive field; how-ever each of the weights will be saturated to either their upper or lower allowed limit as proven by Feng et. al. We do not prove this assertion analytically, instead we will demonstrate it by simulating cases for which we know the exact principal components (see Section 5.3).

5.2.4 *Why are Principal Components not Local*

The environment used for training is usually translationally invariant, that is the distribution at point x is the same as that at point y. This is clearly true when we talk about the distribution of images on the retina, since our eyes move and sample all directions in space. The translational invariance of the environment implies that the correlation function Q is also transla-tionally invariant, that is $Q(\mathbf{r}, \mathbf{r}') = Q(\mathbf{r} - \mathbf{r}')$. This translational invariance of Q forces the receptive fields extracted by a PCA rule to be non-local. In order to show that this is so we will use a simple symmetry argument (such arguments are often used in physics). We will use similar arguments again in the several places in this chapter.

We define the translation operator $T(s)$, such that

$$T(s)d(i) = T(i + s)$$

Note that $T^T(s) = T^{-1}(s) = T(-s)$.

Thus

$$T(s)Q(\mathbf{r} - \mathbf{r}')T^T(s) = < T(s)d(\mathbf{r})d^T(\mathbf{r}')T^T(s) >=$$
$$< d(\mathbf{r} + s)d(\mathbf{r}' + s) > = Q(\mathbf{r} + s - (\mathbf{r}' + s)) = Q(\mathbf{r} - \mathbf{r}').$$

Therefore, as expected, the correlation function is invariant under trans-lation. As seen earlier (Equation 5.6) the receptive fields extracted by this rule are solutions of the eigenvalue equation, which written in operator form has the form

$$Q(\mathbf{r} - \mathbf{r}')\mathbf{m}(\mathbf{r}') = \lambda\mathbf{m}(\mathbf{r}).$$

If we operate on this equation with the translation operator and use the relation $T^T(s)T(s) = 1$, we get

$$T(s)Q(\mathbf{r} - \mathbf{r}')T^T(s)T(s)\mathbf{m}(\mathbf{r}') = \lambda T(s)\mathbf{m}(\mathbf{r}). \qquad (5.8)$$

Therefore $T(s)\mathbf{m}(\mathbf{r})$ is also an eigenvector of Q with the same eigenvalue. In the non degenerate case $\mathbf{m}(\mathbf{r})$ and $\mathbf{m}(\mathbf{r} + s)$ are identical up to a phase, hence $\mathbf{m}(\mathbf{r} + s) = e^{i\alpha s}\mathbf{m}(\mathbf{r})$. In other words the receptive fields are periodic - not local.

5.2.5 *Summary*

Much of the theoretical work on cortical synaptic plasticity stems from Hebb's idea of a correlation based learning rule. We have shown that many of the different ideas proposed can be described as special cases of the covariance rule.

In some cases [Linsker, 1986b; Miller et al., 1989; Erwin and Miller, 1998] the true correlation matrix is replaced by an effective correlation matrix. This change can, under some conditions, produce very different receptive fields.

The simple covariance rule is unstable so that different approaches have been used to stabilize these rules. One approach is to stabilize them by directly normalizing them [von der Malsburg, 1973] or by using a decay term to indirectly normalize them [Oja, 1982]. Another approach is to introduce saturation limits to the synaptic weights.

When weight vectors are normalized they converge to the principal component of the correlation matrix [Oja, 1982]. An exact solution of the dynamics of the Oja rule has also been obtained [Wyatt and Elfadel, 1995]. When saturation limits are used the stable receptive field that is obtained is usually well approximated by a saturated version of the first PC. We will demonstrate this with an example in the next section.

5.3 Orientation Selectivity

Receptive fields in the visual cortex are usually orientation selective. But they receive inputs from LGN cells that are not orientation selective. Can synaptic plasticity account for this transformation?

In this section we review different cases in which the principal components of the input environment can become orientation selective.

Two distinct types of models will be described. In the first part of this section models in which artificial assumptions about the correlation function of the inputs are made in order to produce orientation selectivity, in the second we describe the evolution of orientation selectivity under realistic natural image environments.

We first describe a simple soluble 1D model in which true orientation selectivity can not be obtained; however symmetry breaking analogous to orientation selectivity does appear. This model can give us intuition as to what assumptions about the input environment must be made in order to obtain symmetry breaking. We next describe more elaborate 2D models which under some conditions produce orientation selective PC's; we discuss their symmetry properties as well. We then treat PCA models trained in a realistic natural image environment, display the results of analysis, and show under what conditions orientation selectivity is attained.

5.3.1 *An exactly soluble 1D Model*

This example given a simple demonstration of how symmetry in the correlation function can be broken when principal components do not have the same symmetry as the correlation function. This example is one dimensional (1D) in the sense that x denotes points on a line, in the more realistic two dimensional examples, $\mathbf{x}$ denotes a point on a surface - usually the retinal surface. The 1D case we describe here is analogous to the type of symmetry breaking that occurs when oriented receptive fields arise from radially symmetric correlation function, since both arise from a similar type of symmetry breaking.

Assume a correlation function[‡], Q, of the form

$$Q(x - x') = 1 + q \cos\left(\pi(x - x')\right).$$ (5.9)

The shape of the correlation function changes as a function of q as seen in Figure 5.1.

We will assume that the receptive field is local and is zero outside the range $(-1, 1)$. This locality restriction is essential due to the translationally invariant nature of the correlation function, as explained above.

The PC learning rule finds the highest solution of the eigenvalue equation

$$\int_{-1}^{1} dx' Q(x - x')\mathbf{m}(x') = \lambda\mathbf{m}(x).$$ (5.10)

The correlation function can be written in the equivalent form

$$Q(x - x') = 1 + q\left(\cos(\pi x)\cos(\pi x') + \sin(\pi x)\sin(\pi x')\right).$$

[‡]or pseudo-correlation function

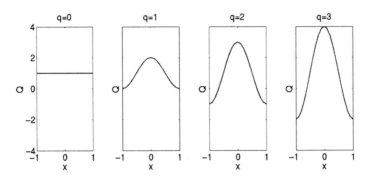

Figure 5.1: Correlation functions used in the 1-D model with different values of q. From left to right: $q = 0$, $q = 1$, $q = q_c = 2$ and $q = 3$

The eigenvectors, $\mathbf{m}$, can be expanded in a Fourier series, so that

$$\mathbf{m}(x) = a_0 + \sum_{l=1}^{\infty} a_l \cos(\pi l x) + \sum_{l=1}^{\infty} b_l \sin(\pi l x).$$

Inserting these into Equation 5.10 produces (due to the orthogonality of the sin's and cos's in this range) the following equation.

$$2a_0 + qa_1 \cos(\pi x) + qb_1 \sin(\pi x) = \lambda \left(a_0 + \sum_{l=1}^{\infty} a_l \cos(\pi l x) + \sum_{l=1}^{\infty} b_l \sin(\pi l x) \right).$$

This implies that for $l > 1$ $a_l, b_l = 0$. Thus, there remain only three possible solutions. The DC solution $\mathbf{m}(x) = $ constant in which $\lambda = 2$, and the two degenerate solutions $m(x) = \sin(\pi x)$ and $m(x) = \cos(\pi x)$ with an eigenvalue $\lambda = q$. Since these two solutions are degenerate, they can be superimposed. Figure 5.2 shows that when $q < 2$ the DC solution dominates, whereas when $q > 2$ the oscillating solutions have a larger eigenvalue. Thus we see a very simple example in which changing the correlation function, which represents the visual environment, results in changing the type of receptive field extracted by the learning rule. It is important to note that in the higher dimensional cases we explore later (Section 5.3.4), all oriented solutions have zero DC. Thus, the simple 1-D case is comparable to the higher dimensional case, with the oscillating (zero-DC) solution representing the oriented solutions and the DC solution representing non-oriented solutions.

The principal component changes abruptly at the critical value, $q_c = 2$, from a constant to a periodic solution. We denote by λ_0 the eigenvalue of the DC solution, and by λ_1 the eigenvalue of the periodic solutions. Due to the degeneracy of the periodic solutions $\sin(\pi x)$ and $\cos(\pi x)$ any solution of

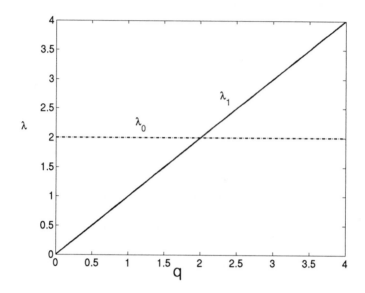

Figure 5.2: A plot of the eigenvalues of the DC and oscillating solutions to the eigenvalue problem. At $q > q_c = 2$ the eigenvalue of the oscillating solution, λ_1, exceeds that of the DC solution, λ_0.

the form $\cos(\pi x + \phi)$ is a principal component. We point out again that this set of degenerate solutions does not have the same symmetry properties as the correlation function. This is similar to what happens in 2D when the correlation function is radially symmetric but the first principal component is orientation selective.

We can also use this simple model in order to demonstrate the effects of using a non-stabilized Hebb rule, as described in Equation 5.3. There are several factors in these equations that may effect the solutions; the saturation limits, the effects of the additional constants (k_1 and k_2) and the initial conditions. In this simple example we ignore the effect of k_1 and k_2 although the correlation function we use can be thought to incorporate the effect of k_2. We also show the effect on the receptive fields obtained with the so-called zero-DC constraint, a key requirement for many of Miller's simulation results[Miller et al., 1989; Miller, 1992].

The effect of saturation limits usually produces a saturated version of the principal component. In Figure 5.3 we have shown several such examples. Results of symmetric saturation limits such that the upper saturation is 2 and the lower saturation is -2 are displayed on the left and center. In these cases the first principal component dominates, this may not be the case if the initial conditions strongly favor one of the lower eigenstates. On

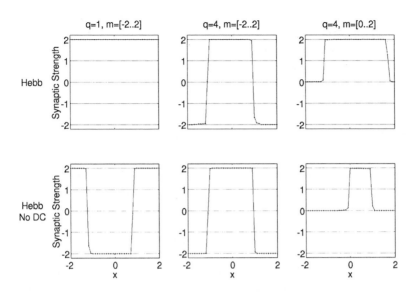

Figure 5.3: Effect of saturation limits and the zero-DC Hebb rule on the receptive field obtained. Above simulations with a simple Hebb rule, below simulations under the same conditions but with the zero-DC Hebb rule. For $q = 1$ the principal component is uniform as a results of the saturated Hebb rule, with saturation limits of [-2..2], converges to the saturation limit (upper left). When the zero DC rule is used an oscillating solution is obtained (lower left) similar to a saturated version of the second principal component. For $q = 4$ the principal component has an oscillating shape as seen in Figure 5.2 above. In this case both the simple Hebb rule (upper, center) and the zero DC rule (lower center) converge to a saturated version of the first principal component. On the right we show the effect of using the more realistic [0..2] saturation limits in the $q = 4$ case. The simple Hebb rule (upper, right) resembles a saturated version of the first principal component. The zero DC rule (lower, right) produces a similar result but a smaller fraction of the weights end up at the upper saturation limit. This happens because with the zero DC rule the final sum of the weights is exactly identical to the initial sum of the weights - thus the initial conditions determine the final outcome.

the right we examine the effect of having only positive weights, resulting in saturation limits of [0..2]. In the example shown here the first principal component dominates, however, if we had started with larger initial weights it would have favored the DC solution.

On the bottom row of Figure 5.3 we show the effect of using the zero-DC rule. It has the effect of favoring eigenstates with lower eigenvectors (lower, left) if they have a lower DC component. It also sets the sum of the final weights to be identical to the sum of initial weights thus determining the number of weights that converge to the upper saturation limit (lower, right).

5.3.2   *Radially symmetric models in 2D*

It is interesting to examine how orientation selectivity can arise in a radially symmetric environment. This is an interesting domain since the real world correlation function seems to deviate only slightly from radial symmetry.

We can use symmetry methods again to show some properties of the receptive fields when the correlation function is radially symmetric, i.e $Q(\mathbf{r}) = Q(|\mathbf{r}|)$. Define the rotation operator $R(\phi)$, such that $R(\phi)\mathbf{m}(r,\theta) = \mathbf{m}(r, \theta + \phi)$. thus, using the same types of arguments as in Section 5.2.4, if $\mathbf{m}(r,\theta)$ is an eigenvector of Q, so is $\mathbf{m}(r, \theta + \phi)$. They have the same eigenvalue and are identical up to a phase. Since $R(2\pi) = 1$, we can that $R(\phi)\mathbf{m}(r,\theta) = \lambda_\phi \mathbf{m}(\mathbf{r})$ and $\lambda_\phi = e^{in\phi}$, where $i = \sqrt{-1}$.

For very small ϕ, $e^{in\phi} \approx 1 + in\phi$. The infinitesimal generator of rotations has the form $R(\Delta\phi) = (1 + \Delta\phi\frac{\partial}{\partial\phi})$. Therefore $(1 + \Delta\phi\frac{\partial}{\partial\phi})\mathbf{m}(\mathbf{r}) = (1 + in\Delta\phi)\mathbf{m}(\mathbf{r})$, hence

$$\frac{\partial}{\partial\phi}\mathbf{m}(\mathbf{r}) = in\mathbf{m}(\mathbf{r}). \qquad (5.11)$$

This has the solution

$$\mathbf{m}(r,\theta) = m(r)e^{in\theta}.$$

For receptive fields, that are by definition real, this means that

$$\mathbf{m}(\mathbf{r}) = m(r)\cos(n\theta + \phi). \qquad (5.12)$$

These solutions are degenerate in ϕ, that is the eigenvalue is independent of ϕ.

5.3.3   *2D correlational Models*

In the two dimensional case, when the coordinates correspond to points on a two-dimensional surface, assumptions made about the correlation function of the visual environment can produce orientation selective receptive fields. Several models for the development of receptive fields with Hebbian learning have been proposed. Some of these models explicitly assume a correlation function for the visual environment[Miller, 1992; Miller, 1994], while in others the shape of the correlation function is influenced by development in earlier layers [Linsker, 1986b].

However, these models use different variants of the learning rule, different stabilization schemes and some of them assume network interactions as well [Linsker, 1986a; Miller, 1992; Miller, 1994]. All of these details have an impact on the results. Much of the behavior of these models can be understood by inspecting the single cell principal components of the pseudo-correlation function.

The model proposed by Miller is a single layer model [Miller, 1992; Miller, 1994]. A translationally invariant, radially symmetric center-surround correlation function $Q(x-x')$ is assumed[§]. In addition a synaptic density function $A(x)$ is assumed; that is the density of synapses is assumed to drop off as a function of the distance from the cell center. The synaptic density function breaks the translational invariance and is therefore essential for forming local receptive fields (see Section 5.2.4 above). In order to produce orientation selectivity it is essential that the correlation function have anti-correlation regions as well. Further, the ratio between the size of the arbor function and the correlation function has a large impact on the receptive fields.

The model proposed by Linsker [Linsker, 1986b] is a multi layer model, that attempts to model the formation of orientation selectivity prenatally. As in the Miller Model the connections to the next layer are restricted by the synaptic density functions. In the appropriate parameter regime all connections from the first to the second layer reach their maximal level.

Due to the overlap between the receptive fields in the second layer, the activity of these cells is correlated. The pseudo correlation function $Q' = Q - k_2 J$ of activities in the second layer therefore can have both a correlation and an anti-correlation regime. The relative sizes and magnitudes of these regions depends on the values of the parameter, k_2. As in the Miller model it is the shape of the pseudo correlation function, the size of the arbor function as well as the ratio between the sizes of the arbor function and correlation function which determine the shape of the receptive fields.

An example of receptive fields obtained when the correlation function is Gaussian is displayed in Figure 5.4. Here we show the effect of different variants of the Hebb rule and how they affect the receptive fields.

How does altering the correlation function affect the receptive fields? The Linsker rule results in the effective correlation function $Q' = Q - k_2 J$ being the driving force of receptive field formation. Altering the correlation function in this manner results in changing the eigenvalues of eigenvectors with a non vanishing DC component, thus changing the identity of the first principal component, as shown in Figure 5.5.

[§]However not every function is a correlation function, see appendix 5B.

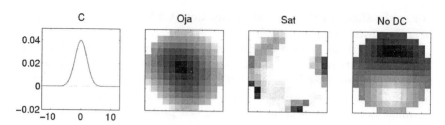

Figure 5.4: An example of receptive fields obtained for a Gaussian correlation function ($\sigma = 2$) (left). The first PC extracted by the Oja rule is radially symmetric (second from left). The saturated Hebb rule results in a radially symmetric receptive field saturated at the upper saturation value (second from right). However, using the zero-DC Hebb rule with saturation limits for stability can result in receptive fields with more structure (right).

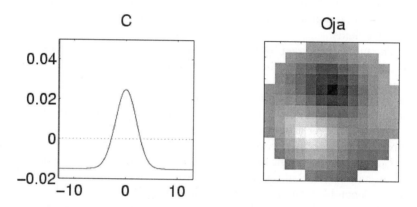

Figure 5.5: The correlation function (Left) has the form $G(0, 2) - k$ where G is a Gaussian correlation function of zero mean and standard deviation of $\sigma = 2$, as in Figure 5.4 and $k = 0.015$. The resulting function has zero mean. The receptive field extracted by the Oja rule (right) has a different shape than the receptive filed extracted when the correlation function is Gaussian.

5.3.4 *Analysis of Linsker's Model*

To some extent, orientation selectivity is present before eye opening. The model proposed by Linsker [Linsker, 1986b] shows how it is possible for such orientation selectivity to self organize, in the absence of visual inputs. Linsker assumes unstructured inputs yet obtains receptive fields in deeper layers that may become orientation selective.

The model consists of several layers. The input layer (Layer $\mathcal{A}$ in Figure 5.6) is spontaneously active. It is assumed that the activity of neurons in this layer is uncorrelated. Therefore the value of activity in this layer is chosen from a random distribution, independently for each neuron. Neurons in the second layer are connected to neurons in the first layer via modifiable synapses. The density of these synaptic connections, that sets the saturation limits of the weights, falls off with distance. The synaptic density function is referred to as the arbor function. The arbor function is essential for the success of this approach, since, as we have shown in Section 5.2.4, the principal components alone are not local. In Linsker's model it is assumed that a neuron located in position $\mathbf{r}$ in layer $\mathcal{B}$ has an arbor function of the form

$$A_{\mathrm{B}}(\mathbf{r} - \mathbf{r}') = e^{-(\mathbf{r} - \mathbf{r}')^2 / 2\sigma_{\mathrm{AB}}^2},$$

where σ_{AB} is the length scale of the arbor function between layers $\mathcal{A}$ and $\mathcal{B}$.

The learning rule used is described above in Equations 5.1 and 5.3. Since the inputs to the first layer are uncorrelated random inputs the correlation function Q in layer $\mathbf{A}$ has the form $Q(\mathbf{r} - \mathbf{r}') = \sigma^2 \delta(\mathbf{r} - \mathbf{r}')$. This implies that as long as $\sigma^2 > k_2$ all weight will grow to reach their maximal value. Therefore, the fully developed synaptic weights, connecting layers $\mathcal{A}$ to layer $\mathcal{B}$, have the form of the arbor function so that receptive fields in layer $\mathcal{B}$ have a radially symmetric, non-oriented form. The arbor here serves to localize the receptive fields which, as we have shown above, would be non-local with Hebbian learning alone. Furthermore, the receptive field shape is determined exactly by the shape of the arbor function.

Due to the local, overlapping receptive fields of neurons in layer $\mathcal{B}$ their responses will be correlated. It is easy to show that the correlation function in layer $\mathcal{B}$ has the form

$$Q(\mathbf{r} - \mathbf{r}') = \int_{-\infty}^{\infty} A_B(\mathbf{r} - \mathbf{r}'') A_B(\mathbf{r}' - \mathbf{r}'') dr''$$
$$= \sqrt{\pi} \sigma_{\mathrm{AB}} e^{-(\mathbf{r} - \mathbf{r}')^2 / (4\sigma_{\mathrm{AB}}^2)}$$

Note that the length scale of the correlation function in layer $\mathcal{B}$ arises solely from the size of the arbor.

The true correlation function observed by neurons in layer C will be affected by the shape of the arbor function from layer $\mathcal{B}$ to layer $\mathcal{C}$. Given that this arbor function, A_C, has the same Gaussian shape as A_B but with a length scale σ_{BC} the effective correlation function for a neuron in layer $\mathcal{C}$

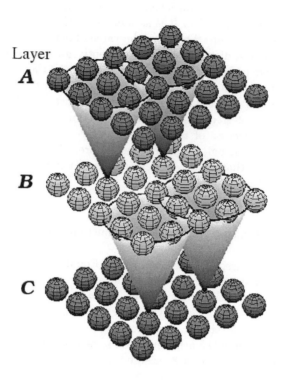

Figure 5.6: A schematic diagram of the architecture of a three layer Linsker type model. The input layer ($\mathcal{A}$) has activity that is assumed to be uncorrelated and random. Subsequent layers are connected to the layer above via modifiable synapses. The maximal synaptic density - the arbor function - varies spatially. This arbor function is depicted schematically by the cones connecting one layer to the previous layer.

has the form

$$Q_B(\mathbf{r}, \mathbf{r}') = e^{\frac{-(r-r')^2}{4\sigma_{\text{AB}}^2}} e^{\frac{-r'^2}{\sigma_{\text{BC}}^2}}.$$

Note further that this correlation function is not translationally invariant, due to the arbor function, and therefore the resulting receptive fields may be local. Mackay and Miller (1990) have found the analytical form of the first three eigenfunctions and eigenvalues of this correlation function.

Name	Eigenfunction	Eigenvalue
1s	$e^{-r^2/2R}$	$2l\sigma_{AB}^2/\sigma_{BC}^2$
2p	$r\cos(\theta + \phi)e^{-r^2/2R}$	$2l^2\sigma_{AB}^2/\sigma_{BC}^2$
2s	$(1 - r^2/r_0^2)e^{-r^2/2R}$	$2l^3\sigma_{AB}^2/\sigma_{BC}^2$

$$R = \sigma_{AB}^2(1 + \sqrt{1 + 2\sigma_{BC}^2/\sigma_{AB}^2})$$
$$l = \frac{R - 2\sigma_{AB}^2}{R}$$
$$r_0^2 = \frac{2\sigma_{BC}^2}{\sqrt{1 + 2\sigma_{BC}^2/\sigma_{AB}^2}}$$

Table 5.1: Eigenfunctions and eigenvalues at layer $\mathcal{C}$ for $k_2 = 0$. The 2p solution is degenerate in the phase ϕ. Note that $l \leq 1$.

The first eigenfunction is radially symmetric and all weights have the same sign, the second eigenfunction has an angular form $\cos(\theta)$ and the third is radially symmetric with a center surround shape. Borrowing notation from physics they have named these functions 1s, 2p and 2s respectively. Table 5.1 shows the exact shape of these eigenfunctions.

But the principal component in layer $\mathcal{C}$ is still radially symmetric, as in layer $\mathcal{B}$. To obtain oriented RF's in layer $\mathcal{C}$ we can choose $k_2 < 0$ so that the radially symmetric solution has an eigenvalue smaller than the oriented solution. In order to see how this happens we need to understand the effect of the term $k_2 J$ on different eigenfunctions. Since J is a matrix of ones then $\sum_i J_{ij}m_i = \sum_i m_i$. The effect of this term is proportional to the DC component of the weight vector. Thus all solutions that have a zero DC component will not be affected by this term. All oriented solutions have zero DC thus the 2p solution will not change its eigenvalue, further it will still be an eigenfunction of $Q' = Q - k_2 J$. The 1s solution has a large DC component, thus as k_2 becomes more negative the eigenvalue of the 1s solution decreases monotonically and at some point goes below the eigenvalue of the 2p solution. This is the regime in which oriented solutions can appear in the Linsker network.

The work by Mackay and Miller accounts for the results Linsker has shown in simulations. The two features that determine exactly the final state of his network are: (i) the shape of the arbor function that localizes the solution and determines the shape of the correlation function of the next layer. (ii) the decay constants that effectively alter the shape of the correlation function, if these are set in a certain range they can favor oriented solutions over radially symmetric solutions.

5.3.5 *Formation of Receptive Fields in a Natural Image Environment*

In cat and ferret a patterned environment is required for attaining sharply tuned cells[Buisseret and Imbert, 1976; Chapman et al., 1999]. Thus it is interesting to know what kind of receptive fields would evolve in a realistic visual environment composed of natural images. The inputs to the cortical cells are influenced by two factors, the visual environment itself and the pre-processing it undergoes in the visual pathway. We have shown that receptive fields extracted by the PCA rule are not localized unless a local arbor function is assumed. In what follows we show that the size of the arbor function is also an important factor in determining the shape of the receptive fields.

If the visual environment, the retinal pre-processing and the arbor function are radially symmetric the receptive field structure is separable to a radial function times an angular function, thus as we have shown above $\mathbf{m}(\mathbf{r}) = m(r)\cos(n\theta + \phi)$. However the visual environment is not exactly radially symmetric. We summarize results about both these cases and show what factors determine the receptive field structure in each case.

(a) The visual environment

In this section we consider a visual environment composed of natural images. One of these images is displayed in Figure 5.7. Later (Chapter 6) we treat this natural image environment in detail; the main topics, however, are summarized here.

We assume that these natural images are pre-processed by a retinal-like filter. Several such filters are used. The standard option in to use a Difference of Gaussians (DOG); we have chosen its parameters to resemble those of a cortical X cell [Linsenmeier et al., 1982]. Another option often used is to perform whitening on the images. Whitening is a linear transformation that will result in a flat power spectrum. Usually a robust type of whitening is performed to prevent exploding the high frequency noise. There are appealing theoretical reasons to choose whitening and it also resembles the effects of retinal filtering to a certain extent [Atick and Redlich, 1992]. For the second order models we are considering, however, it does not make too much sense because whitening eliminates the second order correlations on which these models rely, thus making all solutions degenerate.

Another option used in the analysis below, is local retinal-like filter. The advantage of such a filter is that it is zero outside a given radius. This makes certain types of analysis easier and does not require compensation for finite integration boundaries as required with DOG filters. We will see that an important parameter here is the ratio of the arbor size and the filter size. Another advantage is that a bounded filter has a well defined size.

The local filter we have chosen here is:

$$K(\mathbf{r}) = \frac{1}{g^2} \begin{cases} J_0(q_2^0 r/a) + qJ_0(q_1^0 r/a) & r < ag \\ 0 & r \geq ag \end{cases} \qquad (5.13)$$

where $J_0(qr)$ are Bessel functions of order zero and $q_i^0 = gk_i^0$ are set so that the zeroes of the 0 order Bessel functions will be on the boundary with radius $r = ag$. The coefficient $q = 0.289$ so that $\int K(\mathbf{r})d^2r = 0$. This filter has parameters similar to those of X cells.

In Figure 5.7 we see the effect of this filter on the natural images.

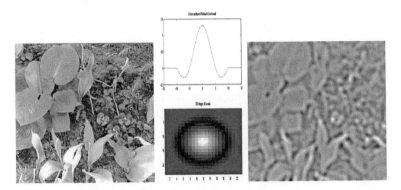

Figure 5.7: One of the natural images used (left) is convolved with the local retinal-like filter (center) to produce the pre-processed image used (right).

The statistics of these images are not radially symmetric. This can easily be seen from the shape of the power spectrum of these images. However since animals can rotate their heads with respect to the horizon, it might be that they do observe a radially symmetric environment, or at least an environment more symmetric than this one. When we simulate a radially symmetric environment we often use an artificially symmetrized environment. We have done this by adding to the image data set, another set of images that are rotated versions of the original images. In this section we have found it is sufficient to rotate them by 90, 180 and 270 degrees.

(b) PCA simulations with natural images

Receptive fields formed from raw natural images are not typically orientation selective. An example can be seen Figure 5.8(left). Is this because the DC component dominates? This can be examined using the zero-DC rule (Figure 5.8(right)), which can produce orientation selective receptive fields under certain conditions.

Retinal pre-processing, as described above, eliminates the DC component of the images (but not necessarily of the eigenvectors), it also alters

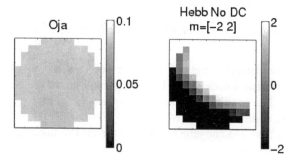

Figure 5.8: Receptive fields obtained from raw natural images. RF diameter 13 pixels. The receptive field obtained by the Oja rule (left) is radially symmetric. The receptive field obtained using the zero-DC Hebb with saturation limits for stability (right) is orientation selective. Note that if the saturation limits are set too high, or too low, the cell will not develop orientation selectivity even with the Zero-DC Constraint.

the structure of the correlation function. Receptive fields obtained from the pre-processed images are presented in Figure 5.9.

Receptive fields in the symmetrized environment have the separable form described above and their preferred orientation can vary and take any value. If the environment is not symmetrized they always have the same preferred orientation. They can also assume a non separable form (see Figure 5.13).

The ratio between the receptive field (or arbor) size and the size of the retinal filter is important in determining the shape of the receptive fields, as seen in Figure 5.10.

(c)   Analysis of receptive fields formed in a Radially Symmetric Environment

Since the power spectrum of natural images is known [Field, 1987] and since Hebbian rules depend only on second order statistics, it is possible to analyze the parameters that determine receptive field formation in a natural image environment. We have done this both for raw natural images [Liu and Shouval, 1994] and for natural images processed by a retinal like filter [Shouval and Liu, 1996], where we have used the local retinal-like filter described above.

In a radially symmetric environment these receptive fields have a separable form as shown above (Section 5.3.2). Simulations displayed in Figure 5.11 show the first 5 solutions obtained with a multiple PCA algorithm [Sanger, 1989]. The environment in these simulations is symmetrized by adding a rotated set of images to the data base. These results are obtained

Symmetrized

Non-Symmetrized

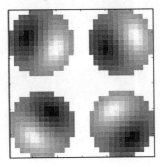 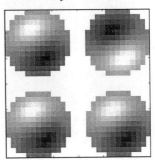

Figure 5.9: Receptive fields obtained from pre-processed natural images as described above. RF diameter 13 pixels. The receptive fields displayed are independent of each other and have different initial conditions. On the left receptive fields that develop in a symmetrized visual environment. They have the separable form expected and are degenerate with respect to phase. When the environment is not symmetrized (right) they all have the same preferred orientations.

Figure 5.10: Receptive fields obtained from pre-processed natural images as described above, for RF diameter 13 pixels (left) and 22 pixels (right). The receptive field structures are quite different in form. However, a word of caution must be added: the eigenvalues of the different solutions are *extremely* close. They are so close, in fact, that repeated simulation may obtain quite different receptive fields, especially with a large arbor.

for a receptive field radius of $a = 10$ pixels and a filter radius of $r = 10$ pixels as well. From these parameters the first principal component is oriented with an angular form of $cos(\theta)$. The first two solutions are degenerate due to the radial symmetry. We find that the critical parameter is the ratio between these two parameters, thus we define a new parameter $g = r/a$.

These results can be accounted for analytically [Shouval and Liu, 1996]. The analysis is based on the scale invariance of the natural image environment. Using these analytical methods we find that the shape and order of

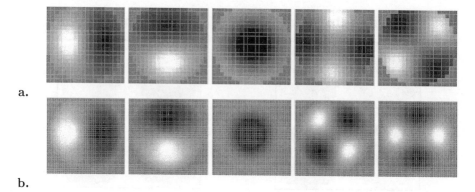

a.

b.

Figure 5.11: a. Simulations results, the inputs are 12 natural scenes which are pre-processed with a center surround filter of radius 10, and in addition each image has been rotated by 90 degrees in order to increase the radial symmetry. The receptive field size used has a radius $a = 10$ thus $g = 1$, and the conditions are identical to those in the theoretical derivation above. b. Theoretical results extracted for the same set of parameters as the simulation results above. We can see considerable similarity between theory and simulation.

the receptive fields is altered by changing the ratio parameter g. In Figure 5.12 we show how the eigenvalues of the different types of solutions change as a function of g.

The types of solutions are denoted by the number of zero crossings in the angular and radial dimensions. The first index stand for the angular zero crossings and the second index the radial zero crossings. Thus λ_{ij} is the eigenvalue of a solution of the form $\cos(i\theta + \phi)f_j(r)$. The index i counts the number of zero crossings of the angular component and the index j counts the number of zero crossings of the radial component. The radial dimension always has a zero crossing at the edge of the arbor function. Thus the smallest radial index is $j = 1$. The smallest angular index is $i = 0$ for a solution not varying in the angular dimension.

The dominant type of receptive field extracted depends of the value of g. At $g = 1$ (Figures 5.11 and 5.12) the dominant eigenfunction is orientation selective, displays a single peak in the tuning curve (within the range 0-180 degrees) and has adjacent inhibitory and excitatory side bands. However it has very broad orientation tuning with half width at half height of ≈ 45 degrees, much broader than for mature cortical cells. In contrast at $g = 0.7$ and below, the dominant eigenfunction has the angular form $\cos(2\theta)$. Its tuning curve has two peaks each of them more narrowly tuned. These double peaks do not resemble those of cortical cells.

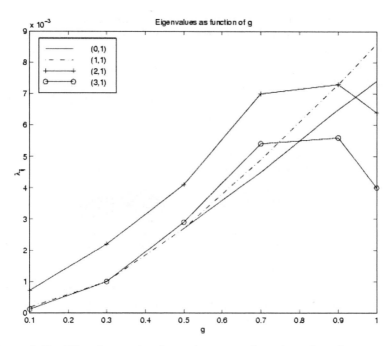

Figure 5.12: The change in eigenvalues as a function of g, for receptive fields with radius a=10. The notation (m, n) implies the n'th solution with angular component m, eg: $(0, 1)$ implies the rotationally symmetric solution with highest eigenvalue. It can be seen the near $g = 1$ the principal component is proportional to $\cos(\theta)$ whereas near $g = 0.7$ the dominant solution becomes the one proportional to $\cos(2\theta)$. For small values of g i.e: $g \leq .3$ the results displayed here are not exact since larger matrices than we have used should be used in order to achieve a good approximation. [for detailed explanation see Shouval and Liu 1996]

In the cortex there is probably not a single value of g, however there is no value of g for which the radially symmetric theory can produce reasonable receptive fields, they are either too broad, or the tuning curves have too many peaks.

(d) Non symmetric environment
The power spectrum of natural images is slightly non-symmetric. The way in which an animal scans the visual environment can effect the degree of asymmetry in the inputs to the cells, if the animal does not rotate its head much while viewing the world some of the asymmetry in the natural world would be preserved in the environment as scanned by the animal. These

slight asymmetries can significantly change the shape of the receptive fields. For different values of g this asymmetry would have a different effect. At $g = 1$ it does not change the shape of the receptive fields but it breaks the degeneracy between the horizontal and vertical solutions; slightly favoring the horizontal RF's (dependent of course on the exact asymmetry in each database). At $g = 0.7$ it has the different effect of changing the structure of the receptive fields as well . In Figure 5.13 we compare receptive fields obtained at $g = 0.7$ for symmetrized and non-symmetrized images.

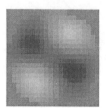 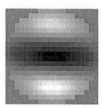

Figure 5.13: Comparison Between Simulations with symmetrized data set (left) and non symmetrized data(right). These simulations were performed at $g = 0.7$. It should be noted that the results of the symmetrized simulations match the theoretical prediction.

The RF extracted from the symmetrized images match our prediction and have the usual separable form (Figure 5.11). The receptive field extracted from the unsymmetrized data can no longer be expressed in a separable form. Its shape and tuning curve, however, resemble more closely those of cortical receptive fields. The problem that arises, in this single cell model, is that the radial asymmetry also favors a single preferred orientation; thus all cells will have exactly the same profile with the same preferred orientation. This too is clearly not biologically realistic.

We have shown [Shouval and Liu, 1996; Liu and Shouval, 1994] that the shape of RF's in a non-symmetric environment be can attained using perturbation theory, that takes into account the non-symmetric portion of the correlation function. The cells will always prefer horizontal directions.

5.3.6 *Summary*

We have shown how orientation selectivity can arise in correlational models in which the correlation function itself is radially symmetric. The receptive field extracted by Hebbian rules is usually dominated by the first PC. In order to attain a first PC that is orientation selective the correlation function must have negative (anti-correlation) regions. In many cases correlation functions that do have a first PC that is oriented are nearly degenerate and often converge to other, possibly non-oriented solutions or even to a mixture of solutions. It is possible to attain oriented solutions even when the correlation function is positive by altering the learning rule. This can be done either by the method proposed by Linsker [Linsker, 1986b] that results in an effective correlation function with negative lobes or by using the zero-DC Hebb rule as proposed by Miller [Miller and MacKay, 1994; Miller, 1994].

We have also shown that for a natural image environment the shape of the receptive fields extracted by the PCA rule depends primarily on the parameter g, the ratio between the receptive retinal filter size and the receptive field size. For values of $g \approx 1$ the receptive fields will be orientation tuned, however the tuning curves will be broad unlike those of cortical cells. For smaller values of g, for instance $g < 0.7$ we get a significantly different shape of the tuning curve. If the environment is radially symmetric the tuning curve would have too many peaks. For a non symmetric environment it will have a single peak, the first PC is always horizontal.

5.4 Ocular Dominance

Neurons in visual cortex of cat and monkey can usually be driven by both eyes, however one of the eyes usually dominates. Many models have tried to account for the development of this ocular dominance segregation.

5.4.1 *Ocular   Dominance   in   Correlational Low-Dimensional Models*

The simplest model in which we can describe ocular dominance, is composed of just two inputs, one for the left eye and one for the right eye. For the type of Hebbian rules examined here the receptive fields are determined by the correlation function. If it is a PCA (Equation 5.5) rule that does not have the Oja normalization term, the dynamics are dominated by the first PC (see Equation 5.4) and the receptive field is the first PC.

In this simple 2D case we have two weights (m_l, m_r) and two inputs (d_l, d_r). The correlation function Q is a two dimensional matrix:

$$\mathbf{Q} = \begin{pmatrix} <d_l d_l> & <d_l d_r> \\ <d_r d_l> & <d_r d_r> \end{pmatrix}$$

where $<>$ denote an average over the input distribution. Due to the symmetry of the two channels $<d_l d_l> = <d_r d_r> = a$ and $<d_l d_r> = <d_r d_l> = b$ where a and b are two constants and $a \geq b$.

Thus Q has the form

$$\mathbf{Q} = \begin{pmatrix} a & b \\ b & a \end{pmatrix}$$

This matrix has two eigenvectors:

$$\mathbf{m}^1 = \frac{1}{\sqrt{2}} \begin{pmatrix} 1 \\ 1 \end{pmatrix} \qquad \mathbf{m}^2 = \frac{1}{\sqrt{2}} \begin{pmatrix} 1 \\ -1 \end{pmatrix},$$

with corresponding eigenvalues

$$\lambda_1 = a + b \qquad \lambda_2 = a - b.$$

In such models ocular dominance emerges if $\lambda_2 > \lambda_1$ in which case the neuron connects with a weight of $1/\sqrt{2}$ to one eye and $-1/\sqrt{2}$ to the other eye[¶]. If synaptic weights are not allowed to become negative the dynamics would result in a neuron that is connected to one eye and not the other eye.

When does λ_2 become larger than λ_1? Obviously this can only happen if $b < 0$. But if the values of activity $\mathbf{d}_i$ are interpreted as firing rates measured from zero, they are always positive numbers. However, measured from some non-zero reference point, d_0, d could have negative values.

Such a reference point might be, for example, the spontaneous firing rate or the mean activity level. If we take it to be the mean activity level, the correlation matrix Q is now the covariance matrix. The off diagonal elements (b) of the covariance matrix can only be negative if the inputs from different (d_l and d_r) channels are anti-correlated. If they are uncorrelated then $b = 0$. Thus for the two eye analogy this is equivalent to assuming that the inputs coming from both eyes are anti-correlated – which does not seem to be a reasonable assumption. However activity levels do not have to be measured with respect to the mean (see Equation 5.1); this results in replacing the correlation function Q by the effective correlation function $Q' = Q - k_2 J$, where J is a matrix of ones and k_2 is a constant defined above. For large values of k_2 the off diagonal elements can indeed become negative, thus favoring the ocular-dominance type of solution. Another option is the use of the zero-DC Hebb rule as described above.

This model can be extended beyond two inputs. If each eye has N different inputs to the cell, supposedly arising from retinotopically adjacent locations, the model becomes $2N$ dimensional. Then the constants a and b above become matrices of dimensions $N \times N$. A simple generalization is to assume that the within-eye and between eye correlation functions differ only by a multiplicative constant, thus $a \rightarrow aQ$ and $b \rightarrow bQ$ where Q is

---

[¶]when $\mathbf{m}^i$ is an eigenvector so is $-\mathbf{m}^i$.

the $(N \times N)$ correlation matrix. This then becomes similar to the model proposed by Miller et. al. (1989) which assumes that the matrix Q has a Gaussian form. If Q has a first eigenvector $\mathbf{m}$ with an eigenvalue λ, then the eigenvectors for the two eye case will have the form:

$$\mathbf{m}^1 = \frac{1}{\sqrt{2}} \begin{pmatrix} \mathbf{m} \\ \mathbf{m} \end{pmatrix} \qquad \mathbf{m}^2 = \frac{1}{\sqrt{2}} \begin{pmatrix} \mathbf{m} \\ -\mathbf{m} \end{pmatrix},$$

with eigenvalues $\lambda_1 = (a + b)\lambda$ and $\lambda_2 = (a - b)\lambda$. If Q has a Gaussian form, its principal component is radially symmetric, and all weights have the same sign. We have schematically drawn the shapes of these eigenfunctions in Figure 5.18.

We have run a set of simulations using these types of two-channel correlation functions.

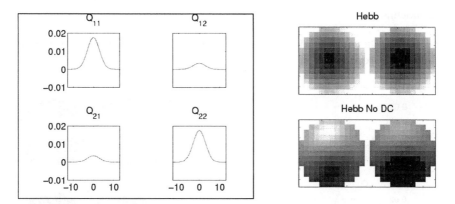

Figure 5.14: A Gaussian model with positive cross-channel correlations, $\eta = 0.2$. On the right the 2 channel correlation functions are shown. On the right receptive files extracted using the simple Hebb rule (upper panel) and the zero-DC rule (lower panel) are shown.

When the cross-channel correlations are positive (Figure 5.14) the simple Hebb rule produces perfectly binocular receptive fields. The zero-DC rule does not change this but produces a binocular oriented solution. This occurs because for this value of the cross channel correlation coefficient, $\eta = 0.2$, the binocular oriented solution (that has zero-DC) has a higher eigenvalue than the 'monocular' radially symmetric solution. If the two channels are anti-correlated (Figure 5.15) the receptive field obtained by the simple Hebb rule is indeed radially symmetric and due to the saturation limits it becomes monocular.

If the positive correlations between the channels are small enough, the

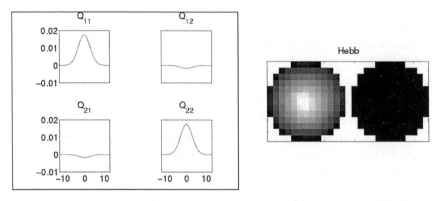

Figure 5.15: A Gaussian model with negative cross-channel correlations, $\eta = -0.1$ (left). Receptive fields produced are radially symmetric and monocular.

zero-DC rule can indeed produce monocular, radially symmetric receptive fields (Figure 5.16).

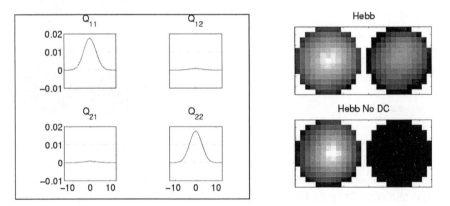

Figure 5.16: Small positive cross channel correlations, $\eta = 0.05$ (left). The simple Hebb rule (upper right) produces binocular receptive fields. The Zero-DC rule (lower right) produces monocular radially symmetric receptive fields.

What will be the effect if a limiting function is imposed on the weights? We do not know how to exactly solve these equations in that case. The analysis proposed by Feng et. al. [Feng et al., 1996], described in Section 5.2.3 can tell us which solutions are stable but not which ones will actually be attained. Any initial weight vector can be written as a superposition of the eigenvectors and therefore initially (before saturation limits are reached) the largest eigenvector would grow the fastest. From simulations displayed above, for simpler cases, we have shown this is often the case; here too it seems that the largest eigenvector will indeed dominate the shape of the receptive field.

Many of these results are very sensitive to the exact parameters used; we therefore urge readers to run these simulations with different parameters to see how sensitive these results are.

5.4.2 *Misaligned inputs to cell*

If the receptive fields of the two eyes are not exactly aligned, that is they do not receive exactly the same input, the functional form of the cross eye correlation function will be different then the form of the within eye correlation function. There are several reasons why inputs received through the two eyes might be different: the eyes are displaced, the lines of sight are not parallel and the angle between them changes as the distance to the focal plane changes. Further there might be a misalignment of the topographic maps from both eyes at the cortical level.

We can examine exactly the shape of the two eye correlation function using a simple variant of the complex situation that arises from binocular viewing of a 3D environment. This variant produces a severe disruption in the form of the two eye correlation function. We use it to demonstrate that in this situation only binocular receptive fields can be produced by the PCA rule. Although it is a simple example, the conclusions drawn from it can be generalized to most scenarios of binocular receptive field formation using a PCA rule.

The simple scenario we examine applies when the input to the two eyes is spatially displaced by a constant. The result is that the inputs a neuron received through the left eye do not perfectly overlap the inputs that neuron receives through the right eye. If the shift is by a vector $\mathbf{s}$ then the input a neuron receives through the left eye at point $\mathbf{r}$ in the receptive field is the same input it receives at point $\mathbf{r} + \mathbf{s}$ from the right eye. Thus, the peak of the cross-eye correlation function would not be at $\mathbf{r} = 0$ but at $\mathbf{r} = \mathbf{s}$. Thus the cross-eye correlation functions are no longer symmetric - although the total two-eye correlation function is symmetric. This scenario is described more precisely in Appendix 5C.

It is shown in Appendix 5C that this correlation function is symmetric under a generalized two-eye parity transform. Further it is shown that when the correlation function is invariant under the parity transform the receptive fields for the two eyes are inverted versions of each other up to a sign. The correlation function for most scenarios in which both channels are equivalent will be invariant to the parity transform, thus under most reasonable conditions this learning rule produces receptive fields that are perfectly binocular.

Since, as shown in Appendix 5C, these results apply to a larger class of correlation functions, including those postulated by Miller et. al. (1989), it raises the question of how they obtained monocular receptive fields? As shown above, they obtained monocularity by choosing a correlation function that produces mono-polar[||], radially symmetric receptive fields and a correlation function in which the cross-eye terms are anti-correlated. Therefore the solution with negative parity ($P = -1$) dominates. Thus by choosing mono-polar weights ($m \geq 0$) they practically set all weights connected from one of the eyes to zero. This method would not apply if the principal component is not mono-polar, as illustrated above.

5.5   Combined Orientation Selectivity and Ocular Dominance

In previous sections we described the emergence of orientation selectivity and of ocular dominance using PCA learning. It is interesting to examine whether it is possible to extract both under the same conditions. Cortical cells exhibit both orientation selectivity and varying degrees of ocular dominance, therefore it is essential that a successful model can develop both concurrently.

5.5.1   *The two-eye 1D soluble Model*

In this section we extend the exactly soluble model described above to the two eye case, this model is also exactly soluble. As before, true orientation selectivity does not emerge from this model because it is a 1D model, however the symmetry breaking which occurs can be thought of as an analog of orientation selectivity. In addition, as shown in Section 5.3.4, in higher dimensional cases all oriented solutions have zero DC. Thus, the simple 1-D case is comparable to the higher dimensional case, with the oscillating (zero-DC) solution representing the oriented solutions and the DC solution representing non-oriented solutions.

In the two eye case we can write down the general form of the two eye correlation function as

$$\mathbf{Q}^2 = \begin{pmatrix} Q_{ll} & Q_{lr} \\ Q_{rl} & Q_{rr} \end{pmatrix} \tag{5.14}$$

[||] All weights from the same eye have the same sign.

	binocular (+)	anti-binocular (-)
oscillating (cos) solutions	$q\pi(1-\eta)$	$q\pi(1+\eta)$
constant (DC) solutions	$(1-\eta)$	$(1+\eta)$

Table 5.2: Different possible eigenvalues of the exactly soluble two-eye problem. The spatial form of the receptive fields is wither the symmetry broken oscillating solutions, which have an arbitrary phase, or the DC for constant solutions. The OD form is either binocular or anti binocular. Note that for binocular solutions the eigenvalue of the parity operator is positive, whereas the anti-binocular solutions have negative eigenvalues.

A simple example has the form $Q_{ll} = Q_{rr} = Q$ and $Q_{lr} = Q_{rl} = -\eta Q$ thus

$$\mathbf{Q}^2 = \begin{pmatrix} Q & -\eta Q \\ -\eta Q & Q \end{pmatrix}. \tag{5.15}$$

We use the same correlation function used in our soluble 1D model and assume that $Q(x) = 1 + q\cos(\pi x)$.

Given that $\mathbf{m}(x)$ is an eigenvector of Q (the one-eye problem) with eigenvalue λ, then $(\mathbf{m}, \mathbf{m})$ and $(\mathbf{m}, -\mathbf{m})$ are both eigenvectors of $\mathbf{Q}$ with eigenvalues $\lambda^- = (1-\eta)\lambda$ and $\lambda^+ = (1+\eta)\lambda$ respectively. The two-eye problem, therefore, has four possible solutions. The eigenvalues of these solutions are shown in Table 5.2.

The schematic shape of these solutions is shown in Figure 5.17.

The bottom part of Figure 5.17 shows schematically the analogous receptive fields that would emerge in a mono-polar model, that is when synaptic weights are restricted to be positive ($m \geq 0$). If no spatial symmetry is broken, then the mono-polar solutions are indeed monocular, that is the neuron connects only to one eye. However, in cases when spatial symmetry is broken, rather than monocularity we obtain subfield reversal due to the $m \geq 0$ constraint. As is demonstrated below, the same logic extended to the 2D models, thus, if the receptive field is a principal component, ocular dominance can occur only if spatially solutions are non-oriented. When solutions do exhibit orientation selectivity, a negative parity would result in subfield reversal.

5.5.2 A Correlational Model of Ocular Dominance and Orientation Selectivity

In previous sections we have shown examples of separate correlational models for orientation selectivity and ocular dominance. In the section above we described an exactly soluble model in 1D. Do the conclusions suggested

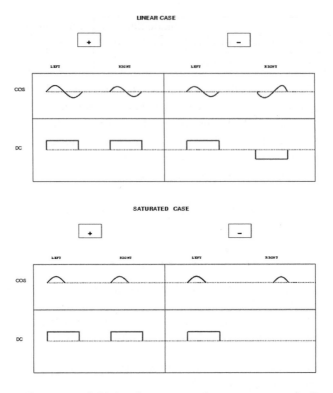

Figure 5.17: Receptive field development in the two-eye case for linear (top) and only-excitatory (bottom) models. The x axis in each subplot represents position in the coordinates of the left and right eyes and the y axis represents synaptic strength. The + and - symbols on top show the different cases when the two eyes receive correlated and anti-correlated inputs. The cos and DC labels on the side show if the oscilatory or constant component of the correlation function is dominant (see Figure 5.2). In each of the two cases (linear and saturated) we get four qualitatively distinct outcomes. (top) Four possible two eye receptive fields are shown for the simple linear model. On the left of each plot the RF's produced when the cross channel correlation has a positive coeffcient ($\eta > 0$) and on the right the RF's produced when it is negative ($\eta < 0$). (bottom) The effect of not allowing weights to become negative is displayed. These are basically truncated versions of the linear case. For the DC RF's this produces monocular RF's. This does not happen in the cos type RF's, which are comparable to the oriented solutions.

by the 1D case hold for true orientation selectivity in 2D?

In order to create such a model we require that minimal conditions for extracting both ocular dominance, and orientation selectivity be met. In order to achieve orientation selectivity we need to choose a single eye correlation function Q and an arbor function A, such that the principal component $\mathbf{m}$ is orientation selective and has an eigenvalue λ_1 (Section 5.3). Using this correlation function we can construct a simple two eye correlation function of the type used for ocular dominance. Thus we propose a two eye correlation function of the form**:

$$Q_2 = \begin{pmatrix} Q_{ll} & Q_{lr} \\ Q_{rl} & Q_{rr} \end{pmatrix} = \begin{pmatrix} Q & -\eta Q \\ -\eta Q & Q \end{pmatrix} \tag{5.16}$$

The principal components in the two eye case depend on the value of η. For $\eta < 0$ the two eye solution $\mathbf{m}_1^2$ takes the form $\mathbf{m}_1^2 = (\mathbf{m}_1, -\mathbf{m}_1)$ with eigenvalue $\lambda = (1 + \eta)\lambda_1$, where $\mathbf{m}_1$ and λ_1 are the eigenvector and eigenvalue or the analogous one eye problem with a correlation function Q. For $\eta > 0$ the solution has the form $\mathbf{m}_1^2 = (\mathbf{m}_1, \mathbf{m}_1)$ with eigenvalue $\lambda = (1 - \eta)\lambda_1$. The case with $\eta < 0$ is the analog of the ocular dominance case. However since the receptive fields are oriented this scenario runs into problems.

Ocular dominance in these models implies that the connections from one eye to the cortical cell are stronger than the connections to the other eye. The linear model assumes bi-modal synapses, that is the synaptic weight can become negative as well. The ocular dominance model described earlier assumes that only positive synapses can evolve. This assumption yields a result similar to setting to zero all synapses that would become negative under the linear assumptions. The ocular dominance model, described above (Section 5.4), assumes a correlation function and arbor function that result in radially symmetric, unimodal receptive fields. Thus the principal component of the linear model that has the form $\mathbf{m}_1^2 = (\mathbf{m}, -\mathbf{m})$ is replaced by the monocular receptive field $\mathbf{m}_1^2 = (\mathbf{m}, 0)$ in the non-linear model (Figure 5.18a.).

When the principal components are oriented, they are no longer unimodal. Saturation limits at zero therefore do not cause a complete disconnection of one of the eyes, rather they disconnect the negative subfields of the eye. This is schematically illustrated in Figure 5.18b. What happens is that one eye connects to one subfield of the RF and the other eye to the complementary subfield.

The conclusion of the arguments above is simple; as long as the receptive

---

**It has often been claimed that assuming anti correlation between the eyes is not realistic. This assumption may be relaxed if appropriate constants are chosen in Equation 5.1 resulting in an anti-correlated pseudo correlation function.

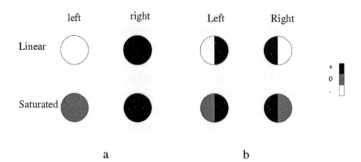

Figure 5.18: On the left formation of ocular dominance is illustrated in the case when receptive fields are unimodal. On the right the situation which arises when receptive fields are orientation selective is illustrated.

field structure of linear models is anti-symmetric and receptive fields are oriented, saturation limits would not induce monocularity.

What would happen if the cross correlation component had a more complex structure, that is $Q_{lr} \neq \eta Q_{rr}$. Symmetry under the two eye parity transform, described in the Appendix 5C ensures that as long as the two eyes are symmetric, the two eye receptive fields would also be symmetric under parity. For a $P = +1$ parity, this would imply simply that the left-eye RF ($\mathbf{m}^l$) is a mirror image of the right-eye RF ($\mathbf{m}^r$), producing a binocular RF. When $P = -1$ the left-eye RF ($\mathbf{m}^l$) is also sign inverted on top of the mirror symmetry. When synaptic weights are restricted to be positive, the $P = -1$ can produce ocular dominance, if the dominant PC of a single eye is mono-polar. However, if the dominant PC is orientation selective, restricting weights to be positive would only result in subfield inversion, as illustrated in Figure 5.18. This result is consistent with the intuition gained from the 1D model.

5.5.3   *Four Channel Models*

The retina and LGN have several distinct types of neurons. One of the major distinctions is the difference between ON type cells that are excited by light falling on the center of their receptive fields and OFF type cells that are inhibited by light falling on their center.

Would assuming a four channel model, which includes also OFF and ON channels for each eye overcome the difficulties encountered by the 2 channel model? The general form of this four channel correlation function [tt] can be reduced to the following form:

$$Q^4 = \begin{pmatrix} Q^{ss} & Q^{so} & Q^{os} & Q^{oo} \\ Q^{so} & Q^{ss} & Q^{oo} & Q^{os} \\ Q^{os} & Q^{oo} & Q^{ss} & Q^{so} \\ Q^{oo} & Q^{os} & Q^{so} & Q^{ss} \end{pmatrix} \qquad (5.17)$$

Where Q^{ss} denotes the correlation function between same type of channel (eg: ON-ON or OFF-OFF) and same eye (eg: left-left or right-right), Q^{so} means same channel different eye, Q^{os} means different channel same eye and Q^{oo} denotes different channel different eye. This form is based on several simplifying assumption of equivalent eyes and equivalent channels. It follows that the correlation function within the right eye are identical to those within the left eye and that the correlation function within the ON channel is the same as within the OFF channel.

Making the additional assumption that input from the OFF channel is the negative of the input from the ON channel, the four channel correlation function has the form

$$Q^4 = \begin{pmatrix} Q & -Q & Q^c & -Q^c \\ -Q & Q & -Q^c & Q^c \\ Q^c & -Q^c & Q & -Q \\ -Q^c & Q^c & -Q & Q \end{pmatrix} \qquad (5.18)$$

Where Q_c is the cross eye correlation function between the same type of channels. If we assume further that the cross eye correlation function Q_C has the simple form $Q_c = -\eta Q$, then the PC for $\eta > 0$ has the form

---

[tt] left-ON, left-OFF, right-ON, right-OFF

$$\mathbf{m} = \begin{pmatrix} \mathbf{m}_l^+ \\ -\mathbf{m}_l^- \\ -\mathbf{m}_r^+ \\ \mathbf{m}_r^- \end{pmatrix} = \begin{pmatrix} \mathbf{m} \\ -\mathbf{m} \\ -\mathbf{m} \\ \mathbf{m} \end{pmatrix}. \tag{5.19}$$

With an eigenvalue $\lambda = 2(1+\eta)\lambda_1$. Thus, as in the two channel model, monocularity is not achieved for oriented $\mathbf{m}$ instead a reversal of subfields is achieved. In the analogous monopolar case $(m \geq 0)$ a cell connected to the ON channel of one eye subfield would be connected to OFF channel inputs from the other eye in the same subfield. The inverse would be true for the other subfields.

5.5.4 *Mixing Principal Components*

In Appendix 5C, below, the Parity Transform is used to elucidate the symmetry properties of two-eye receptive fields. We have demonstrated that principal components are symmetric to the parity transform. Some have a $p = +1$ parity and others a $p = -1$ parity. When the receptive fields are radially symmetric the $p = -1$ case can be used for producing monocular receptive fields if synaptic weights have a lower saturation bound. This no longer holds for oriented receptive fields as illustrated in the soluble example of Section 5.5.1 and as seen schematically in Figure 5.18. However, combinations of different principal components, some with $p = +1$ and others with $p = -1$, are no longer symmetric under parity.

If a Hebbian rule with saturating bounds is used rather than the Oja rule, the resulting receptive fields could be well approximated by a combinations of several of the major PC's. This is so since, as can be seen from Equation 5.4, all PC's present in the initial state grow exponentially with an exponent proportional to the eigenvalue; thus the eigenvectors with the larger eigenvalues quickly come to dominate the solution. A four channel model has been proposed [Erwin and Miller, 1995; Piepenbrock et al., 1997; Erwin and Miller, 1998] that obtains both orientation selectivity, and ocular dominance. These receptive fields are obviously not principal components but combinations of principal components. In such a model it is essential to choose both the correlation functions and the saturation limits carefully in order to obtain just the right combination of principal components. Furthermore the assumption that inputs from the ON-channel are the negative of the OFF-channel inputs must be abandoned; nevertheless it is still assumed that these two channels have the same within-channel correlation functions despite having different probability distributions. This correlation function has the general form described in Equation 5.17.

Due to the symmetries it is possible to block diagonalize this function with the transformation matrix U [Piepenbrock et al., 1997; Erwin and Miller, 1998]

$$U = \frac{1}{2} \begin{pmatrix} 1 & 1 & 1 & 1 \\ 1 & 1 & -1 & -1 \\ 1 & -1 & 1 & -1 \\ 1 & -1 & -1 & 1 \end{pmatrix} \tag{5.20}$$

where the ones here stand for unit matrices with the appropriate dimension.

After diagonalizing, the correlation function has the form

$$Q_d^4 = \begin{pmatrix} Q^s & 0 & 0 & 0 \\ 0 & Q^{od} & 0 & 0 \\ 0 & 0 & Q^{or+} & 0 \\ 0 & 0 & 0 & Q^{or-} \end{pmatrix}, \tag{5.21}$$

where the subscript d refers to the block-diagonalized form. It is important to note the principal component of this correlation function is still the single PC with the highest eigenvalue. It is therefore an eigenstate of one of the sub-correlation functions $Q^s, Q^{od}, Q^{or+}, Q^{or-}$.

We denote the eigenstates of each of the correlation functions in this space as $\mathbf{m}_i^s$, $\mathbf{m}_i^{od}$, $\mathbf{m}_i^{or+}$, $\mathbf{m}^{or-}$ and their eigenvalues as λ_i^s, λ_i^{od}, λ_i^{or+}, λ^{or-} respectively.

The dynamics of the non-saturating Hebb rule in the original, non-transformed, four channel space are then

$$\mathbf{m}(t) = \sum_i \left(\begin{pmatrix} 1 \\ 1 \\ 1 \\ 1 \end{pmatrix} \mathbf{m}_i^s a_i^s e^{\lambda_i^s t} + \begin{pmatrix} 1 \\ 1 \\ -1 \\ -1 \end{pmatrix} \mathbf{m}_i^{od} a_i^{od} e^{\lambda_i^{od} t} \right.$$
$$\left. + \begin{pmatrix} 1 \\ -1 \\ 1 \\ -1 \end{pmatrix} \mathbf{m}_i^{or+} a_i^{or+} e^{\lambda_i^{or+} t} + \begin{pmatrix} 1 \\ -1 \\ -1 \\ 1 \end{pmatrix} \mathbf{m}_i^{or-} a_i^{or-} e^{\lambda_i^{or+} t} \right)$$

$$= \sum_i \left(\begin{pmatrix} 1 \\ 1 \\ 1 \\ 1 \end{pmatrix} \mathbf{m}_i^s a_i^s(t) + \begin{pmatrix} 1 \\ 1 \\ -1 \\ -1 \end{pmatrix} \mathbf{m}_i^{od} a_i^{od}(t) \right.$$

$$\left. + \begin{pmatrix} 1 \\ -1 \\ 1 \\ -1 \end{pmatrix} \mathbf{m}_i^{or+} a_i^{or+}(t) + \begin{pmatrix} 1 \\ -1 \\ -1 \\ 1 \end{pmatrix} \mathbf{m}_i^{or-} a_i^{or-}(t) \right)$$

where the a are the coefficients at time 0, and a(t) the coefficients at time t. As usual we see that asymptotically the eigenstate with the largest eigenvalue will dominate. Therefore the state converges to be either orientation selective or monocular, not both.

How then can this model be used to create receptive fields that are both orientation selective and have ocular dominance? This is done by terminating the dynamics early enough so that several of the larger principal components are still of relatively similar magnitudes. It is important therefore to choose the correlation functions so that the eigenvalues of Q^s are very small in order to depress the growth of binocular solutions[‡‡], and that the eigenvalues of Q^{od} and Q^{or+} (or Q^{or-}) are of the same magnitude. Furthermore it is essential that Q^{or+} be chosen such that its first eigenstate is indeed orientation selective, that is that it have large enough negative lobes that fall within the arbor function range (Section 5.3).

In Figure 5.19 we have displayed the correlation functions used by Erwin and Miller to obtain states that are both orientation selective and have ocular dominance. For this choice of correlation functions $\lambda_1^{or+}/\lambda_1^{od} = 0.8$. It is interesting to see what these correlation functions look like in the original, non-diagonalized, space. This is displayed in the upper part of Figure 5.19

Looking at the correlation functions in the original space (Figure 5.19-top) Erwin and Miller (1998) stated conditions under which monocular oriented receptive fields will appear. They have stated that the correlation function within the channel (that is ON-ON or OFF-OFF) must be stronger than those between different channels (that is between ON and OFF) at small distances but smaller at large distances. Further the cross-eye correlation functions must be smaller than those between different channels. Indeed the receptive fields extracted from this correlation function, with the zero-DC rule have the desired characteristics; they are monocular oriented and the ON subfield is complimentary to the OFF subfield.

It is possible however to create a correlation function that adheres to

---

[‡‡]Miller in much of his work uses a hard form of subtractive normalization, in which the sum of the change in the synaptic strengths is always zero - this is done to eliminate the growth of the DC component but is implemented in a non-local way.

the same set of requirements but which does not produce the desired shape of receptive fields. Such a correlation function is shown in Figure 5.21 and the resulting receptive fields are shown in Figure 5.22.

Therefore the conditions described in Erwin and Miller (1998) might be necessary but they are not sufficient. The most prominent effect observed when running such simulations is how sensitive the results are to the exact parameters of the model. Therefore we urge readers to run these simulations, using the simulation package, while slightly varying the parameters of the correlation functions used.

Erwin and Miller (1995, 1998) often make the simplifying assumption that Q^{or-} and Q^s are negligible, thus the eigenvectors of Q^{od} and Q^{or+} would dominate the solutions. On the average the ratio between the coefficients of these two states in the receptive field is $< a_1^{or+}(t)/a_1^{od}(t) >= \exp\left((\lambda_1^{or+} - \lambda_1^{od})t\right)$. This fraction is time dependent. The dynamics in this model are terminated at a different times for each synapse due to the saturation limits of the synapses and sticky bounds. However the situation is qualitatively similar to freezing the dynamics at the same time t_f for all the synapses.

We devise a dominance measure (DM) such that

$$DM = \left(\frac{a_1^{od}(t) - a_1^{or+}(t)}{a_1^{od}(t) + a_1^{or+}(t)}\right) = \frac{1 - \exp^{(\lambda_1^{or+} - \lambda_1^{od})t}}{1 + \exp^{(\lambda_1^{or+} - \lambda_1^{od})t}}.$$

This measure is 1 when the monocular non oriented solution completely dominates and -1 when the binocular oriented solution dominates.

Demanding that the correlational model explain both ocular dominance and orientation selectivity has put strong constraints on the possible underlying assumptions of the model. In order to get the combined model to work it is essential that;

(a) Q^{od} have a radially symmetric unipolar PC with eigenvalue λ_1^{od},

(b) that Q^{or} have an orientation selective PC with λ_1^{or},

(c) that λ_1^{od} and λ_1^{or} are of the same order of magnitude,

(d) that Q^{sum} has eigenvalues λ^{sum} that are much smaller than those of Q^{od} and of $Q^{or\pm}$,

(e) that the dynamics terminate early (t_f is small enough or saturation limits low enough) enough so that the two leading components have a significant contribution.

In order to do this, a very particular form of the correlation functions has to be assumed, as illustrated in Figure 5.19. The most important assumption that goes into these models is that although the ON and OFF models have the same second order statistics, their statistics in general differ from each other since the cross-correlation of these two channels is not simply the negative of the auto-correlation, but has a quite different shape. This is a constraint that needs to be examined experimentally as well as theoretically. Both the activities of the ON channel and OFF channel are functions of the inputs, that is $\mathbf{d}^{ON} = K^{ON}(I)$ and $\mathbf{d}^{OFF} = K^{OFF}(I)$ and for a non singular K, $\mathbf{d}^{OFF} = g(\mathbf{d}^{ON})$. It is interesting to see what kind of functions K indeed perform this transform such that $Q_{ij}^{ss} \neq \pm Q_{ij}^{os}$, that is $< d_i^{ON} d_j^{ON} > = < d_i^{OFF} d_j^{OFF} > = < g(d^{ON})_i g(d^{ON})_j >$ but that also $< d_i^{ON} d_j^{OFF} > \neq \pm < d_i^{ON} g(d^{ON})_j >$.

Further the cross-channel correlation must have a very specific shape, as shown in Figure 5.19. It is possible to show that g can not be a linear transformation, so it would be interesting to know what kind of transformation it could be, and whether this corresponds to known properties of the OFF and ON channels.

Recently direct measurements of correlations between different cells in the LGN of ferrets have been carried out [Weliky and Katz, 1999]. The results have been obtained in vivo before eye opening. These results show that under normal conditions there are positive correlations between the two eyes and even stronger positive correlations between the ON and OFF channel within the same eye. These results are **not** consistent with the assumptions made by these correlational models[Miller et al., 1989; Erwin and Miller, 1998]. In order to attain separate ON and OFF subfields, these models require that the activity of ON and OFF neurons be anti-correlated. When animals are viewing a patterned visual environment the responses of ON and OFF cells are indeed anti-correlated. This can possibly account for sub-field segregation occurring *after* eye opening, but cannot account for the segregation *before* eye opening predicted by these correlation models. These recent experimental results pose a serious challenge to the correlational model described above.

5.5.5   *Local External Symmetry Breaking*

In order to create real ocular dominance concurrently with orientation selectivity, in a single principal component, we must postulate correlation functions which are not symmetric under the parity transform. This is very easy to do, consider for instance the diagonal correlation function:

$$Q_2 = \begin{pmatrix} Q & 0 \\ 0 & \mu Q \end{pmatrix} \tag{5.22}$$

If $\eta < 1$ the PC is $\mathbf{m} = (\mathbf{m}_1, 0)$ with eigenvalue λ and if $\mu > 1$ it is $\mathbf{m} = (0, \mathbf{m}_1)$ with eigenvalue $\mu\lambda$. In this case monocular RF's do appear however it is based on assuming an asymmetry between the eyes. Furthermore the resulting asymmetry between the eyes is reduced by assuming a positive cross correlation between the eyes.

Assuming a local asymmetry between the eyes, i.e: that the signals coming from the left eye to a cortical cell are larger than those coming from the right may be reasonable. Making such assumptions however shifts the responsibility for the formation of ocular dominance from the learning rule to other external factors. A relatively realistic scenario of such external symmetry breaking can be discussed in the context of the perturbation analysis [Dayan and Goodhill, 1992]. One of the assumptions examined there is of weak local symmetry breaking between the two eyes.

As we have shown the final state in case of external symmetry breaking is perfectly monocular. We should thus expect that the time evolution of receptive fields should lead from a relatively binocular initial state to a monocular final state. The data indicate the opposite: initially there is a strong contra-lateral bias of the ocular dominance histogram, during postnatal development the cortex becomes more balanced as time passes [Crair et al., 1998].

5.5.6 *A two eye model with Natural Images*

We have shown that symmetry to the parity operator implies that only binocular neurons are produced by the PCA rule. Here we display simulation results in a natural image environment as described above (Section 5.3.5, using a binocular input sampled from the images with different degrees of overlap.

The PCA results of partially overlapping receptive fields are presented in Figure 5.24. The degree of overlap between receptive fields does not alter the optimal orientation, so that whenever a cell is selective its orientation is in the horizontal direction. The degree of overlap does affect the shape of the receptive fields, and the degree of orientation selectivity that emerges under PCA: orientation selectivity decreases as the amount of overlap decreases. However, when there is no overlap at all, one again gets higher selectivity. For PCA, there is a symmetry between the receptive fields of both eyes that imposes binocularity. This arises from the invariance of the two-eye correlation function to a parity transformation (see Appendix 5C).

We also study the possibility that under the PCA rule, different orientation selective cells could emerge if the misalignment between the two eyes is in the vertical direction. This tests the effect of a shift orthogonal to the preferred orientation. The results (Figure 5.25, bottom) show that there is no change in the orientation preference; even in this case only horizontal receptive fields emerge.

The PCA results described above are quite robust to introduction of non-linearity in cell's activity; there is no qualitative difference in the results when a non symmetric sigmoidal transfer function is used. Further we have shown [Shouval et al., 1996a] that a linear network of interacting

PCA neurons is still perfectly binocular. It can also be shown that the parity transform applies to such networks as well. We conclude that using second order learning rules it is not easy to attain receptive fields that are orientation selective and not binocular.

5.6 Deprivation Experiments

The best demonstration of plasticity in visual cortex is provided by deprivation experiments in which input to cortex are disrupted by some artificial manipulation. It has been shown already by Hubel and Wiesel [Wiesel and Hubel, 1962] that such manipulations can alter receptive fields of cortical neurons. The best examples are those in which the binocular properties of neurons are altered by depriving one of the eyes of normal visual inputs. In this section we examine what the effect is of such deprivation experiments on a PCA neuron. We discuss the following conditions:

- Normal Rearing (**NR**), The baseline condition in which animals are reared normally with both eyes open. This results in an ocular dominance histogram in which most cells are driven by both eyes.
- Monocular Deprivation (**MD**) Inputs from one eye are altered. This is typically done by suturing the eye lid: a procedure that results in shifting the ocular dominance histogram so the most cells become dominated by the open eye.
- Reverse Suture (**RS**). This procedure follows MD; the previously sutured eye is opened and the other eye is sutured. This results in reversing the effect of MD - most cells become dominated by newly opened eye.
- Binocular Deprivation (**BD**). Both eyes are sutured - this results in a slow loss of orientation selectivity. This processes is much slower than MD.

5.6.1 *A Simple Correlational Model using Exact PCA Dynamics*

In this section we use the Wyatt solution (Equation 5.23) to determine the time dynamics of a neuron following Oja's learning rule in an environment modeling the classical visual cortical plasticity experiments.

Since this is a second order learning rule all we have to know is the correlation function and the initial conditions. The solution shown by Wyatt and Elfeldel [Wyatt and Elfadel, 1995] has the form

$$m(t) = \frac{e^{Qt}\mathbf{m}_0}{||(e^{Qt}\mathbf{m}_0||^2 + 1 - ||\mathbf{m}_0||)^{\frac{1}{2}}}, \tag{5.23}$$

where $\mathbf{m}_0 = \mathbf{m}(t = 0)$ is the initial state of the weight vector.

The basic assumption we make is that during lid suture, the output of the deprived channel is uncorrelated noise. Thus the correlation function of the deprived channel has the form:

$$Q^{deprived} = \begin{pmatrix} \sigma^2 & 0 & 0 & \cdots & 0 \\ 0 & \sigma^2 & 0 & \cdots & 0 \\ \vdots & \vdots & \vdots & & \vdots \\ 0 & 0 & 0 & \cdots & \sigma^2 \end{pmatrix}.$$

No assumptions are necessary about the form of Q_{open}; however we usually assume that the largest eigenvalue of Q_{open} is larger than σ^2. The basic methodology is to expand the initial conditions in terms of the eigenvectors of the correlation function Q_{open}, insert them into the Wyatt solution and produce the result.

(a) Normal Rearing (NR)

Assume, for convenience, that both eyes have exactly the same input. The correlation function, Q^{NR}, then has the form

$$Q^{NR} = \begin{pmatrix} Q_{open} & Q_{open} \\ Q_{open} & Q_{open} \end{pmatrix}$$

We expand the initial weight vector $\mathbf{m}(0)$ in terms of the eigenvectors of the correlation matrix $(\mathbf{m}_j)$.

$$\mathbf{m}(0) = \begin{pmatrix} \mathbf{m}^l(0) \\ \mathbf{m}^r(0) \end{pmatrix} = \sum_j \begin{pmatrix} a_j^l \mathbf{m}_j \\ a_j^r \mathbf{m}_j \end{pmatrix}$$

where $\mathbf{m}_j$ the $j'th$ eigenvector of the correlation function Q^{open}, has the eigenvalue λ_j and a_j^l, a_j^r are the expansion coefficients for left and right eye respectively. We assume that eigenvectors and eigenvalues are arranged in a descending order, that is $\lambda_1 > \lambda_2 > \cdots \lambda_N$. Inserting this into the Wyatt formula produces the generic solution for the dynamics of normal rearing

$$\mathbf{m}^{NR}(t) = \frac{\sum_j \frac{1}{2} \begin{pmatrix} \mathbf{m}_j \left[(a_j^l + a_j^r)e^{2\lambda_j t} + (a_j^l - a_j^r) \right] \\ \mathbf{m}_j \left[(a_j^l + a_j^r)e^{2\lambda_j t} + (a_j^r - a_j^l) \right] \end{pmatrix}}{\left(\frac{1}{2} \sum_j \left[(a_j^l + a_j^r)^2 e^{4\lambda_j t} + (a_j^l - a_j^r)^2 \right] + 1 - \sum_j \left[(a_j^l)^2 + (a_j^r)^2 \right] \right)^{1/2}}$$

$$(5.24)$$

The $t \to \infty$ limiting case, needed for the calculations in the next few sections, is straightforward to obtain. If the largest eigenvalue is non-degenerate, then **m** will become

$$\mathbf{m}^{NR}(t \to \infty) = \sqrt{\frac{1}{2}} \begin{pmatrix} \mathbf{m}_1 \\ \mathbf{m}_1 \end{pmatrix}$$

Thus the solution converges to a state in which both eye receptive fields are eigenvectors of Q_{open}. The higher the ratio between λ_1 and the smaller eigenvalues the faster it will converge.

(b)   Monocular Deprivation (MD)

We assume that one eye is open and generates a structured input to the cortical cell, whereas the other eye is closed and generates noise. The noise is uncorrelated, thus the closed eye correlation matrix is diagonal, which implies that the cross eye correlations vanish.

Thus the correlation function has the form

$$Q^{MD} = \begin{pmatrix} Q^{open} & 0 \\ 0 & Q^{deprived} \end{pmatrix}$$

We assume that MD is started after a NR phase in which the solution has already converged to the binocular fixed-point.

Thus

$$\mathbf{m}^{MD}(0) = \sqrt{\frac{1}{2}} \begin{pmatrix} \mathbf{m}_1 \\ \mathbf{m}_1 \end{pmatrix}$$

which yields

$$\mathbf{m}^{MD}(t) = \frac{\begin{pmatrix} e^{\lambda_1 t} \mathbf{m}_1 \\ e^{\sigma^2 t} \mathbf{m}_1 \end{pmatrix}}{(e^{2\lambda_1 t} + e^{2\sigma^2 t})^{1/2}} \tag{5.25}$$

If the magnitude of the noise from the closed eye σ^2 is smaller than the largest eigenvalue of the visual inputs, that is $\lambda_1 > \sigma^2$, then the $t \to \infty$ limiting case becomes

$$\mathbf{m}^{MD}(t \to \infty) = \begin{pmatrix} \mathbf{m}_1 \\ 0 \end{pmatrix}$$

Hence, as observed experimentally, the neuron will eventually disconnect from the closed eye. Notice that the rate of the disconnection is *slowed* as the level of noise *increases*.

(c)   Reverse Suture (RS)
This processes follows MD: the deprived and normal channels are reversed. Thus we assume the correlation function has the form:

$$Q^{RS} = \begin{pmatrix} Q^{deprived} & 0 \\ 0 & Q^{open} \end{pmatrix}$$

Reverse suture is the procedure that starts at the end of an MD protocol. However if we assume that the initial conditions of RS are the final conditions of MD as $t \to \infty$ we run into an immediate problem. This happens because an eye which is totally disconnected, can never reconnect. To alleviate this, we assume that the monocular deprivation experiment did not achieve $t = \infty$, but just some large number T. In that case the initial weight vector for RS is

$$\mathbf{m}^{RS}(0) = \begin{pmatrix} \mathbf{m}_1 \\ \epsilon \mathbf{m}_1 \end{pmatrix}$$

where $\epsilon \sim e^{(\sigma^2 - \lambda_1)T} \ll 1$

We put this into the Wyatt solution (Equation 5.7) to obtain $\mathbf{m}(t)$. This yields

$$\mathbf{m}^{RS}(t) = \frac{\begin{pmatrix} e^{\sigma^2 t}\mathbf{m}_1 \\ e^{\lambda_1 t}\epsilon\mathbf{m}_1 \end{pmatrix}}{(e^{2\sigma^2 t} + \epsilon e^{2\lambda_1 t})^{1/2}} \tag{5.26}$$

(d)   Binocular Deprivation (BD)
In this condition both channels are deprived; thus the correlation function has the form:

$$Q^{BD} = \begin{pmatrix} Q^{deprived} & 0 \\ 0 & Q^{deprived} \end{pmatrix}$$

As in MD, the initial weight vector is

$$\mathbf{m}^{BD}(0) = \sqrt{\frac{1}{2}} \begin{pmatrix} \mathbf{m}_1 \\ \mathbf{m}_1 \end{pmatrix}$$

which yields

$$\mathbf{m}^{BD}(t) = \sqrt{\frac{1}{2}} \begin{pmatrix} \mathbf{m}_1 \\ \mathbf{m}_1 \end{pmatrix} \tag{5.27}$$

The Wyatt solution is a solution for the deterministic analog of the stochastic learning rule proposed by Oja. Therefore Equation 5.27 implies that a neuron following Oja's rule, experiencing binocular deprivation following normal rearing, performs a random walk about the normal reared state.

5.6.2 *Simulation results with natural images*

The same type of deprivation experiments can be performed for an environment composed of natural images. As in the analysis above, inputs from the deprived eye are assumed to generate random independent noise. The results of such simulations are shown in Figure 5.26.

Qualitatively these ocular dominance results are identical to those obtained from the simple model outlined above. In Normal Rearing (NR) both eyes develop nearly identical receptive fields (Figure 5.26, top), although the cells are only marginally selective. Monocular Deprivation (MD) leads to a disconnection of the deprived eye with an approximately exponential time course (Figure 5.26, second from top). Reverse Suture (RS), reversed the effect of MD (Figure 5.26, second from bottom); the open eye reconnects to the neuron and the newly deprived eye disconnect. Binocular Deprivation (BD) does not produce a significant change in the receptive fields of the neuron.

5.7 Discussion

Most theoretical learning rules, derived from Hebb's original postulate, depend primarily on the second order statistics of the input. In this chapter we investigated this family of learning rules, and show that there is a simple common methodology for studying them. This methodology is used to explain how orientation selectivity, ocular dominance, and many deprivation experiments are accounted for by models based on these learning rules.

As observed long ago for this family of plasticity rules to be stable, additional constraints must be imposed. Some of these constraints such as normalization [von der Malsburg, 1973] or the more biologically plausible decay term [Oja, 1982] produce receptive fields that are the principal component of the inputs. Other constraints such as saturation bounds or subtractive decay terms [Miller, 1992; MacKay and Miller, 1994], produce receptive fields that are combinations of several of the largest principal components. Additional constraints are important not only for stabilization of learning but also for producing receptive fields with interesting structure or with structure resembling that found experimentally. For example, a decay term that subtracts the DC projection from the weight growth, might be necessary in many cases in order to reduce the growth rate of principal components with a strong DC component.

We have also shown how orientation selectivity can be produced, by choosing an appropriate correlation function, or from natural images by choosing the appropriate retinal filter. Both of these approaches produce oriented receptive fields that are quite broadly tuned. More significantly, these results are not robust, as small parameter changes significantly alter the receptive field structure.

Ocular dominance segregation can also be obtained by an appropriate choice of a correlation function. For ocular dominance to develop it is necessary that the effective correlation function have negative cross-correlations between the two-eye channels. This does not arise simply in a natural two eye environment. In addition it is not possible to obtain a principal component that is both orientation selective and that is driven differently by the two eyes. Second order models that can produce both orientation selectivity and ocular dominance depend on a combination of several principal components with a similar eigenvalue magnitude. Further, the parameters under which both ocular dominance and orientation selectivity can emerge are very finely tuned, so that the results are not robust to small changes in the parameters.

We have also analyzed and simulated different types of deprivation experiments, such as monocular and binocular deprivation. The results obtained are not always consistent with experiment. For example with a PCA rule, binocular deprivation causes no change in receptive fields and no reduction in response magnitudes.

In all, these second order learning rules, with sometimes delicate and sometimes unrealistic constraints, can account for different subsets of the data. However there does not seem to be a single such rule and set of constraints (even delicate or unrealistic) consistent with available experimental results that can, with one set of parameters, account for all of the data.

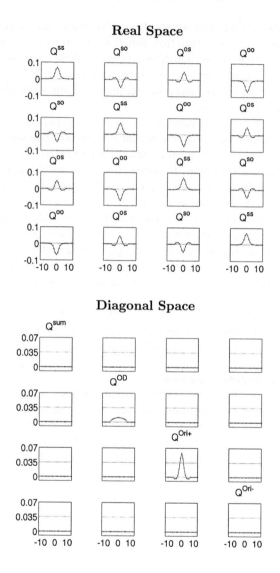

Figure 5.19: The 4-channel correlation functions similar to those used in Erwin and Miller 1998, which produce both orientation selectivity and ocular dominance. Above they are displayed in the original space and below in block diagonal space. We chose $Q^{sum} = 0$ and $Q^{ori-} = 0$. $Q^{OD} = 1.5 * G(0, 3 * 0.24 * 6.5)$ and $Q^{ori+} = G(0, 1 * 0.24 * 6.5) - G(r, 0, 3 * 0.24 * 6.5)$. These numbers were taken to exactly replicate the assumptions and results presented by Erwin and Miller, 1998.

Hebb No DC

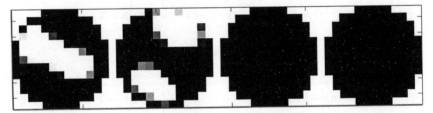

Figure 5.20: Receptive fields obtained using the zero-DC Hebb rule from the correlation function of Figure 5.19. The right eye is completely disconnected, the receptive field is orientation selective and the ON and OFF subfields do not overlap.

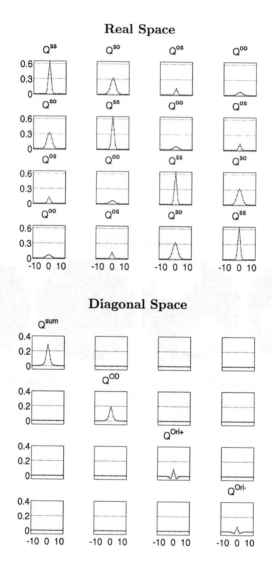

Figure 5.21: A 4-channel correlation function in real and diagonal space (above and below, respectively). It is most convenient to describe this correlation function in real space where $Q^{ss} = G(0,1)$, $Q^{so} = G(0,3)$, $Q^{os} = 0.2G(0,1)$ and $Q^{oo} = 0.2 * G(0,3)$.

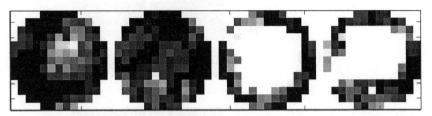

Figure 5.22: Receptive fields obtained using the zero-DC Hebb rule from the correlation function of Figure 5.21. These receptive fields do not become orientation selective

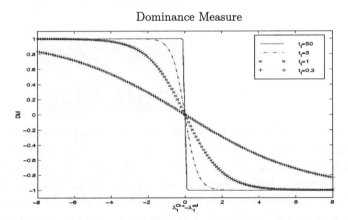

Figure 5.23: The DM measure as a function of $(\lambda_1^{or+} - \lambda_1^{od})$. The different plot correspond to different time for termination of the dynamics t_f.

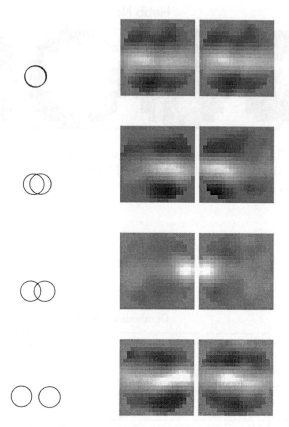

Figure 5.24: Receptive fields for partially overlapping inputs using the PCA rule. Receptive field for an overlap value of $O = .6$ (top left). Receptive field for a small overlap, $O = .2$ (top right). Receptive field for no overlap , $O = -.2$ (bottom left). Receptive field for shift in the vertical direction between the visual inputs when $O = .5$ (bottom right). In all cases the cell is binocular and horizontal. The symmetry property evident in these receptive fields is analyzed in Shouval et. al. (1995).

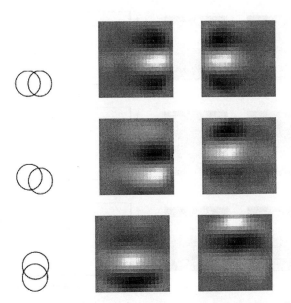

Figure 5.25: Shift in non-horizontal direction does not alter the horizontal preference, and binocularity of the PCA neuron receptive fields. The overlap value $O = 0.5$ in these simulations, and the shift angles from top down are $0, 36$, and 90 degrees.

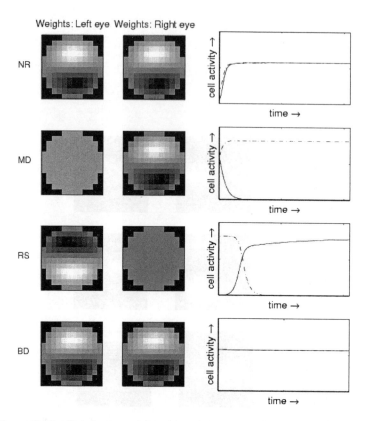

Figure 5.26: Simulation of deprivation experiments. Top row- normal rearing (NR), both eyes develop nearly identical receptive fields. Feed-forward
receptive fields are shown on two left hand side panels. On the right responses from both eyes as they develop in time. In this case the responses
are identical. Second row from top - Monocular Deprivation (MD). Responses from deprived eye monotonically decrease in time. The receptive
field of the deprived eye becomes weak and loses its structure. Third row -
Reverse Suture, the previously deprived eye receptive field reconnects and
responses form that eye increase. The responses from the deprived eye
decrease and the synaptic connections become weak. Bottom row - Binocular deprivation. Responses and synaptic weights stay constant despite
deprivation.

Appendix 5A

Representing the Correlation Matrix in a Bessel Function Base

Since the spectrum of the correlation function has the form, $Q(\mathbf{k}) = c/\mathbf{k}^2$ where c is a constant [Field, 1987], $Q(\mathbf{r})$ satisfies

$$\nabla^2 Q(\mathbf{r}) = -c\delta(\mathbf{r}), \qquad (5A.1)$$

This can be easily shown by taking Fourier transformation of both sides of this equation. In principle, a gauge $g(\mathbf{r})$ which satisfies $\nabla^2 g(\mathbf{r}) = 0$, can be added to $Q(\mathbf{r})$. But the only such gauge, which is radially symmetric, is a constant (denoted as b).

A representation for the radially symmetric form of the $\delta(r)$ function in terms of Bessel functions, is

$$\delta(\mathbf{r}) = \frac{1}{2\pi a^2} \sum_i \frac{J_0(k_1^0 r/a)}{N_0(k_i^0)}$$

where J_l is the lth order Bessel function, k_i^0 is the ith zero of J_0, r and θ are the polar coordinates of $\mathbf{r}$, and $N_0(k_j^0) = \int_0^1 rdr[J_0(k_j^0 r)]^2$ is the normalization constant of $J_0(k_j^0 r)$. Therefore it can be seen that

$$Q(\mathbf{r}) = -c\left[\frac{1}{2\pi} \sum_i \frac{J_0(k_i^0 r/a)}{(k_i^0)^2 N_0(k_i^0)} + b\right],$$

since it solves Equation 5A.1. Using an addition theorem for Bessel functions, we obtain a representation for the correlation function $Q(\mathbf{r} - \mathbf{r}')$

$$Q(\mathbf{r} - \mathbf{r}') = c\left[\sum_{jl} \frac{J_l^*(k_j^0 r/a)J_l(k_j^0 r'/a)}{2\pi(k_j^0)^2 \; N_0(k_j^0)} e^{il(\theta-\theta')} + b\right]. \qquad (5A.2)$$

We shall rewrite this correlation function in terms of the normalized Bessel-Fourier basis W_{mi}. These functions are zero on the boundary and take the form [Jackson, 1975]

$$W_m(k\mathbf{r}/a) = \begin{cases} \frac{J_m(kr/a)}{a\sqrt{2\pi N_m(k)}}e^{im\theta} & \text{for } r \leq a \\ 0 & \text{for } r > a \end{cases}$$

In which $N_m(k)$ is the normalization constant, and is equal to

$$N_m(k) = \frac{1}{2}[J_{m+1}(k)]^2.$$

From now on, for simplicity, we will set $a = 1$.

These W functions are solutions of the differential equation,

$$\nabla^2 W_m = -k^2 W_m. \tag{5A.3}$$

These functions are set to be zero on a circular boundary of radius 1: thus the solutions for k are quantized; they take discrete values k_i^m where i denotes the ith zero of the function.

We can rewrite $J_l(k_n^0 r)e^{il\theta} = \sum_j \varepsilon_{lnj} W_l(k_j^l \mathbf{r})$, where the value of the coefficients are

$$\varepsilon_{lnj} = \int J_l(k_n^0 r)e^{il\theta} W_l(k_j^l \mathbf{r})d^2r$$

$$= \begin{cases} \sqrt{2\pi N_0(k_i^0)}\delta_{jn} & \text{for } l = 0 \\ \sqrt{\frac{2\pi}{N_l(k_j^l)}}\left(\frac{k_j^l}{(k_n^0)^2-(k_j^l)^2}\right) J_l(k_n^0)J_{l+1}(k_j^l) & \text{for } l > 0 \end{cases}$$

We can now obtain a representation of the correlation function in terms of the Bessel-Fourier set,

$$Q(\mathbf{r} - \mathbf{r}') = c\left[\sum_{ljj'}[Q(l)]_{jj'} W_l(k_j^l \mathbf{r})W_l^*(k_{j'}^l \mathbf{r}') + b\right],$$

where

$$[Q(l)]_{jj'} = \sum_i \frac{\varepsilon_{lij}\varepsilon_{lij'}}{2\pi N_0(k_i^0)\,(k_i^0)^2}.$$

This representation of $Q(\mathbf{r} - \mathbf{r}')$ is unique only up to a constant b; this adds the term $\delta_{l0}V_jV_{j'}$ to the representation of the correlation matrix, where $V_j = \int W_0(k_j^0 \mathbf{r})d^2r = 2\sqrt{\pi}/k_j^0$.

Putting this form of the correlation function into the eigen-Equation 5.6; representing the eigenfunctions as a sum of this complete set, or, $\psi(\mathbf{r}) =$

$\sum_{mn} A_{mn} W_m(k_n^m \mathbf{r})$, and using the orthogonality relations, we obtain the matrix equation,

$$\sum_j [Q(l)]_{ij} A_{lj} = \lambda A_{li}.$$

In this appendix we have set the boundary $a = 1$. In order to take the parameter a into account, the simple transformation $\mathbf{r} \to \mathbf{r}/a$ must be performed on the representation of the correlation function. It is important to note that the value of the constant b is dependent on the value of a.

Including a non-zero b results in

$$[Q(l)]_{jj'} = \sum_i \frac{\varepsilon_{lij} \varepsilon_{lij'}}{2\pi N_0(k_i^0) \, (k_i^0)^2} + b\delta_{l0} V_j V_{j'} \tag{5A.4}$$

where

$$\varepsilon_{lnj} = \int J_l(k_n^0 r) e^{il\theta} W_l(k_j^l \mathbf{r}) d^2 r$$

$$= \begin{cases} \sqrt{2\pi N_0(k_i^0)} \delta_{jn} & \text{for } l = 0 \\ \sqrt{\frac{2\pi}{N_l(k_j^l)}} \left(\frac{k_j^l}{(k_n^0)^2 - (k_j^l)^2} \right) J_l(k_n^0) J_{l+1}(k_j^l) & \text{for } l > 0 \end{cases}$$

and

$$V_j = \frac{2\sqrt{\pi}}{k_j^0}.$$

and N_m is the normalization constant, which takes the value $N_m(k) = (\frac{1}{2})[J_{m+1}(k)]^2$.

5A.1 The correlation function for the pre-processed images.

The correlation function

$$Q^p(\mathbf{r} - \mathbf{r}') = \int d^2x \int d^2y K(\mathbf{r} - x) Q(x - y) K(y - \mathbf{r}')$$

Using the addition formula for Bessel functions we get

$$K(\mathbf{r} - \mathbf{r}') = \frac{1}{g^2} \sum_i \alpha_i J_0(k_i^0(\mathbf{r} - \mathbf{r}')) = \frac{1}{g^2} \sum_i \alpha_i \sum_n J_n(k_i^0 \mathbf{r}) J_n(k_i^0 \mathbf{r}') e^{in(\theta - \theta')}$$

Thus

$$\int W_l(k_j^l \mathbf{r}') K(\mathbf{r} - \mathbf{r}') d^2 r = \frac{1}{g^2} \sum_i \alpha_i \varepsilon_{lij} J_l(k_i^0 r) = \frac{1}{g^2} \sum_{in} \alpha_i \varepsilon_{lij} \varepsilon_{lin} W_l(k_n^l \mathbf{r})$$

and therefore

$$Q^p(\mathbf{r} - \mathbf{r}') = \sum_{lmn} [Q^p(l)]_{mn} W_l(k_m^l \mathbf{r}) W_l(k_n^l \mathbf{r}')$$

where

$$[Q^p(l)]_{nm} = \frac{1}{g^4} \sum_{jj'ip} [Q(l)]_{jj'} \alpha_i \alpha_p \varepsilon_{lij} \varepsilon_{lpj'} \varepsilon_{lin} \varepsilon_{lpm}. \tag{5A.5}$$

Appendix 5B

Properties of Correlation Functions
And
How to Make Good Ones

A correlation function is by definition positive semi-definite. This implies that every projection of the correlation function is positive. Mathematically any vector $\mathbf{v}$ with the same dimensionality as the correlation function Q has the property that

$$\mathbf{v}^{\mathrm{T}} Q \mathbf{v} > 0$$

Therefore all eigenvectors have positive eigenvalues. It follows that not every function is a correlation function and some of the functions used by different researchers are indeed not correlation functions. In some of these cases, for instance in the papers by Linsker, this comes about since he creates a pseudo-correlation function $Q' = Q - k_2 J$ which may have some negative projections.

As part of our software package, we can create environments from a specified correlation function. These environments have Gaussian statistics with a pre-specified covariance matrix. However this can be done only if the specified function is positive definite. Since simulations of second order learning rules are affected only by several eigenvectors – those with the highest eigenvalues – this problem can be overcome by creating instead an equivalent positive definite correlation function.

How is this done? Assuming a matrix Q is specified, that is symmetric and real. Such a matrix can be diagonalized by a rotation matrix R such that

$$R^{\mathrm{T}} Q R = \Lambda,$$

where Λ is a diagonal matrix composed of the eigenvalues of Q:

$$\Lambda = \begin{pmatrix} \lambda_1 & 0 & \dots & 0 \\ 0 & \lambda_2 & \dots & 0 \\ \vdots & \vdots & & \vdots \\ 0 & 0 & \dots & \lambda_n \end{pmatrix}.$$

We assume that eigenvalues are arranged in descending order, $\lambda_1 > \lambda_2 > ... > \lambda_n$. The rotation matrix R is composed of the eigenvectors of Q, hence $R = (\mathbf{u}_1, \mathbf{u}_2, ..., \mathbf{u}_n)$ where $\mathbf{u}_i$ is the eigenvector of Q with eigenvalue λ_i.

Given a set of eigenvalues and their corresponding eigenvectors the matrix Q can be reconstructed by $Q = R\Lambda R^{\mathrm{T}}$.

Let us now assume now that for all $i < k$, $\lambda_i \geq 0$ and for $j \geq k$, $\lambda_j < 0$. We replace this set of eigenvectors by a new set in which all the negative eigenvalues are replaced by small positive eigenvalues. We choose the new set of eigenvalues λ_j^* such that for every $j > k$ such $0 < \lambda_j^* < \lambda_k$. This set of eigenvalues is used to create a new eigenvalue matrix Λ^*.

We now replace the original matrix Q by the true correlation matrix Q^* that is created by

$$Q^* = R\Lambda^* R^{\mathrm{T}}. \tag{5B.1}$$

This new matrix Q^* is now positive definite and can be used to create an environment. It will produce results nearly identical to those produced by training directly with Q since all the principal components with large positive eigenvalues have not been altered.

Equation 5B.1 can also be used to create an environment with principal components to our liking. If we choose the basis vectors $\mathbf{u}_i$ we can give the one we want to dominate, say $\mathbf{u}_k$ the largest eigenvalue such that $\lambda_k \gg \lambda_{i \neq k}$. In order to insure a radially symmetric environment, the basis chosen must have a separable form $\mathbf{u}_i(r) = f(r) \cos(l\theta + \phi)$ and the eigenvalues for $\mathbf{u}_i(r) = f(r) \cos(l\theta)$ and $\mathbf{u}_j(r) = f(r) \cos(l\theta + \pi/2)$ must be the same.

Appendix 5C

The Parity Transform: Symmetry Properties of the Eigenstates of the Two Eye Problem

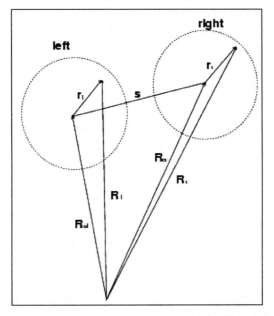

Figure 5C.1: Coordinates for the two eyes. For a shift $\mathbf{s}$ between the two eyes, $R_{0l} + \mathbf{s} = R_{0r}$. Therefore $R_r - R_l = R_{0r} - R_{0l} + \mathbf{r}_r - \mathbf{r}_l = \mathbf{s} + \mathbf{r}_r - \mathbf{r}_l$

The evolution of neurons in a binocular environment under the PCA learning rule, according to Equation 5.5 reaches a fixed point when

$$\mathbf{Q}^2 \mathbf{m} = \lambda \mathbf{m}. \tag{5C.1}$$

where $\mathbf{m}^T = (\mathbf{m}^l, \mathbf{m}^r)$, the left and right eye synaptic strengths; the two-eye correlation function $\mathbf{Q}^2$ has the form:

$$\mathbf{Q}^2 = \begin{pmatrix} Q_{ll} & Q_{lr} \\ Q_{rl} & Q_{rr} \end{pmatrix} \tag{5C.2}$$

where Q_{ll} and Q_{rr} are the correlation functions within the left and right eyes respectively, and Q_{lr} and Q_{rl} are the correlation functions between the left-right and right-left eyes. We denote by upper case $R's$ the coordinates in each receptive field with respect to a common origin, and by lower case $r's$ the coordinates from the centers of each of the receptive fields (Figure 5C.1). Thus R_{0l} and R_{0r} are the coordinates of the centers of the left and right eyes, R_l and R_r are the coordinates of points in both receptive fields, and $\mathbf{r}_l$ and $\mathbf{r}_r$ are the coordinates of the same points with respect to the centers of the left and right receptive field centers. For a misalignment $\mathbf{s}$ between receptive field centers, $R_{0l}+\mathbf{s} = R_{0r}$, therefore $R_r - R_l = R_{0r} - R_{0l} + \mathbf{r}_r - \mathbf{r}_l = \mathbf{s} + \mathbf{r}_r - \mathbf{r}_l$ (see Figure 5C.1).

Using translational invariance, it is easy to see that

$$Q_{ll} = E\left(d(\mathbf{r}_l)d(\mathbf{r}'_l)\right) = Q(\mathbf{r} - \mathbf{r}')$$
$$Q_{rr} = E\left(d(\mathbf{r}_r)d(\mathbf{r}'_r)\right) = E\left(d(\mathbf{r}_l + \mathbf{s})d(\mathbf{r}'_l + \mathbf{s})\right) = Q(\mathbf{r} - \mathbf{r}')$$
$$Q_{lr} = E\left(d(\mathbf{r}_l)d(\mathbf{r}'_r)\right) = E\left(d(\mathbf{r}_l)d(\mathbf{r}'_l + \mathbf{s})\right) = Q(\mathbf{r} - \mathbf{r}' + \mathbf{s})$$
$$Q_{rl} = E\left(d(\mathbf{r}_r)d(\mathbf{r}'_l)\right) = E\left(d(\mathbf{r}_l + \mathbf{s})d(\mathbf{r}'_l)\right) = Q(\mathbf{r} - \mathbf{r}' - \mathbf{s})$$

where E denotes an average with respect to the environment and where, occasionally, for simplicity, we replace $\mathbf{r}_l$ by $\mathbf{r}$. Since $Q(\mathbf{r}-\mathbf{r}') = E\left(d(\mathbf{r}_l)d(\mathbf{r}'_l)\right)$ then $Q(\mathbf{r} - \mathbf{r}') = Q(\mathbf{r}' - \mathbf{r})$.

We thus obtain a two-eye correlation function of the form

$$\mathbf{Q}^2 = \begin{pmatrix} Q(\mathbf{r} - \mathbf{r}') & Q(\mathbf{r} - \mathbf{r}' + \mathbf{s}) \\ Q(\mathbf{r} - \mathbf{r}' - \mathbf{s}) & Q(\mathbf{r} - \mathbf{r}') \end{pmatrix}. \tag{5C.3}$$

We now introduce a two-eye parity operator $\mathbf{P}$, which inverts the coordinates, as well as the two eyes:

$$\mathbf{P} : \begin{cases} \mathbf{r}_l \Rightarrow (-\mathbf{r}_l) \\ \mathbf{r}_r \Rightarrow (-\mathbf{r}_r) \\ \mathbf{s} \Rightarrow (-\mathbf{s}) \end{cases} \tag{5C.4}$$

It follows that under $\mathbf{P}$, $\quad R_l - R_r = \mathbf{r}_r - \mathbf{r}_l + \mathbf{s} \Rightarrow -\mathbf{r}_r + \mathbf{r}_l - \mathbf{s}$

The two-eye parity operator can also be written in matrix form in terms of the one eye parity operator P, thus

$$\mathbf{P} = \begin{pmatrix} 0 & P \\ P & 0 \end{pmatrix}. \tag{5C.5}$$

The effect $\mathbf{P}$ on the two-eye receptive fields $\mathbf{m}$ is

$$\mathbf{P} \begin{pmatrix} m^l(\mathbf{r}_l) \\ m^r(\mathbf{r}_r) \end{pmatrix} = \begin{pmatrix} m^r(-\mathbf{r}_l) \\ m^l(-\mathbf{r}_r) \end{pmatrix}$$

Any correlation function that is invariant to a two-eye parity transformation $\mathbf{P}$, has eigenfunctions $\mathbf{m}^T(\mathbf{r}) = (m^l(\mathbf{r}_r), m^r(\mathbf{r}_l))$, that are also eigenfunctions of $\mathbf{P}$. This imposes symmetry constraints on the resulting receptive fields that force them to be binocular.

Any correlation function * of the form

$$\mathbf{Q} = \begin{pmatrix} Q(\mathbf{r} - \mathbf{r}') & Q'(\mathbf{r} - \mathbf{r}' + \mathbf{s}) \\ Q'(\mathbf{r} - \mathbf{r}' - \mathbf{s}) & Q(\mathbf{r} - \mathbf{r}') \end{pmatrix} \tag{5C.6}$$

is invariant to the two-eye parity transform $\mathbf{P}$ (that is $\mathbf{PQP} = \mathbf{Q}$), as long as $Q(d) = Q(-d)$ and $Q'(d) = Q'(-d)$.

Thus the eigenfunctions of $\mathbf{Q}$, are also eigenfunction of $\mathbf{P}$. The eigenvalue is ± 1, Since $P^2 = 1$.

Therefore we deduce that

$$\begin{pmatrix} m^l(\mathbf{r}_l) \\ m^r(\mathbf{r}_r) \end{pmatrix} = \pm \begin{pmatrix} m^r(-\mathbf{r}_l) \\ m^l(-\mathbf{r}_r) \end{pmatrix}. \tag{5C.7}$$

Thus

$$\mathbf{m}(\mathbf{r}) = \begin{pmatrix} m^l(\ \mathbf{r}_l) \\ \pm m^l(-\mathbf{r}_r) \end{pmatrix}. \tag{5C.8}$$

This means that the receptive fields for the two eyes are inverted versions of each other up to a sign. Therefore for this learning rule the receptive fields are always perfectly binocular.

---

*This class includes the type of correlation function described in equation 5C.2, as well as the type postulated by Miller [Miller et al., 1989], in which $s = 0$ and $Q' = \eta Q$. There monocularity is attained by choosing $\eta < 0$ and restricting weights to be positive.

Chapter 6

Receptive Field Selectivity in a Natural Image Environment

Selectivity is a feature displayed by many cortical cells. In visual cortex (V1) this manifests itself most strikingly as selectivity to preferred orientations. There is substantial evidence that the normal development of this orientation selectivity requires rearing in a patterned visual environment[Wiesel and Hubel, 1965; Blakemore, 1976]. In previous chapters we used mostly low dimensional input environments in our explorations. In this chapter we employ more realistic visual environments in order to investigate how and why such selectivity develops, comparing BCM and several related statistically derived learning algorithms.

In what follows we present simulations of single cells in realistic environments composed of natural scene images to explore the normal development of orientation and direction selectivity. In subsequent chapters we introduce environments to represent the input activity to the cortex in deprived scenarios, such as monocular and binocular deprivation.

6.1 Modeling Orientation Selectivity

In this section we investigate a simple single cell model for developing monocular, orientation selective cells. Inputs $\mathbf{d}$ are chosen from pre-processed natural images. The output of the cell c, is a sigmoid of the weighted sum of inputs $c = \sigma(\sum_i m_i d_i)$. By convention the output activity c is measured with respect to the level of spontaneous activity, such that $c < 0$ represents firing below spontaneous. Typically we choose a non-symmetric sigmoidal, this asymmetry is a reasonable assumption for cortical neurons with a low level of spontaneous activity, which can have an output rate high above spontaneous but can not have negative firing rates, as we see below it is also a necessary assumption. The learning rule used is the quadratic BCM rule, described in previous sections.

6.1.1   *The input environment*

We employ a simple model of the visual pathway. Figure 6.1 shows the architecture of our model and Figure 6.2 shows the environment used for our simulations. Patches are taken from 12 images of natural scenes and presented to the retinal cells in a random order. The results do not change significantly with a larger number of images. A smaller set of images could be used, but the environment would not be as rich, and the number of orientations found by the neurons could potentially be smaller*.

These cells have an ON-center, OFF-surround response, modeled here as a difference of Gaussians (DOG) filter. A difference of Gaussians is given by

$$DOG(r) \equiv \frac{1}{2\pi\sigma_c^2}e^{-r^2/2\sigma_c^2} - \frac{1}{2\pi\sigma_s^2}e^{-r^2/2\sigma_s^2} \qquad (6.1)$$

where σ_c^2 and σ_r^2 are the variances of the center and surround Gaussians, respectively. This filter is commonly used to model the processing done in the retina [Law and Cooper, 1994]. The LGN in this model serves only to relay the signals from the retina to the cortex, so the inputs to the cortex are the retinally processed patches taken from the images. Typically we use $\sigma_c = 1$ ans $\sigma_s = 3$; however these can vary. At each simulation step a small circular patch is chosen randomly from one of the pre-processed images. This patch serves as the input vector **d** to the BCM neuron.

6.1.2   *Sufficient conditions for obtaining orientation selectivity*

With the above assumptions selective receptive fields develop. These can be visualized by making a gray-scale image of the weights, m_i. If white denotes strong responses and black denotes weak responses, then the pattern of this image shows the response of the cell to a spot of light at that position. Negative weights imply that light falling on that location in the retina produces a response from the output neuron that is *below spontaneous activity*. Sample receptive fields from training with the BCM rule in this natural scene environment, are shown in Figure 6.3. These oriented receptive fields are compatible with those observed by Hubel and Wiesel. Note that in the simulations, we have allowed the synaptic weights to change polarity during learning, so the final weights include both positive and negative values. The weights can be interpreted as *effective* synapses in a mean-field approximation of a network of BCM neurons (Chapter 4), rather than single-cell

---

*In some cases we introduce rotated versions of the same images to make the environment rotationally symmetric. Most of the results do not depend on this, but some of the network simulations (explored in Chapter 8) are sensitive to it.

synapses, or a combination of ON and OFF cells. In the lower panel of Figure 6.3 we represent the receptive fields as polar tuning plots, in which the magnitude represents the firing rate in response to a grating with the given orientation and direction of movement. In these simplified simulations the response to both directions of movement is always equal and independent of the speed of movement. The technical details for the test stimuli are given in Appendix 6A.1.

A necessary condition for such receptive fields to develop is the use of a non-symmetric sigmoidal output function, as shown in Figure 6.1. If a linear or symmetric sigmoidal is used then orientation selective receptive fields do not develop. This is because the odd moments of these natural images are essentially zero, due to symmetry in the natural images. Since BCM depends on the third moment (Equation 3.2), if a linear neuron is used it would not develop selective RF's. The non-symmetric neuron breaks the symmetry in the images, resulting in oriented RF's. Below we show that plasticity rules that depend on even moments do not require the non-symmetric output function.

The RF's we have shown were produced using retinally pre-processed images, as described above. However oriented receptive fields develop for many different forms of retinal pre-processing and can even develop from raw natural images. To achieve orientation selectivity using BCM, the specifics of the retinal preprocessing are not crucial.

6.1.3 *Dependence on RF size and localization*

The properties of the receptive fields can be affected by many factors other than the learning rule, such as the receptive field size and the parameters of the pre-processing DOG filter (see Equation 6.1). The receptive field's maximal size is determined by the size of the input patches, however the developed receptive fields might localize to a smaller region and its properties might not depend strongly on the size of patches chosen.

In Figure 6.4 we show the effect of the input patch size on the RF structure. The subfield bands of the receptive field tend to extend the full length of the receptive field for small RF's, but become more localized for larger RF's. The width of the subfields seems to be independent of the patch size.

6.1.4 *Spatial frequency of receptive fields*

Since the statistical properties of the inputs are affected by the retinal-like pre-processing, it is likely that receptive field properties would also be affected by properties of the filtering. To see the effect of the size of the filter on the RF's, we trained a neurons using images filtered with difference of Gaussians of various sizes. Examples of such retinal filters and resulting pre-processed images are shown in Figure 6.5. With a smaller DOG filter, the retinal cells respond to higher spatial frequencies in the images. The details are described in Appendix 6A.2.

All the trained neurons achieved oriented receptive fields. Sample RF's from small- and large-DOG cells are shown in Figure 6.6. These, and the other RF's found, differed primarily in *spatial frequency*. Figure 6.7 shows the dependence of the resulting spatial frequency on the center and surround sizes of the retinal DOG. Those retinal cells which have a *smaller* receptive fields yield cortical cells with *higher* spatial frequency. In the visual system there are various types retinal cells with different receptive field sizes and properties. Two such types characterized in cat are called X and Y cells [Linsenmeier et al., 1982]. X cells have smaller receptive fields, and respond slowly to moving stimuli. Y cells have larger receptive fields, and respond rapidly to moving stimuli.

In order to quantify this we can estimate the dominant spatial frequency of the different receptive fields. The method we use is described in Appendix 6A.2. In Figure 6.7 we show how the properties of retinal filters determine the spatial frequency of the cortical cells. We have marked two specific retinal filters that correspond to average X and Y cells. As expected pre-processing by X cells produces RF's with significantly higher spatial frequencies than pre-processing with Y cells. The existence of retinal cells with different properties could be a simple strategy for ensuring representation of images at different scales.

6.2 Orientation Selectivity with Statistically Defined Learning Rules

The quadratic form of BCM, used in the previous section to obtain orientation selectivity in only one of many possible plasticity rules. In Chapter 5 we have extensively surveyed second order learning rules and under what conditions they can produce orientation selective cells. We find that even when they do produce orientation selective cells, their properties are not very realistic. In Section 3.5 we derived a family of statistically motivated plasticity rules. These rules, like quadratic BCM, depend on higher moments of the input environment. The rules we have extracted are referred to as S_1, S_2 which maximize the multiplicative and subtractive forms of skewness, respectively, and K_1, K_2 that maximize the multiplicative and subtractive forms of Kurtosis. In this section we compare orientation selectivity produced by these different plasticity rules. We have performed a detailed study of the receptive fields for the different projection indices described above, in the natural scene environment.

The resulting receptive fields formed are shown in Figures 6.8 and 6.9 for both the DOGed and whitened images, respectively (recall from Chapter 5 that whitening is a linear transformation that will result in a flat power spectrum). To some extent, every learning rule developed oriented receptive fields, although some were more sensitive to the pre-processing than others. This behavior, as well as the resemblance of the receptive fields to those obtained from PCA [Shouval and Liu, 1996], suggest that the corresponding measures have a strong dependence on the second moment. The multiplicative versions of kurtosis and skew, as well as Quadratic BCM, show selectivity to many orientations regardless of the pre-processing suggesting that they did not have as strong a dependence on second order statistics. The multiplicative skewness rule gives receptive fields with lower spatial frequencies than either Quadratic BCM or the multiplicative kurtosis rule. This also disappears with the whitened inputs, which implies that the spatial frequency of the receptive field is related to the strength of the dependence of the learning rule on the second moment. Sample receptive fields using Oja's fixed-point ICA algorithm[Hyvarinen and Oja, 1997] are also shown in Figure 6.9, and look qualitatively similar to those found using the stochastic maximization of subtractive kurtosis.

Quadratic BCM and the multiplicative version of kurtosis are less sensitive to the second moments of the distribution and produce oriented receptive fields even when the data is not whitened. This is clear from the results from DOG-processed vs. whitened inputs. The reduced sensitivity follows from the built in second order normalization that these rules have, kurtosis via division and BCM via subtraction. The subtractive version of kurtosis is strongly sensitive to the second moment and produces oriented RF only after sphering the data [Friedman, 1987; Field, 1994]. The quadratic BCM learning rule, that has been proposed as a projection index for finding multi-modality in high dimensional distribution, can find projections emphasizing high kurtosis when no clusters are present in the data.

The rectified skewness rule can also find oriented RF's; these however seem to be dominated by lower spatial frequencies than QBCM or Kurtosis rules. The single cell ICA rule we considered, used the subtractive form of kurtosis as a measure for deviation from Gaussian distributions, achieved receptive fields qualitatively similar to other rules discussed.

It is important to note that for learning rules with odd moments, the non-symmetric sigmoid is necessary to obtain oriented receptive fields since the nearly symmetric input distributions, cause odd moments to vanish. This sigmoid is not needed for rules dependent only on the even powered moments, such as kurtosis. Figure 6.10 demonstrates both that the removal of the sigmoid and the removal of the mean from the moments calculations does not substantially affect the resulting receptive fields of the kurtosis rules. Note that the choice of 13 by 13 receptive fields was made only for computational efficiency. Figure 6.11 shows some 21 by 21 receptive fields and it is clear that little difference is made.

All the learning rules we have used found projections with kurtotic output distributions (depicted on the right of Figures 6.8 and 6.9). This should not come as a surprise as there are suggestions that a large family of linear filters can find kurtotic distributions in a natural image environment [Ruderman, 1994].

6.3   What Drives Orientation Selectivity

Learning rules that are dependent on large polynomial moments, such as Quadratic BCM and kurtosis, tend to be sensitive to the tails of the distribution. This property implies that neurons are highly responsive, and sensitive, to the outliers of the input distribution.

We now investigate what fraction of the input patches are responsible for the formation of these selective receptive fields. The procedure we have chosen is to first train our neurons with the complete data set. Once the RF's converge we delete from the data-set those patterns from the environment for which the neuron responds strongly. The number of deleted input patterns needed to be removed in order to cause a change in the receptive field gives a direct measure of what fraction of the input is responsible for the stability of each receptive field. The process of training a neuron, deleting patterns that yield high responses, and retraining can be done recursively to sequentially remove the structure from the input environment, and to pick out the most salient features in the environment. The results of this are shown in Figure 6.12.

Both Quadratic BCM and kurtosis are sensitive to the tails of the output distribution. This sensitivity is so high that the RF changes due to elimination of the upper 1% portion of the distribution (Figure 6.12). The change in RF is gradual; at first, removal of some of the inputs results in RF's that have the same orientation but a different phase, once more patterns from the upper portion of the distribution are removed, different RF orientations are found. This finding gives some indication of the kind of inputs the cell is most selective to (values below its highest 99% selectivity); these are inputs with the same orientation but with different phase (different locality of RF). The sensitivity to small portions of the distribution represents the other side of the coin of sparse coding. It should be further studied as it may reflect some fundamental instability of kurtotic approaches.

When the small, but important, part of the input distribution is deleted (namely, the tails of the distribution), the neuron seeks a different RF. This occurs in both the BCM and kurtosis learning rules, and most likely occurs in other rules that seek kurtotic projections. It is important to note, however, that patterns must be deleted from *both* sides of the distribution for any rule that does not use the rectifying sigmoid because the strong *negative* responses carry as much structure as the strong positive ones. Such responses are not biologically plausible, so they wouldn't be part of the encoding process in real neurons.

It is also interesting to observe that the RF found after structure removal is initially of the same orientation, but of different spatial phase. Once enough input patterns are removed, the RF becomes oriented in a different direction. If the process is continued, all of the orientations and phases would be obtained.

These results are related to the issue of sparse coding [Olshausen and Field, 1996b]. We see that only a small fraction of the inputs drives the formation of the highly selective receptive fields, especially in the case of QBCM and Kurtosis. This probably arises because of the polynomial moments in these learning rules. A different approach[Olshausen and Field, 1996b] has shown that if a sparse code is enforced on the network, through internal network dynamics, then a plasticity rule dependent in this sparse output activity would develop orientation selective receptive fields, that are qualitatively similar to ours.

6.4 ON/OFF inputs

The receptive field of the cortical cell shows adjacent excitatory and inhibitory subfields. There is evidence that these subfields are projections from ON-center and OFF-center LGN cells, respectively [Reid and Alonso, 1995]. In the previous sections we assumed only ON-center cells. In this section we expand our results to include both ON- and OFF-center cell inputs. The input consists of two channels, one representing ON center cells and the other OFF center cells, each receiving identical input. The two channels (ON and OFF) do not interact at the level of the LGN but converge in the cortex. We represent the total input to the BCM neuron by $\mathbf{d} = [\mathbf{d}^{ON}, \mathbf{d}^{OFF}]$, the synaptic weights by $\mathbf{m} = [\mathbf{m}^{ON}, \mathbf{m}^{OFF}]$. The response of the cortical cell is given by $c = \sigma_c(\mathbf{m} \cdot \mathbf{d})$ where $\sigma_c(\cdot)$ is a rectifying sigmoid, which sets the minimum and maximum values of the postsynaptic response.

The vectors $\mathbf{d}^{ON}$ and $\mathbf{d}^{OFF}$ are related according to

$$\begin{cases} d_i{}^{ON} = \sigma(D_i) + K + N_i^{ON} \\ d_i{}^{OFF} = \sigma(-D_i) + K + N_i^{OFF} \end{cases} \tag{6.2}$$

where the values D_i define the input pattern after retinal processing with an *excitatory*-center DOG filter, and the offset K is related to the level of LGN spontaneous activity. Thus here we are deviating from our convention of measuring activity with respect to the level of spontaneous activity. We find that the results do not depend strongly on K, so the level chosen for spontaneous activity is unimportant. The variable N_i^{ON} and N_i^{OFF} represent independent (Gaussian) noise added to each channel independently. This additive noise becomes critical only in the non-symmetric LGN case, explored below.

We define the LGN activation function σ as:

$$\sigma(D_i) = \begin{cases} D_i & \text{if } D_i \geq D_{\min} \\ D_{\min} & \text{if } D_i < D_{\min} , \end{cases} \qquad (6.3)$$

where the lower cut-off $D_{\min}$ is negative.

The variables $\mathbf{d}$, $\mathbf{m}$, and c obey the standard BCM equations;

$$c = \sigma_{\text{cortical}} \left(\mathbf{m}^{ON} \cdot \mathbf{d}^{ON} + \mathbf{m}^{OFF} \cdot \mathbf{d}^{OFF} \right)$$
$$\begin{cases} \dot{m}_i^{ON} = \mu \phi(c, \theta_M) d_i^{ON} \\ \dot{m}_i^{OFF} = \mu \phi(c, \theta_M) d_i^{OFF} , \end{cases} \qquad (6.4)$$

where we have used $\phi = c(c - \theta_M)/\theta_M$ [Law and Cooper, 1994].

Now we explore the segregation of the ON and OFF channels into different subfields of the simple cell receptive field. Specifically, we look at two cases of the Equation 6.3; this allows us to determine the relation between some of the basic statistics of the LGN activity and the segregation of the ON/OFF receptive fields. The two cases are

- **Symmetric LGN**

  In this case, we assume that LGN cells operate in the linear region, where $-|D_{\min}| < D_i < |D_{\min}|$, and that LGN activities are measured relative to spontaneous activities, where $K = 0$. Since the results do not strongly depend on the value of K, we present the simplest case. Thus Equation 6.2 reduces to:

$$\begin{cases} d_i^{ON} = D_i \\ d_i^{OFF} = -D_i , \end{cases} \qquad (6.5)$$

where D_i are the input values after retinal pre-processing with an ON-center DOG filter. Note that ON and OFF cells that see the same part of the retina display exactly opposite responses to light of *any* intensity, and that the input distribution is symmetric.

Simulation results for the two channel model, under the linear LGN assumption (activity in the symmetric region), is shown in Figure 6.13. The final configurations of the effective synapses $\mathbf{m}^{ON}$ and $\mathbf{m}^{OFF}$ display adjacent "excitatory" and "inhibitory" bands (cf. subregions of strong and weak synaptic weights).

We define two new variables the "sum" and "difference" configurations $\mathbf{m}^+$ and $\mathbf{m}^-$, such that:

$$
\begin{cases}
\mathbf{m}^+ = \frac{1}{\sqrt{2}}\left(\mathbf{m}^{\mathrm{ON}} + \mathbf{m}^{\mathrm{OFF}}\right) \\
\mathbf{m}^- = \frac{1}{\sqrt{2}}\left(\mathbf{m}^{\mathrm{ON}} - \mathbf{m}^{\mathrm{OFF}}\right) .
\end{cases}
\tag{6.6}
$$

These variables are displayed in Figure 6.14, for the same examples shown in Figure 6.13. The summed configuration $\mathbf{m}^+$ lacks any significant structure and has a zero mean. This means that $m_i^{\mathrm{ON}} \approx -m_i^{\mathrm{OFF}}$, i.e. the effective synapses from ON and OFF cells that see the same part of the retina are of opposite type ("excitatory" versus "inhibitory").

We would like to point out that *restricting the weights to positive values* by, for example, imposing hard bounds on the weight values, has no noticeable effect on the receptive field arrangement. It is merely simpler to consider the case where the weights are allowed to be negative.

We make a variable substitution on the inputs in the BCM equation, defining the "sum" and "difference" input configurations $\mathbf{d}^+$ and $\mathbf{d}^-$, respectively, with the linearity constraint in Equation 6.5. It is straightforward to show that

$$
\mathbf{m}^-(t) \propto \mathbf{m}^{\mathrm{single}}(t)
\tag{6.7}
$$

$$
\mathbf{m}^+(t) = \mathbf{m}^+(t = 0)
\tag{6.8}
$$

where $\mathbf{m}^{\mathrm{single}}$ is the weight configuration for a single channel model. The relation predicts that (1) the final ON and OFF receptive fields display the same type of elongated subregions of strong and weak connections as in previous single-channel models, and (2) subregions of strong ON synapses overlap subregions of weak OFF synapses and vice versa. This is consistent with the simulation results in Figures 6.13 and 6.14.

- **Non-Symmetric LGN**
The linear assumption cannot be valid for light of any intensity, since the *absolute* LGN cell activity must be positive. For example, assume that the absolute spontaneous activity is, say, 14 Hz for all LGN cells (these numbers are not meant to be realistic, but only serve as an example). If an ON (OFF) cell fires with frequency 24 Hz, the OFF (ON) cell that sees the same part of the retina fires with frequency 4 Hz. However, light that leads to a response above 30 Hz of an ON (OFF) cell, will inhibit *all* activity of the corresponding OFF (ON) cell. LGN cells operate in the symmetric region when $D_{\min} < D_i < |D_{\min}|$, and in the non-symmetric region when $D_i > |D_{\min}|$ or $D_i < -|D_{\min}|$. With the LGN activation function σ is defined by Equation 6.3, the magnitude of the lower cutoff $D_{\min}$ can be interpreted as the difference between the spontaneous activity and the minimal activity of the LGN cells.

To investigate the effect of the non-symmetric region, we perform simulations with a cut-off at $D_{\min}$ for different values. Note that whereas the input distributions are almost symmetrical around spontaneous activity for linear cells, they are *asymmetrical* with this cut-off. The results of simulations, for several values of the cut-off, are shown in Figure 6.15.

One observes that the stronger asymmetry yields a change in the results, from *reversed* weight configurations $\mathbf{m}^{ON} \approx -\mathbf{m}^{OFF}$ (or $\mathbf{m}^+ \approx \mathbf{0}$) to *equal* weight configurations $\mathbf{m}^{ON} \approx \mathbf{m}^{OFF}$ (or $\mathbf{m}^- \approx \mathbf{0}$).

The results from the ON/OFF channel model imply that, if the BCM learning rule is valid, and we accept the experimental evidence for the segregation of ON/OFF receptive fields [Reid and Alonso, 1995], then the input distribution from LGN to cortex should be almost symmetrical. *There is a relation between the organization of simple cell receptive fields and the shape of the input distribution*; the mean of the input distribution, on the other hand, seems to be less important. If, however, the input distribution is very asymmetrical, we do not obtain the proper segregation of the ON/OFF receptive fields.

6.5   Direction Selectivity

Most simple and complex cells in the cat striate cortex are both orientation[Hubel and Wiesel, 1959; Hubel and Wiesel, 1962] and direction selective[Hammond, 1978; Reid et al., 1991; Deangelis et al., 1995]. At the preferred orientation, a cell which is direction selective responds to a drifting grating moving in one direction more strongly than the opposite direction. The ability of the cell to detect the direction of motion depends on the interaction of responses to at least two different points in the visual field at different times. This is to say, that it depends on the *spatio-temporal* receptive field of the cell[Reid et al., 1991].

A cell which is not direction selective (non-DS) has a maximum response to a sine grating moving in one direction equal to its maximum response to a sine grating moving in the opposite direction. In a linear approximation, the response of a cell, $c(t)$, can be written as a convolution between the spatio-temporal input pattern, $I(x,t)$, and a spatio-temporal receptive field kernel, $K(x,t)$, giving

$$c(t) = \int_{-\infty}^{+\infty} dx' \int_{-\infty}^{t} dt'\, I(x',t') K(x', t - t') \qquad (6.9)$$

It is easy to show that, in this approximation, a direction selective cell must have a spatio-temporally (ST) inseparable receptive field, that is, the kernel cannot be expressed as $K(x,t) = F(t)G(x)$, where $F(t)$ and $G(x)$ are functions which depend only on time and only on space, respectively.

There are many models of direction selectivity[Barlow and Levick, 1965; Burr, 1981; Adelson and Bergen, 1985; Watson and Ahumada, 1985]. In all of the models, the response of the cell is determined by receptive fields that have different temporal response properties at different spatial locations (i.e. spatiotemporal inseparable). This can be realized by the appropriate spatial positioning of the receptive fields, and the introduction of temporal shifts. These temporal shifts could possibly arise from delays caused by cortical loops[Suarez et al., 1995; Maex and Orban, 1996], phase advances caused by depressing synapses[Chance et al., 1998], or by lagged responses in the LGN[Mastronarde, 1987; Saul and Humphrey, 1990].

We introduce a feed-forward model of the development of direction selectivity which includes the effects of two types of LGN cells, called lagged and non-lagged cells, that differ only in their response timing. This is similar to a previous model[Feidler et al., 1997], but differs significantly in the input environment used. The previous model uses a neuron with three inputs each with sinusoidally varying activations governed by a single parameter. In our case, we use a natural scene environment, providing a more realistic correspondence with biology and a more direct connection to experiment. The primary difference between this model and the binocular model discussed earlier comes from the temporal relationship between the two channels.

There are two possible factors contributing to motion in the visual environment: movements of the eyes and head and movements of objects in the world. To model the former, input patches are chosen using a sequence of random *saccades* and *drifts*[Carpenter, 1977]. A saccade is a large jump to a random part of an image, and a drift is a continuous motion within an image in a particular direction at a particular velocity. In the model, the drift velocity is kept constant, and the drifts last a time interval that is random. In between drifts are saccades to a different image or part of the same image. Although this is a simplification of both the temporal properties of lagged and non-lagged cells, and of the true input structure available to an animal in a dynamic environment composed of moving objects in addition to eye and head movements, the added complexities make no noticeable difference in the results[Blais et al., 2000].

Sample receptive fields and their orientation tuning, for a velocity of 2 pixels per iteration, are shown in Figure 6.16. The orientation tuning was obtained using drifting oriented sine gratings. We observe that the lagged RF is a shifted version of the non-lagged RF, which yields a spatiotemporal *inseparable* receptive field.

6.5.1 *Strobe Rearing*

Some experiments use rearing in visual environments in which the ability to perceive motion is restricted. This disrupts the development of normal direction selectivity. Rearing kittens in an environment illuminated by a low frequency (1 Hz) strobe has severe effects, producing an almost complete loss of both direction and orientation selectivity [Cynader et al., 1973]. Rearing in a higher rate strobe light reduces the proportion of direction selective cells, leaving the spatial receptive field unaltered [Cynader and Chernenko, 1976; Humphrey and Saul, 1998]. It has been shown that this elimination of direction selectivity occurs because the strobe rearing prevents the convergence of inputs with different response timings onto the cortical cells.[Humphrey et al., 1998]

Cats reared in an environment with motion restricted to one direction showed a bias in direction selectivity [Cynader et al., 1975]. The cells in V1 were more responsive to stimulation in the biased direction than in normally reared cats. Rearing in a moving striped environment produces a bias in both direction and orientation selectivity [Tretter et al., 1975].

To examine the effects of strobe rearing, we modify the environment used to obtain direction selectivity earlier, in order to determine the development of direction selectivity in an environment with very high velocities; this has a similar effect of disrupting correlations between lagged and non-lagged inputs as strobe rearing. The flash from the strobe gives the retina a normal input pattern instantaneously and then dark for the rest of the time. Roughly speaking, because of the time lag in the lagged channel, the cortical cell experiences one of two input scenarios: 1) normal input on the non-lagged channel and noise on the lagged channel and 2) noise input on the non-lagged channel and normal input on the lagged channel. This temporally decorrelates the channels, and is comparable to the high-velocity case described below, where the two channels are not receiving the same input and are thus decorrelated.

We measure direction selectivity using the DS index, defined as

$$\text{DS} \equiv \frac{R_{(\text{preferred})} - R_{(\text{nonpreferred})}}{R_{(\text{preferred})} + R_{(\text{nonpreferred})}} \tag{6.10}$$

where $R_{(\text{preferred})}$ and $R_{(\text{nonpreferred})}$ are the responses to a sine grating, at optimum orientation and spatial frequency, moving in the *preferred* direction and *non preferred* direction, respectively. Figure 6.17 shows the direction selectivity index as a function of eye drift velocity, for a constant LGN lag of 1 iteration. Sample receptive fields from the BCM learning rule for each velocity are shown. Neurons following the BCM rule show some tuning to eye drift velocity: they develop direction selectivity for some velocities, but all lose it for either velocities which are too high or too low.

At very low velocities, the lagged and non-lagged RF's are identical (ST separable), and at very high velocities only the lagged or the non-lagged develops while the other RF is small and random (also ST separable). This is analogous to the strobe light environment [Cynader et al., 1973], at high velocity temporal correlations are lost, and at low velocity there is the strongest correlation between the channels at time zero.

Mathematically there is a parallel between these results and the results on binocular cortical misalignment[Shouval et al., 1996b], which will be treated in Chapter 7. In the misalignment work, we show that the BCM rule in a natural scene environment, with varying degrees of binocular overlap, develops either identical receptive fields (for complete overlap), *monocular* receptive fields (for no overlap), or receptive fields formed only in the overlap region (for intermediate overlap). In the current work, if the lag time of the LGN lagged cells is kept constant, then a constant velocity would imply a constant amount of overlap of input patterns during eye drift. Thus, zero velocity would yield identical lagged and the non-lagged RF's, yielding no direction selectivity. Likewise, high velocity would give no overlap of input patterns during eye drift, and would yield either a completely lagged or a completely non-lagged receptive field, and again no direction selectivity. The high velocity case is analogous to the strobe light environment[Cynader et al., 1973; Cynader and Chernenko, 1976; Humphrey and Saul, 1998], because in both situations the temporal correlations are lost. In the experiment, direction selectivity was lost but orientation selectivity remained; this is reproduced by the simulations for the high velocity case. In addition, there is evidence[Humphrey et al., 1998] that strobe rearing prevents the convergence of the lagged and non-lagged inputs onto the cortical cell, i.e. the cortical receptive field is affected by either lagged or non-lagged, but not both. This result is reproduced completely in the simulations.

6.6   Conclusions

We have presented simulations of BCM neurons in a natural image environment that develop orientation and direction selectivity, as well as the proper segregation of ON- and OFF-subfields. The BCM learning rule is robust to many changes in the environment, including most preprocessing. It is shown to develop orientation selectivity even in raw natural images. Changes in the preprocessing affects the spatial frequency of the receptive fields, and possibly the particular set of orientations found, but not the level of selectivity: the cell becomes responsive to a small set of patterns in the environment. Restricting the weights to positive values by, for example, imposing hard bounds on the weight values, has no noticeable effect on the receptive field arrangement.

There is a relation between the organization of simple cell receptive fields and the shape of the input distribution; the mean of the input distribution, on the other hand, seems to be less important. If, however, the input distribution is very asymmetrical, we do not obtain the proper segregation of the ON/OFF receptive fields. For direction selectivity to develop, there must be motion in the environment which cannot be either extremely slow or fast, and there must be some temporal difference between sets of LGN cells. All of these simulation results are consistent with the results in lower dimensional environments, explored in earlier chapters.

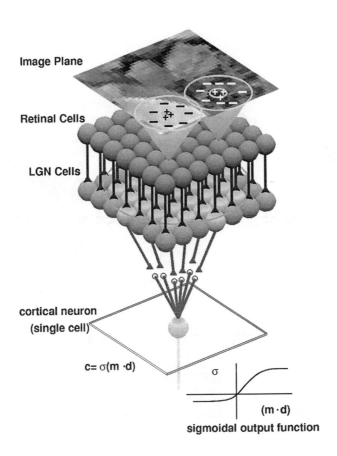

Image Plane

Retinal Cells

LGN Cells

cortical neuron
(single cell)

$c = \sigma(\mathbf{m} \cdot \mathbf{d})$

σ

$(\mathbf{m} \cdot \mathbf{d})$

sigmoidal output function

Figure 6.1: Model Architecture. Shown are the image plane (top), the (single eye) retinal cells, LGN cells, and the single cortical cell (bottom). Sample center-surround receptive fields are drawn in the image plane for the retinal cells highlighted. Nearby retinal cells see nearby points in the image plane. Retinal cells project directly to LGN cells, on a one-to-one basis. A circular patch of LGN cells projects to the single cortical cell. These projections form the input vector, $\mathbf{d}$, for which there is a corresponding weight vector, $\mathbf{m}$. The output of the cell is given as $c = \sigma(\mathbf{m} \cdot \mathbf{d})$, where σ is an asymmetric, sigmoidal function shown in the lower right.

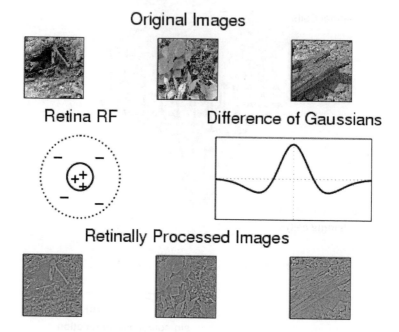

Figure 6.2: Input Environment. Shown are the original images (top) and the retinally processed images used as the actual inputs to the neuron (bottom). The images are processed with a difference of Gaussians (DOG) filter (center, right), which is used as a model of the receptive field properties of the retinal cells (center left).

Weights

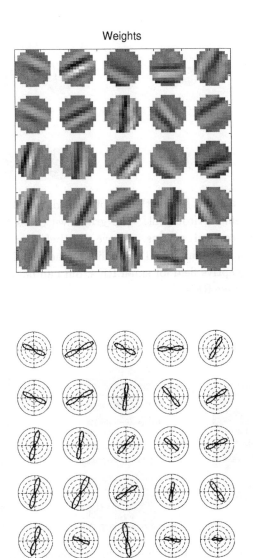

Figure 6.3: Sample Receptive Fields (above) and Polar Tuning Plots (below) from a BCM neuron trained in a natural scene environment. The gray level codes for the magnitude of the thalamo-cortical weights. The polar tuning plots (below) indicated response magnitude as a function of test stimulus angle.

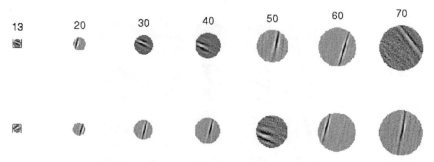

Figure 6.4: The effect of size on the receptive fields of a BCM neuron trained in a natural scene environment. The gray level codes for the magnitude of the thalamo-cortical weights. Above and below are two independent examples for each patch size. The subfield bands tend to extend the full length of the receptive field for small RF's, but can be somewhat localized, especially for larger RF's.

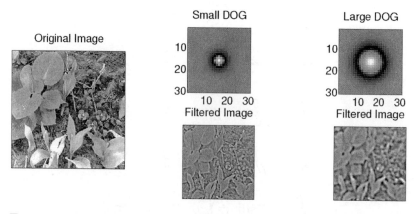

Figure 6.5: Filters and filtered images for retinal cells employing small and large DOG filters. Shown is the original image (left), and two different sized difference of Gaussian (DOG) filters (above center and right). The center and surround values used are $c = 0.83, s = 3.2$ for small-DOG cells and $c = 2.9, s = 4.3$ for large-DOG cells. Shown also are the images resulting from the application of these filters (below center and right). The small-DOG cells respond to much higher spatial frequencies in the images than the large-DOG cells.

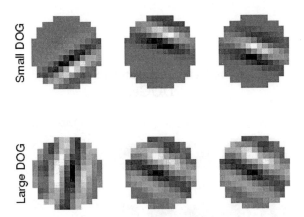

Figure 6.6: Sample receptive fields from neurons trained with images filtered with a small- (above) and a large-DOG (below).

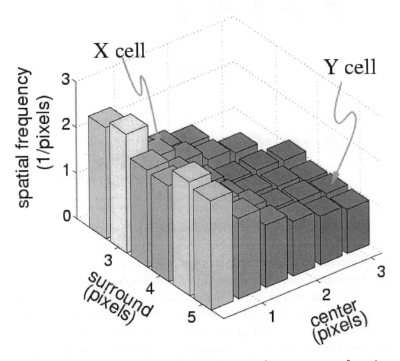

Figure 6.7: Spatial frequency of trained cortical neurons, as a function of the center and surround sizes of retinal receptive fields. The values measured for X and Y cells (Linsenmeier et. al. 1982) are labeled.

Receptive Fields from Natural Scene Input:
DOGed

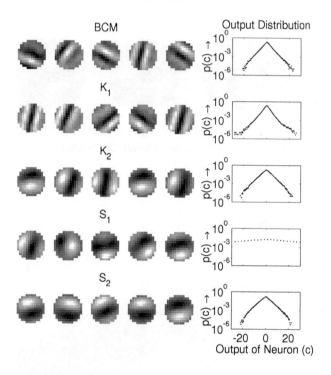

Figure 6.8: Receptive fields using DOGed image input, obtained from learning rules maximizing (from top to bottom) the Quadratic BCM objective function, Kurtosis(multiplicative), Kurtosis (additive), Skew (multiplicative), and Skewness (additive). Shown are five examples (left to right) from each learning rule as well as the normalized output distribution, before the application of the rectifying sigmoid. Plotted is the probability of a pattern in the environment, $p(c)$, yielding an output, c. Note that the plot is a log plot, and that the distributions are approximately double-exponential.

Receptive Fields from Natural Scene Input:
Whitened

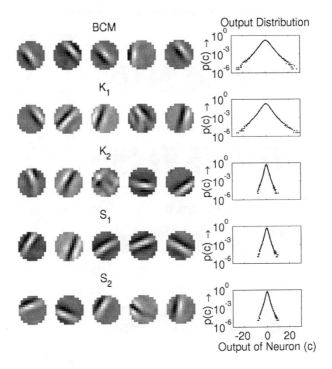

Figure 6.9: Receptive fields using whitened image input, obtained from learning rules maximizing (from top to bottom) the Quadratic BCM objective function, Kurtosis (multiplicative), Kurtosis (additive), Skew (multiplicative), Skewness (additive), and Oja's ICA rule based on the additive kurtosis measure. Shown are five examples (left to right) from each learning rule as well as the log of the normalized output distribution, before the application of the rectifying sigmoid. Plotted is the probability of a pattern in the environment, $p(c)$, yielding an output, c. Note that the plot is a log plot, and that the distributions are approximately double-exponential.

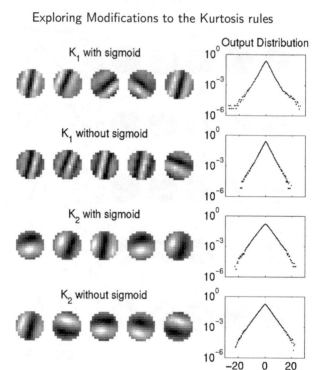

Figure 6.10: Receptive fields using DOGed image input, obtained from learning rules maximizing (from top to bottom) multiplicative form kurtosis with rectified outputs, non-rectified outputs, additive form kurtosis with rectified outputs, and non-rectified outputs respectively. Shown are five examples (left to right) from each learning rule and the corresponding output distribution.

Effects of Larger Receptive Fields

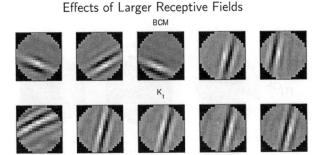

Figure 6.11: Large receptive fields using DOGed image input, obtained from the Quadratic BCM learning rule and the rule maximizing the multiplicative form of kurtosis.

Structure Removal for BCM, Kurtosis, and Skew

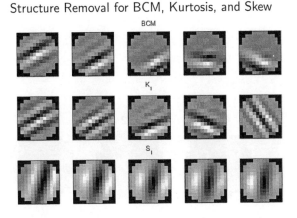

Figure 6.12: Receptive fields resulting from structure removal using the Quadratic BCM rule, the rule maximizing the multiplicative form of kurtosis and skewness. The RF on the far left for each rule was obtained in the normal input environment. The next RF to the right was obtained in a reduced input environment, whose patterns were deleted that yielded the strongest 1% of responses from the RF to the left. This process was continued for each RF from left to right, yielding a final removal of about five percent of the input patterns.

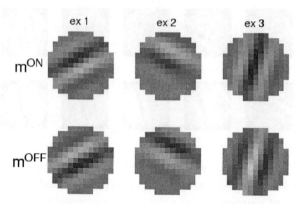

Figure 6.13: Weight configurations $\mathbf{m}^{ON}$ (*top row*) and $\mathbf{m}^{OFF}$ (*bottom row*) developed according to the ON/OFF channel model; each column represents an example. The brightness codes for the strengths of the synaptic weights.

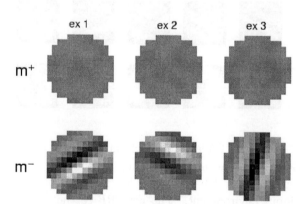

Figure 6.14: The "sum" and "difference" weight configurations $\mathbf{m}^{+}$ (*top row*) and $\mathbf{m}^{-}$ (*bottom row*) for the examples in Figure 6.13.

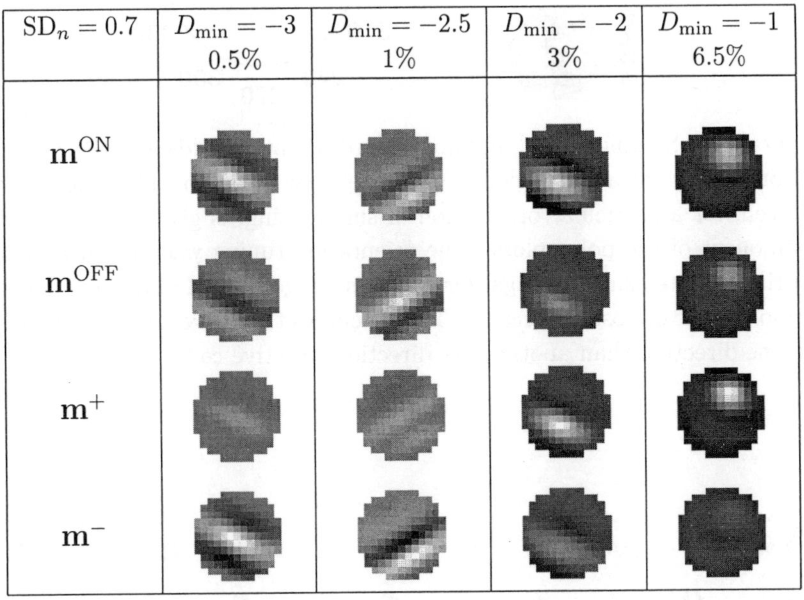

SD$_n$ = 0.7	$D_{\min} = -3$ 0.5%	$D_{\min} = -2.5$ 1%	$D_{\min} = -2$ 3%	$D_{\min} = -1$ 6.5%
$\mathbf{m}^{ON}$				
$\mathbf{m}^{OFF}$				
$\mathbf{m}^{+}$				
$\mathbf{m}^{-}$				

Figure 6.15: Simulations results for cutoff at different values of $D_{\min}$; the percentage shows the fraction of the inputs that are cut-off at $D_{\min}$. The figure shows that a stronger asymmetry in the inputs yields a change in the results, from *reversed* ON/OFF configurations $\mathbf{m}^{ON} \approx -\mathbf{m}^{OFF}$ or $\mathbf{m}^{+} \approx \mathbf{0}$ (see, for example, $D_{\min} = -3$) to *equal* ON/OFF configurations $\mathbf{m}^{ON} \approx \mathbf{m}^{OFF}$ or $\mathbf{m}^{-} \approx \mathbf{0}$ (see, for example, $D_{\min} = -1.5$). The noise level SD$_n$ = 0.7.

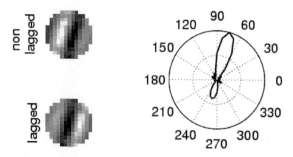

Figure 6.16: Sample lagged and non-lagged receptive fields and their orientation tuning, for a drift velocity of 2 pixels per iteration. The response of the cell, for a particular orientation of sine grating, is given by the radial component of the polar plots. The orientation tuning was obtained using drifting oriented sine gratings. Orientations larger than 180 degrees denote motion in the opposite direction. Tuning curves that have a larger response for one direction than another are direction selective cells.

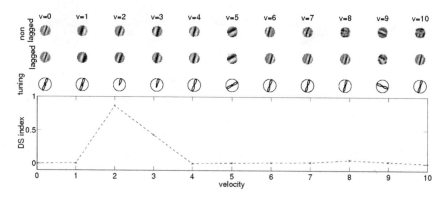

Figure 6.17: Sample receptive fields with polar tuning plots (above) for BCM, for several eye drift velocities. The direction selectivity index as a function of velocity (below). The neurons show some velocity tuning: they all lose direction selectivity for either velocities which are too high or too low. The LGN lagged cells had a constant 1 iteration lag.

Appendix 6A

Technical Remarks Concerning Simulations of Selectivity

6A.1 Testing Orientation and Direction

6A.1.1 *Orientation Selectivity*

To investigate cell responses, we test with sine gratings. We would like to optimize over spatial frequency, angle of orientation, and phase. We could use a Fast Fourier Transform (FFT) procedure to get the spatial frequency by simply looking at the peak in frequency space of the weight vector. Unfortunately, this is very sensitive to noise. What we do in practice is to use a spatial frequency, k, determined empirically, for all BCM simulations of $4.4\pi/(\text{rf diameter})$.

Optimizing over angle requires a programming loop*, but the optimization over phase can be done in the linear region, using the following trick.

We first introduce rotated coordinates

$$x' = x\cos\theta + y\sin\theta \tag{6A.1}$$

$$y' = -x\sin\theta + y\cos\theta \tag{6A.2}$$

$$\text{weights:} \quad m(x,y) \tag{6A.3}$$

$$\text{sine grating: } f(x,y) = \sin(ky' + \phi)$$

$$= \sin\left(ky\cos(\theta) - kx\sin(\theta) + \phi\right) \tag{6A.4}$$

$$\text{cell output: } c(\phi) = \int m(x,y)f(x,y,\phi)dxdy \tag{6A.5}$$

Now we maximize with respect to ϕ.

---

*Loops in a program are inherently slow. Using analysis to by-pass the necessity for a loop can improve efficiently greatly

$$\frac{dc(\phi)}{d\phi} = 0 \tag{6A.6}$$

$$= \int m(x,y) \cos\left(ky\cos(\theta) - kx\sin(\theta) + \phi\right) dxdy \tag{6A.7}$$

$$= \int m(x,y) \left[\cos\left(ky\cos(\theta) - kx\sin(\theta)\right)\cos\phi \right. \tag{6A.8}$$

$$\left. - \sin\left(ky\cos(\theta) - kx\sin(\theta)\right)\sin\phi\right] dxdy \tag{6A.9}$$

$$\Rightarrow \tan\phi = \frac{\int m(x,y) \cos\left(ky\cos(\theta) - kx\sin(\theta)\right) dxdy}{\int m(x,y) \sin\left(ky\cos(\theta) - kx\sin(\theta)\right) dxdy} \tag{6A.10}$$

We then use this phase in Equations 6A.4 and 6A.5 in order to find the maximum response (over phase), at a particular angle. We then need only to calculate the response of the cell to a sine grating (zero phase) and a cosine grating (zero phase).

6A.1.2　*Direction Selectivity*

For direction selectivity, in a two channel model, we follow a similar procedure.

The cell is tested with gratings of spatial frequency, k, and temporal frequency, ω. The two channels are offset by a delay, τ. Thus the response is

$$c(t) = \int m_1(x,y) \sin\left(ky' + \omega t\right) dxdy \tag{6A.11}$$

$$+ \int m_2(x,y) \sin\left(ky' + \omega(t - \tau)\right) dxdy$$

Since we are maximizing with respect to time and temporal frequency, we can treat the problem as follows. We find the phase which maximizes each term independently using Equation 6A.10,

$$c(t) = \int m_1(x,y) \sin\left(ky' + \phi_1\right) dxdy \tag{6A.12}$$

$$+ \int m_2(x,y) \sin\left(ky' + \phi_2\right) dxdy \tag{6A.13}$$

$$\tan\phi_1 = \frac{\int m_1(x,y) \cos(ky')}{\int m_1(x,y) \sin(ky')} \tag{6A.14}$$

$$\tan\phi_2 = \frac{\int m_2(x,y) \cos(ky')}{\int m_2(x,y) \sin(ky')} \tag{6A.15}$$

This gives the optimum *difference* in phase $\delta\phi \equiv \phi_1 - \phi_2$, which is the optimum phase $\omega\tau$ from Equation 6A.11, and allows us to find the response in the optimum direction. Once we have this, we can then optimize for time using the grating moving in the opposite direction $(\delta\phi \rightarrow -\delta\phi)$.

$$c(t) = \int m_1(x,y) \sin(ky' + \phi) \, dxdy \tag{6A.16}$$

$$+ \int m_2(x,y) \sin(ky' + \phi - \delta\phi) \, dxdy \tag{6A.17}$$

$$\frac{dc(t)}{d\phi} = \int m_1(x,y) \cos(ky' + \phi) \, dxdy \tag{6A.18}$$

$$+ \int m_2(x,y) \cos(ky' + \phi - \delta\phi) \, dxdy \tag{6A.19}$$

$$\tan\phi = \frac{\int [m_1 \cos(ky') + m_2 \cos(ky') \cos\delta\phi + m_2 \sin(ky') \sin\delta\phi] \, dxdy}{\int [m_1 \sin(ky') - m_2 \cos(ky') \sin\delta\phi + m_2 \sin(ky') \cos\delta\phi] \, dxdy}$$

where we have abbreviated $m_i(x,y)$ as simply m_i.

6A.2 Spatial Frequency of Receptive Fields

To see the effect of the size of the filter on the RF's, We trained neurons with images filtered with difference of Gaussians of various sizes. The receptive fields were fit to Gabor filters [Jones and Palmer, 1987], shown in Figure 6A.1, which are sine gratings restricted by a Gaussian window

$$\text{Gabor}(x, y, \theta) = \sin(kx\cos(\theta) + ky\sin(\theta)) \cdot \frac{1}{2\pi\sigma^2} e^{-((x-x_o)^2 + (y-y_o)^2)/2\sigma^2}$$

These, and the other RF's found, differed primarily in *spatial frequency*.

In the visual system there are at least two different types of retinal cells, called X and Y cells [Linsenmeier et al., 1982]. X cells have smaller receptive fields, and respond slowly to moving stimuli. Y cells have larger receptive fields, and respond rapidly to moving stimuli. This could be a simple way for the visual system to ensure that the cortex has a representation of many scales from the environment. Figure 6.7 shows the dependence of the resulting spatial frequency on the center and surround sizes of the retinal DOG. Those retinal cells which have a *smaller* receptive fields yield cortical cells with *higher* spatial frequency.

6A.3   Displaying the Weights

In an experiment, one does not have direct access to the values of the synaptic weights. One can only probe with visual stimuli, e.g. points of light, look at responses and *infer* the synaptic weights. In simulation, we have access to the weights directly. The effect of presenting points of light, which may provided stimulus to more than one input, is to give a smoother version of the receptive field that would be obtained if one had direct access to the weights themselves. For this and for aesthetic reasons, we pass the weights through a smoothing DOG filter before displaying them (in the package you can turn this off to look at the weights directly). An example of this is shown in Figure 6A.2.

6A.4   Different Forms of BCM Modification

There are several different versions of the BCM equations that are commonly used, and have been explored in previous chapters. In this section we outline some of the practical differences between three forms of BCM when using them for simulations. The three forms are the following

1 **Intrator and Cooper (Objective Function) BCM**[Intrator and Cooper, 1992]. This form of BCM has been analyzed in detail in Chapter 3.

$$c = \sigma(\mathbf{m} \cdot \mathbf{d})$$
$$\dot{\mathbf{m}} = \phi\mathbf{d} = c(c - \theta_M)\mathbf{d}\sigma'$$
$$\theta_M = E[c^2]$$

where σ' is the derivative of the sigmoidal output function.

2 **Quadratic BCM**. The quadratic BCM is the simplest form of BCM that meets the requirements for BCM modification (see Section 1.4). It is identical to Intrator and Cooper BCM with a the derivative of the sigmoid, $\sigma' = 1$. All of the simulations in this book, unless specified otherwise, use this form.

$$c = \sigma(\mathbf{m} \cdot \mathbf{d})$$
$$\dot{\mathbf{m}} = \phi\mathbf{d} = c(c - \theta_M)\mathbf{d}$$
$$\theta_M = E[c^2]$$

3 **Law and Cooper BCM**[Law and Cooper, 1994]. This form of BCM is introduced in Law and Cooper, 1994, and has been used in most of the papers on networks of BCM neurons[Shouval et al., 1997b; Goldberg

et al., 1999; Shouval et al., 2000]. It is identical to the Quadratic BCM, except for a variable learning rate proportional to $1/\theta_M$.

$$c = \sigma(\mathbf{m} \cdot \mathbf{d})$$
$$\dot{\mathbf{m}} = \phi \mathbf{d} = c(c - \theta_M)\mathbf{d}/\theta_M$$
$$\theta_M = E[c^2]$$

The Law and Cooper form contains an extra $1/\theta_M$ and has *all of the same fixed points* as the Quadratic form. It has different dynamics, however, that results in a specific practical consequence: it tends to converge somewhat faster. The $1/\theta_M$ can be understood as a dynamic learning rate. It speeds up the learning when the threshold is low (presumably at the beginning of a simulation) and slows the learning when the threshold is high. As a result, it makes the system somewhat more stable to fluctuations, and allows one to use a higher learning rate than normal. It will often start with a wildly oscillating threshold that stabilizes rapidly. It is the convergence time advantage that often makes it useful in network simulations, that can take quite a long time to perform.

The Objective Function BCM contains an extra σ' compared with the Simple Quadratic form. It has the *same fixed points* for a linear sigmoidal output function, or an environment where the outputs all fall within the linear region of the sigmoid. It does have the feature of making the neuron less sensitive to outliers: very large (or small) responses, which saturate the sigmoidal output function, result in $\sigma' = 0$ and the weights do not change. This form is particularly useful in an environment with many outliers.

6A.4.1 Evaluation of the Objective Function using Newton's Method

In this section we use Newton's Method to evaluate the objective function (see Chapter 3) and show that this leads to the Law and Cooper,1994 form of BCM. This method has been used in [Hyvarinen, 1998] to derive a fast fixed-point method for ICA using Subtractive Kurtosis as a projection index.

In order to solve the vector equation $\mathbf{f}(\mathbf{m}) = \mathbf{0}$ with the Newton's method, one first solves the equation

$$(\nabla \otimes \mathbf{f}(\mathbf{m})) \mathbf{D} = -\mathbf{f}(\mathbf{m})$$

for the direction $\mathbf{D}$,

$$\mathbf{D} = -(\nabla \otimes \mathbf{f}(\mathbf{m}))^{-1} \mathbf{f}(\mathbf{m})$$
$$= -\mathbf{J}^{-1}\mathbf{f}(\mathbf{m})$$

where $\mathbf{J}$ is the Jacobian matrix. One then updates the weight vector in that direction

$$\mathbf{m} \to \mathbf{m} + \mathbf{D}$$

The equation we need to solve for BCM is

$$c = \sigma(\mathbf{m}^{\mathrm{T}}\mathbf{d})$$
$$E\left[\mathbf{d}\phi(c)\sigma'(c)\right] = 0$$

where $\sigma(c)$ is a sigmoid. If we take the very simple sigmoid

$$\sigma(c) = \begin{cases} c \text{ if } c > 0 \\ 0 \text{ if } c \le 0 \end{cases}$$

then

$$\sigma'(c) = \begin{cases} 1 \text{ if } c > 0 \\ 0 \text{ if } c < 0 \end{cases}$$
$$\sigma''(c) = 0$$

The Jacobian matrix is then given by

$$\mathbf{J} = E\left[\mathbf{d}\mathbf{d}^{\mathrm{T}}\left(\phi'(c)\sigma'(c) + \phi'(c)\sigma''(c)\right)\right]$$
$$= E\left[\mathbf{d}\mathbf{d}^{\mathrm{T}}\phi'(c)\right]$$

For quadratic BCM, we have

$$\phi(c) = c(c - E[c^2])$$
$$\phi'(c) = 2c(1 - E[c]) - E[c^2]$$

So we arrive at the BCM fixed point learning rule

$$\mathbf{m} \to \mathbf{m} - \mathbf{J}^{-1}E\left[\mathbf{d}\phi(c)\right]$$
$$\mathbf{J} = E\left[\mathbf{d}\mathbf{d}^{\mathrm{T}}\phi'(c)\right]$$

We use the approximation (used in [Hyvarinen, 1998]) $E\left[\mathbf{d}\mathbf{d}^{\mathrm{T}}\phi'(c)\right] \sim E\left[\mathbf{d}\mathbf{d}^{\mathrm{T}}\right]E\left[\phi'(c)\right]$, and also assume that the data are whitened so that $E\left[\mathbf{d}\mathbf{d}^{\mathrm{T}}\right] = 1$. We now obtain

$$\mathbf{m} \to \mathbf{m} - E\left[\mathbf{d}\phi(c)\right] / \left(2E[c] - 2E^2[c] - E[c^2]\right]$$

If we make the further assumption that $E[c] \ll E[c^2]$ (ie. the mean of the output is small compared with the variance), then we retrieve the Law and Cooper form of BCM

$$\mathbf{m} \to \mathbf{m} + E\left[\mathbf{d}\phi(c)\right] / E[c^2]$$

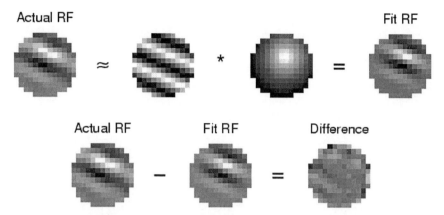

Figure 6A.1: Fitting a receptive field to a Gabor filter. Shown is an example receptive field (upper left), the best fit sine grating (upper right), the best fit Gaussian window (lower left), and the product of the sine grating and the Gaussian window.

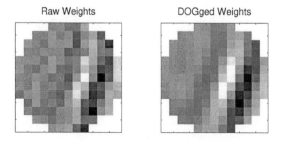

Figure 6A.2: Raw weights (left) and the smoothed weights (right), presented to more reasonably account for the presentation of points of light to infer the receptive field.

Chapter 7

Ocular dominance in normal and deprived cortex

The shift in ocular dominance in monocular deprivation is probably the most robust result of deprivation during the critical period. This experience dependent plasticity of binocular vision during the critical period is an important reason for choosing the visual system as a model system for theories of synaptic plasticity.

Most cortical cells in kittens are *binocular*, this means that they respond to stimuli from either eye [Hubel and Wiesel, 1962]. There are a few cells which are *monocular* (respond to only one eye), but they are far fewer in number. The amount by which a cell responds to one eye or another is called *ocular dominance*. Traditionally these cells have been categorized into 5 or 7 categories[Hubel and Wiesel, 1965]. In a normal cortex this results in ocular dominance distributions as seen in Figure 7.1.

Although most cortical cells are binocular, the majority of such cells are dominated by inputs from one of the eyes. Cells with similar ocular dominance are usually clustered together in the cortex, in elongated bands, that are referred to as ocular dominance columns.

There has been a long ongoing dispute as to how much the development of the ocular dominance distributions and ocular dominance columns is activity or experience dependent[Crowley and Katz, 2002]. There exists evidence for a strong initial bias in the OD distribution and cortical architecture. However, there exists a period, termed the critical period, in which these distributions can be changed by altering visual experience. Ocular dominance plasticity during the critical period is one of the best studied examples of developmental plasticity, and therefore is a good model system for testing theories of synaptic plasticity.

7.1 Development of normal ocular dominance

In this section we show that BCM neurons trained in a binocular natural image environment produce the experimentally observed normal ocular

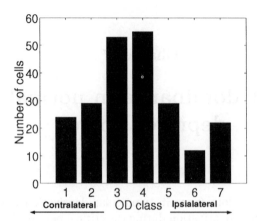

Figure 7.1: The normal distribution of ocular dominance in kitten visual as measured by Hubel and Wiesel, 1965. The cortex displays a range of cells dominated by responses to the left and right eyes, with many cells responding equally to both.

dominance distributions. In the next chapter we show that when embedded in a network of interacting neurons, ocular dominance columns are produced as well. Although some of the formation of normal OD distributions occurs prior to the critical period[Crowley and Katz, 2002], it is important to show that this can be accomplished by activity dependent mechanisms. For example, a learning rule could produce purely binocular receptive fields (or purely monocular ones) irrespective of the initial conditions. The condition of the cortex at the beginning of the critical period might be regarded as an initial condition, and such a rule would create a perfectly binocular (or monocular) cortex, irrespective of the initial conditions.

Traditionally the categorization into ocular dominance groups is made subjectively; simply by listening to the spike trains elicited by stimulation of each eye. Alternatively a quantitative measure can be used. We use an ocular dominance index defined as:

$$OD = \frac{R^{\text{left}} - R^{\text{right}}}{R^{\text{left}} + R^{\text{right}}} \tag{7.1}$$

where $R^{\text{left/right}}$ is the response of the cell to stimulation using oriented gratings through the left/right eye, at an orientation which yields the largest binocular response. When $OD = 1$ the cell is driven only by the left eye, when $OD = -1$ it is driven only by the right eye, and when $OD = 0$, it is a perfectly binocular cell. In order to display the ocular dominance distribution we discretize the OD index into 5 equal groups, this produces ocular dominance (OD) distribution in a form similar to those usually presented by experimentalists (Figure 7.1), enabling a comparison between theory and experiment.

In mature animals, raised under normal conditions, cortical cells display sharp orientation and direction tuning, as well as a range of ocular dominance (Figure 7.1) We have developed a model of a binocular visual environment, to emulate normal binocular rearing, and the synapses modified via the BCM learning rule. This two-eye model is almost identical to the one-eye model presented earlier. Patches are taken from images of natural scenes and presented to left and right retinal cells. When in perfect alignment, the eyes in these simulations see the same patch of the image. This assumption is relaxed below, where the eyes see a slightly shifted version of the same patch or versions of the same patch corrupted by noise. The cells have the same DOG properties as the single-eye model, and the LGN again relays the retinal signals unmodified to the cortex, this is depicted in Figure 7.2.

In normal development, the alignment of the left and right eye fields of vision may not be identical. We therefore introduce a model of binocular misalignment, where the left and right receptive fields have an overlap region. This is a simplification of the general case of misalignment, but the robustness of results indicates that the conclusions are general. In order to examine the effect of varying the overlap between the receptive fields, we define an overlap parameter $O = s/2a$, where a is the receptive field radius in pixels, and s is the linear overlap in pixels (Figure 7.3). Thus, $O = 1$ when the left and right receptive fields are completely overlapping and $O \leq 0$ when they are completely separated. We use the ocular dominance index defined in Equation 7.1.

When the input patches are completely overlapping (i.e identical) nearly identical oriented receptive fields develop in both eyes (Figure 7.3, top). This produces OD distributions that are perfectly binocular (Figure 7.3, top-right). When receptive fields are misaligned, various ocular dominance preferences may occur even for the same overlap (Figure 7.3 bottom three panels). As the overlap decreases, more monocular cells appear. Finally when there is no overlap (Figure 7.3 bottom panel) only monocular cells appear. This visual misalignment does not decrease the orientation selectivity in the dominant eye, but might decrease or even eliminate orientation selectivity in the non-responsive eye. The case of no overlap ($O < 0$) is similar to the condition known clinically as strabismus. This condition prevents binocular vision and when induced experimentally in kittens it produces only monocular cells, in agreement with our results.

It is reasonable to expect that in normal animals there will be a distribution of cortical ocular misalignments. Depending on the distribution of the misalignments we would expect that the OD distributions in kittens

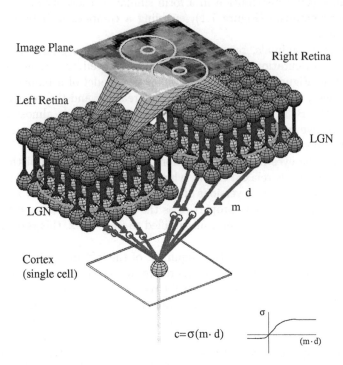

Figure 7.2: Model Architecture for 2 Eyes. Shown are the image plane (top), the left and right retinal cells, LGN cells, and the single cortical cell (bottom). Sample center-surround receptive fields are drawn in the image plane for the retinal cells highlighted. Nearby retinal cells see nearby points in the image plane. Retinal cells project directly to LGN cells, on a one-to-one basis. A circular patch of LGN cells from each eye projects to the single cortical cell. These projections form the input vector, $\mathbf{d}$, for which there is a corresponding weight vector, $\mathbf{m}$. The output of the cell is given as $c = \sigma(\mathbf{m} \cdot \mathbf{d})$.

could be produced by a weighted sum of the different OD histograms on the right of Figure 7.3.

A summary of the results is

- for *complete* overlap ($O = 1$), the neurons developed *identical* receptive fields.
- for *no* overlap ($O \leq 0$), the neurons developed *monocular* receptive fields
- for *partial* overlap ($0 < O < 1$), the cortical receptive fields developed *in the overlap region*, as well as in one of the single-eye receptive fields

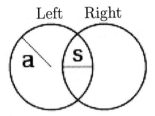

Figure 7.3: Overlap between Left and Right input patches in a model of binocular misalignment.

The partial correlation between the two eye channels is analogous to the partial correlation between lagged and non-lagged channels during the development of direction selectivity (Section 6.5). Consistent with this, the loss of direction selectivity (DS) in strobe rearing is similar to the case of complete misalignment.

7.2 Deprivation of Normal Binocular Inputs

Rearing young animals in altered visual environments can yield significant changes in the OD distributions. In this section, we review the experimental results where the input environment is changed in specific ways to yield changes in ocular dominance and direction selectivity.

The simulations we discuss in detail can be compared with experiments that give robust effects and are straightforward in their implementation and interpretation. These include binocular and monocular deprivation, reverse suture, and strabismus. There are many variations, and different protocols, that are either not quite as straightforward to implement or interpret. These experiments often seem very suggestive and can be understood, at least qualitatively, from our theoretical results, but they are not the focus of the comparison we wish to make with experiment. Examples include rearing in a striped [Blakemore and Cooper, 1970; Stryker et al., 1978] or spotted [Pettigerew and Freeman, 1973] environments, monocular deprivation of *particular* orientations [Cynader and Mitchell, 1977; Rauschecker and Singer, 1979].

We continue using the two-eye model presented in the previous section to simulate normal binocular rearing and typically assume perfect overlap for these conditions. The time course of the development of orientation selectivity during normal rearing is presented in Figure 7.5 (top). The simplifying assumption of perfect alignment during NR does not significantly effect the results of the subsequent deprivation experiments.

Modeling deprivation requires an assumption about the signals from the visually deprived eye. We use uncorrelated noise to correspond to the random firings of deprived eyes to simulate the different deprivation protocols: monocular deprivation (MD), binocular deprivation (BD), and reverse suture (RS). For BD, we follow normal rearing (NR) by presenting noise to both eyes, simulating the deprivation of visual experience to each eye. MD, likewise, is simulated by following NR, with noise presented to one eye while the other receives patterned input from the natural scene environment. Reverse suture (RS) follows MD, but then the previously deprived eye subsequently receives patterned input, and the previously open eye is produces uncorrelated noise.

7.2.1 *Binocular Deprivation*

Rearing animals in environments completely deprived of patterns, such as total darkness or binocular lid suture, has been shown to alter the development of the receptive field properties of visual cortical cells. For up to 3 weeks from eye opening, such deprivation produces receptive fields that are very similar to those of normally reared animals [Buisseret and Imbert, 1976; Frégnac and Imbert, 1978]. This is at least partially due to the time it takes for the optics to clear. However, long term deprivation results in a large percentage of unselective cells. Most responsive cells remain binocularly activated, but the remaining selective cells tend to be monocular [Blakemore and van Sluyters, 1974; Frégnac and Imbert, 1978; Levental and Hirsh, 1980]. There is some anecdotal evidence for a significant differences between the effects of total deprivation (dark rearing) and pattern deprivation (bilateral lid suture).

It has also been shown [Wiesel and Hubel, 1962; Freeman et al., 1981] that binocular deprivation, on the order of 3 or 4 days, causes deterioration of the responses and orientation selectivity in normally reared cats. The cells, however, remain binocular and direction selective . It is unclear, however, what the exact time course of the loss of response is. Chronic experiments might give a better idea of the time course of the deprivation.

An example simulation of binocular deprivation (BD) is shown in Figure 7.5 (bottom). For BD, we follow normal rearing (NR) by presenting noise to both eyes, simulating the deprivation of visual experience to each eye. We observe a decrease in the responsiveness of the cells, and eventually orientation selectivity itself is lost, but the time course tends to be slower than that of MD.

7.2.2 *Monocular Deprivation*

There is a very striking difference between the effects of monocular and binocular deprivation. When one eye of a previously normally reared kitten is deprived of patterned input, cells in kitten's visual cortex change from mostly binocular to almost exclusively monocular: in as little as 24 hours most cells lose their response to stimulation through the deprived eye and can only be driven through the eye that remains open [Wiesel and Hubel, 1963; Mioche and Singer, 1989]. This ocular dominance shift is not caused simply by the atrophy of neurons connected to the closed eye, because there is no measured decrease in the number of neurons which are visually responsive.

It appears that the lack of *patterned* visual input to the eye is required to attain these deprivation effects. Using a translucent contact lens, and keeping the total flux into both eyes the same, produces the same striking ocular dominance shift [Wiesel and Hubel, 1965; Blakemore, 1976]. Merely reducing the total amount of light entering the eye, while maintaining patterned vision, does not produce a significant effect [Blakemore, 1976].

The very fast change in the ocular dominance of the cells during monocular deprivation (MD) is likely to be due to the change of the efficacy of synapses from the closed eye. An example of a MD simulation is shown in Figure 7.5 (top). We see here that the deprived eye responses drop quickly, and that open eye responses increase. The time course of deprivation in MD (Figure 7.5 (top)) is significantly faster than during BD (Figure 7.5 (bottom)).

Because the effects of binocular deprivation (BD) are much less severe than those observed for monocular deprivation[Wiesel and Hubel, 1962; Freeman et al., 1981], many have been led to the hypothesis that a *spatially competitive* process is at work. However, BD can also be produced by a homosynaptic mechanism. In the BCM theory the difference between the rates of disconnection in BD and MD is the result of a moving threshold. This effect is illustrated in Figure 7.6. During monocular deprivation, the patterned input into the open eye keeps the modification threshold, θ_M, high resulting in a large depression region of the modification function (Figure 7.6A). In binocular deprivation, the unpatterned activity entering both eyes is insufficient to maintain the threshold at a high value, resulting in a significantly reduced depression (Figure 7.6B). Eventually, binocularly deprived cells lose orientation selectivity, but the time scale is much longer than that for the loss of response to the closed eye in MD.

7.2.3 *Recovery from Monocular Deprivation*

Another experiment, that supports the claim that the OD shifts are likely to be due to the change of the efficacy of synapses from the closed eye, uses a procedure called reverse suture (RS). In this procedure, there is an initial period of monocular deprivation: after the cortical neurons have become monocular, the deprived eye is opened and the other eye closed. In this situation the cortical neurons lose responsiveness to the newly closed eye, and become responsive to the newly opened eye [Blakemore and van Sluyters, 1974]. At least 24 hours of RS is required before the responses to the deprived eye reappears [Mioche and Singer, 1989]. The time it takes to lose the response in monocular deprivation, and to recover it after the reverse suture is probably too short to be entirely due to the addition or subtraction of new synapses [Jacobson et al., 1985]. The change in efficacy of synapses, whatever the mechanism is, is likely to be primarily responsible for these changes. The exact speed at which the deprivation effects occur is a function of where we are in the critical period. After five weeks of age, a constant deprivation period has a smaller effect.

A sample simulation of RS is shown in Figure 7.5 (middle). Reverse suture (RS) follows MD, but the eye previously given noise now receives patterned input, and the previously open eye receives noise. The BCM rule is consistent with the ocular dominance shifts described in both experiments.

Recovery from MD can also be accomplished by opening *both* eyes after deprivation. Recent evidence[Kind et al., 2002] suggests that binocular rearing (BR) following MD results in a faster, more robust recovery than the recovery that results from reverse suture. This is difficult to reconcile with competitive learning rules, such as PCA and the subtractive forms of kurtosis and skewness, but is consistent with BCM. Examples of simulations of this kind, using BCM, are shown in Figure 7.5 (bottom).

For BCM, the recovery times for RS and BR depend most critically on the noise from the deprived eyes. As we have seen before, for RS the *more* noise from the closed eye the *faster* the recovery (as a result of a faster decay of the newly deprived eye responses). For BR it is necessary for there to be some noise from the eye receiving patterned input. Otherwise, both eyes receive the same input, and the left and right eye weights will have *exactly* the same changes every iteration. No recovery is possible in this case. However, if there is independent noise from each eye, then the change in the weights is different for the two eyes, and recovery can take place. The more noise, the faster the recovery. Figure 7.7 compares the recovery times for RS and BR for values of the open and closed-eye noise variances. Except for very small open-eye noise (slow BR), and small closed eye noise (slow MD resulting in fast RS), the binocular recovery is faster than reverse suture.

7.2.4 *Strabismus*

Hubel and Wiesel (1965) perform an experiment where the eyes of the kitten are artificially misaligned. After rearing with this condition, a drastic reduction in binocularity in the cortical cells is found, with most cells re-

Parameters for BCM Simulations	
Learning Rule	$\dot{\mathbf{m}} = \eta c(c - \theta)\mathbf{d}$ $\dot{\theta} = \frac{1}{\tau}(c^2 - \theta)$
Activation Rule	$c = \sigma(\mathbf{m} \cdot \mathbf{d})$
cortical sigmoid	$\begin{cases} \sigma(-\infty) = -1 \\ \sigma(+\infty) = 50 \end{cases}$
Initial threshold	$\theta_o = 0.73$
Input mean	$\langle \mathbf{d} \rangle = 0$
Input variance	$\mathrm{var}(\mathbf{d}) = 1.0$
RF Diameter	13 pixels
Retinal DOG ratio	3:1
Learning rate	$\eta = 5 \cdot 10^{-7}, ..., 5 \cdot 10^{-5}$
Memory constant	$\tau = 10, ..., 3510$
Noise Levels	uniform noise$=$ $[-.25:.25], ..., [-2.5, 2.5]$

Table 7.1: Parameters for BCM Deprivation Simulations

maining responsive to one or the other eye. This result has been widely reproduced [Blakemore, 1976; van Sluyters, 1977; van Sluyters and Levitt, 1980]. A common interpretation of this result is that the lack of correlation between the two eyes is responsible for the degradation of the binocular connections.

One way to perform a simulation of strabismus is to eliminate the overlap between the right and left channels, so that the eyes see completely different parts of the visual field. The effects of this is shown in the bottom of Figure 7.4, where the overlap between the eyes is set to $O = -0.2$. What is found is an ocular dominance distribution of purely monocular cells, consistent with the experimental observations.

7.2.5   *Robustness to Parameters*

The main parameters of the model are the learning rate, η, the memory constant, τ, and the noise level from the closed eye, σ^2. Other parameters that can significantly affect the timing include the RF size, the bottom value of the sigmoid on the output, the input variance and mean, and the form of the retinal preprocessing. The RF size increases the number of inputs, but does not seem to alter the receptive field structure significantly (except for very large or very small RF's), as explored in Section 6.1.3. This increase can be thought of as a simple increase in the learning rate. The input variance can be thought of as a simple scaling of the learning rate and the threshold. The mean of the inputs, the form of the retinal preprocessing, and the lower limit of the sigmoid cannot be seen as a simple scaling of model parameters. We have discussed some of this earlier. Here we focus on the two parameters τ and σ^2, because these parameters have significant biological interpretations. The memory constant, τ, determines the time scale over which the sliding threshold is averaged, and thus may give an indication of the cellular and molecular mechanisms underlying the sliding threshold. The noise level, σ, corresponds to the level of the spontaneous activity in the LGN during unpatterned stimulus. We will see that the dependence on this parameter leads to an unintuitive[Blais et al., 1999], yet experimentally verified [Rittenhouse et al., 1999], phenomenon. All of the simulations, unless otherwise specified, have the parameter values given in Table 7.1.

In order to investigate the dynamics of cell response, we measure the response $Y(t)$ of the neurons using oriented stimuli. Of particular interest is the characteristic half-rise (half-fall) time for the growth (decay) of neuronal response, referred to as either $t_{1/2}$ or simply T.

For each learning rate, η, there is a valid range for τ. If τ is too large, then oscillations occur and the weights may not converge. Normal rearing is more sensitive to this than the various deprivation simulations. We could choose the stability of normal rearing as the criterion for setting the upper bound on τ. This upper bound, however, may be misleading because the stability of a simulation depends on the initial conditions, for which we have very little detailed knowledge in the case of normal rearing. For instance, if there is a partially orientation selective receptive field *before* eye opening, stability may be enhanced and we could use a larger value for τ. We choose, then, to use the stability of the deprivation protocols to set the upper bound on τ.

The lower bound for τ is more difficult to set from simulations, because in many cases a very quickly moving threshold (τ small) still converges. This, however, leads to rapid fluctuations of the threshold, that may be difficult to embody biologically. In vivo LTD and LTP experiments as well as an understanding of underlying cellular mechanisms will probably help us to determine the value of τ.

The dependence of the half-fall times, $T_{\text{fall}}^{\text{MD}}$, $T_{\text{fall}}^{\text{BD}}$, and $T_{\text{fall}}^{\text{RS}}$ on the memory constant τ within the stable range is shown in Figure 7.8. It is clear that there is little dependence of these half-times over a wide range of values of the memory constant. This is somewhat surprising, given that the memory constant determines the time scale over which the threshold averages the neural activity. This suggests that there is limited sensitivity of the threshold to the averaging of the environment.

This may indicate a striking difference between the natural scene environment and the one dimensional oscillations results, where the memory constant played a more important role in the timing. This is not merely an effect of added dimensionality, because previous work modeling deprivation using higher dimensional inputs[Clothiaux et al., 1991] showed a strong dependence on the memory constant. There, the input environment was not taken from the natural scene images, but were high dimensional linearly independent vectors with added noise. We find here an indication that the *statistics* of the input environment has a dramatic effect on the behavior of the model.

Another outcome of the lack of dependence on the memory constant, τ, is that the deprivation experiments cannot give us any *detailed* information about this parameter. The range of valid τ is determined completely by the stability of the simulations, and has no obvious measurable effect on the time course of deprivation. We can establish an upper bound, but that is all we can state with any degree of confidence. Thus, we have some freedom in establishing the mechanisms behind the moving threshold. The range that we do find is consistent with mechanisms such as gene expression and protein synthesis.

7.3 Time Course of Deprivation: Simulation Time Versus Real Time

We require that the consequences of the BCM theory be consistent with *many* biological experiments, using *one set of parameters*. This is crucial to determining validity because it provides the most strict tests, and highlights potential problems.

One straightforward way to compare difference models with experiment is to compare the *relative* timing of the ocular dominance shifts during deprivation. For instance, we can measure from simulations the time for the closed eyes to lose responsiveness in binocular, monocular deprivation and reverse suture, and the time for the recovery of the newly open eye in reverse suture. Since we do not know the conversion between simulation time units (iterations) and real time units (seconds) we cannot directly compare the absolute timings of these simulations. Below, however, we make estimates by comparing the "time" periods of the simulations with experiment at some point in the critical period. We can compare *ratios* of these simulation times to the same ratios found in experiment, because ratios are not dependent on units.

Some of the questions we would like to answer are *What can the biological deprivation experiments tell us about the possible range of the parameters in the theory?*, *Within this restricted parameter regime, how does the time course of the deprivation experiments depend on the parameters?*, and

Summary of Experimental Results		
Exp't	Reference	Half-Time T
MD	• OD changes were observed as **early as 6 h**[Freeman and Olson, 1982; Mioche and Singer, 1989] • **complete loss** of response to closed as early as **12 h**[Mioche and Singer, 1989] • moderate increase of response to the normal eye occasionally[Mioche and Singer, 1989]	$T_{\text{fall}}^{\text{MD}} \approx$ 6-12 h
BD	• cortical response reduced **within 3 d**[Freeman et al., 1981]	$T_{\text{fall}}^{\text{BD}} <$ 3 d
RS	• the time course for the reduction of response to the newly deprived eye was **similar to monocular deprivation**[Mioche and Singer, 1989] • **At least 24 h** of reverse suture is required before the responses to the deprived eye reappear[Mioche and Singer, 1989]	$T_{\text{fall}}^{\text{RS}} \approx T_{\text{fall}}^{\text{MD}}$ $T_{\text{rise}}^{\text{RS}} \approx$ 1-4 d

Table 7.2: Summary of Experimental Results in Deprivation

Can we use this dependence to propose experimental measurements of the parameters?

Table 7.2 summarizes the experimental results from the deprivation literature. The exact results depend on when in the critical period the experiments were done, and the most appropriate experiments using chronic recording have not been done yet. The results shown in the table allow us to roughly estimate the values of the activity half-rise time, T_{rise}, or half-fall time, T_{fall}, whichever is appropriate for the particular experiment. The ratios of these times, from experiment, are simply

- $T_{\text{fall}}^{\text{RS}}/T_{\text{fall}}^{\text{MD}} \approx 1$
- $1 < T_{\text{fall}}^{\text{BD}}/T_{\text{fall}}^{\text{MD}} < 12$
- $2 < T_{\text{rise}}^{\text{RS}}/T_{\text{fall}}^{\text{MD}} < 16$
- $0.33 < T_{\text{rise}}^{\text{RS}}/T_{\text{fall}}^{\text{BD}} < 16$

It is unclear whether the $T_{\text{rise}}^{\text{RS}}$ time is a good number to use for a comparison, because it depends on how long the preceding MD was performed. If, for instance, one performed MD for weeks and then followed with RS, one would expect a slower recovery than RS following a day of MD. Therefore, we will use the $T_{\text{rise}}^{\text{RS}}$ only as a very rough test of consistency.

We do find a range of parameters for BCM over which the deprivation simulations are consistent with experiment. This range has an upper-bound on the learning rate at $\eta = 4.5 \cdot 10^{-6}$, and a possible lower bound at around $\eta = 7 \cdot 10^{-6}$. The lower bound may be extended using faster computers. For this range of learning rate, the upper bound on the value of τ is determined to be $\tau = 8500$ for stability with the deprivation experiments. As stated before, there is no strong lower bound on τ. The value of the standard deviation of the noise is restricted to the range $0.8 < \sigma < 1.4$, in order to be consistent with experiment. This range is around the value 1, the standard deviation of the natural scene environment.

Given a valid parameter regime for the deprivation experiments, and half-times for those deprivation experiments within this range, we can obtain a conversion between the simulation time units (iterations) and the real time units (seconds). Monocular deprivation, within the parameter regime found, takes about $2 \cdot 10^5$ iterations. In experiment, the half-time is around 12 hours. This makes one iteration about a 0.2 sec.

We then note that for monocular deprivation (and other deprivation protocols), using a noise standard deviation of $\sigma = 0.8$, the maximum consistent memory constant is as high as $\tau \sim 8500$ iterations, which is around 30 minutes. We are not certain what mechanisms govern the motion of the threshold, but this time scale is consistent with protein synthesis which can occur on the order of minutes[Alberts et al., 1994]. The upper limit set by normal rearing is $\tau \sim 3500$ iterations, or 13 minutes, but it may be altered by the initial conditions which are not known precisely. The lower bound on τ is quite small, on the order of a few iterations, which is equivalent to a second or more. Basically, τ is on the order of minutes or a few seconds, but not on the order of milliseconds or hours. This places constraints on the possible mechanisms involved.

Although these results are *reasonable*, the conclusions are still tentative for the following reasons:

- the experimental results are quite rough, so that it is difficult to make the time comparisons
- other forms of the BCM learning rule may have quite different dynamics, and may shift the valid parameter range considerably

These results show, however, that there is at least one set of parameters that is consistent with all of the experimental results. They also suggest the necessity for further experiments such as chronic deprivation experiments. Careful chronic measurements could determine these time scales quantitatively.

7.4   Dependence of Deprivation on Spontaneous Activity or Noise

Figure 7.9 shows the dependence of the half-fall times, $T_{\text{fall}}^{\text{MD}}$, $T_{\text{fall}}^{\text{BD}}$, and $T_{\text{fall}}^{\text{RS}}$ on the variance of the noise, σ. For all types of deprivation experiments we see a strong dependence of the rate of loss of response for the deprived eye, or eyes, on the noise level. Specifically we see that *higher levels of noise* from a closed eye during any of the deprivation protocols, produces *faster* loss of response (smaller T_{fall} time).

In addition we notice that the half-fall times of both reverse suture (RS) and binocular deprivation (BD) have a steeper dependence on the noise than monocular deprivation (MD). We can understand why this might be the case for binocular deprivation, because noise is all that is being presented to the cell. For RS we expect that, at first, it should have similar timings to BD. In both cases, the cell is essentially receiving noise from both eyes, but perhaps with different variance. In BD we have noise from both eyes, whereas in RS we have structured input entering an initially noisy receptive field and noise entering an initially oriented receptive field. Naturally we would expect a stronger dependence on the noise in these two cases.

The specific dependence of deprivation experiments is different for different families of learning rules [Blais et al., 1999]. Referring to the learning rules in Chapter 3, we divide the learning rules into two classes based on their sensitivity to the closed-eye noise level in monocular deprivation:

Homosynaptic Class

- Quadratic BCM
- Skewness 1
- Kurtosis 1

Heterosynaptic Class

- linear and non-linear PCA (Hebbian)
- Skewness 2
- Kurtosis 2

We have introduced the terms "homosynaptic class" and "heterosynaptic class" to denote the primary mechanism of depression of the deprived-eye synapses in monocular deprivation: homosynaptic (uses temporal competition) and heterosynaptic (uses spatial competition), respectively. As shown in Figures 7.10 and 7.11, these two classes of rules have the *opposite* dependence on the noise for the time-course of MD. The homosynaptic class of learning rules show a *faster* loss of response to the closed eye for higher presynaptic activity levels in the closed eye channel. The heterosynaptic class of learning rules show the opposite behavior.

The dependence of deprivation experiments on noise levels for BCM (homosynaptic class), can be explained using a simple example of BCM in an environment composed of clusters (for an analysis in a non-cluster environment see Appendix 3A.2. The same conclusions are found in both environments). If we assume that the cell is initially selective to one of the clusters, as it is after normal rearing, then most of the responses will either be around $c \approx 0$ or $c \approx \theta_M$. We can then approximate the modification function, $\phi(c, \theta_M)$, around those points (see Figure 7.12). In monocular deprivation, patterned input comes into the open eye and noise comes from the closed eye. We then have two cases for the open eye inputs:

- non optimum patterns into open eye: $c \approx 0$
- optimum patterns into open eye: $c \approx \theta_M$

This immediately leads to two cases for synaptic modification; (we assume, for simplicity, that the mean of the noise is zero, $\bar{n} = 0$)

- non optimum patterns into open eye

$$\frac{d\mathbf{m}^{\text{closed}}}{dt} \approx \eta(-\epsilon_2)\bar{n}^2\mathbf{m}^{\text{closed}} \qquad \text{(weights decrease)}$$

- optimum patterns into open eye

$$\frac{d\mathbf{m}^{\text{closed}}}{dt} \approx \eta(+\epsilon_1)\bar{n}^2\mathbf{m}^{\text{closed}} \qquad \text{(weights increase)}$$

The net effect, over the entire environment of N_{opt} optimal patterns and $N_{\text{non-opt}}$ non-optimal patterns is then

$$\log \mathbf{m}^{\text{closed}}(t) \propto -\bar{n}^2(\epsilon_2 N_{\text{non-opt}} - \epsilon_1 N_{\text{opt}})t \qquad (7.2)$$

This implies that, for a selective neuron, $N_{\text{non-opt}} \gg N_{\text{opt}}$, the closed eye weights decrease and they decrease *faster* for increased presynaptic activity[*]. In addition there should be a correlation between selectivity and the ocular dominance shift – less selective cells shifting less.

7.5   Conclusions

We have shown that the BCM neurons can develop varying degrees of ocular dominance with only the additional assumption of misalignment of the retinal inputs. For extreme misalignments, the BCM neuron becomes

---

[*]See Chapter 9 for a comparison with the experimental results of Rittenhouse et. al. 1999

monocular as in strabismus, due to the lack of correlations between the two eyes. Using inputs taken from Gaussian or uniform noise, the deprivation protocols are all simulated and consistent with results of experiment. The effects of binocular deprivation (BD) are less severe than for monocular deprivation (MD), without the addition of a spatial competition mechanism. This is the result of the BCM temporal competition between patterns exhibited.

This temporal competition also leads to the result that in monocular deprivation, the homosynaptic class of learning rules (e.g. BCM) have a *faster* loss of response to the closed eye, for higher presynaptic activity levels in the closed eye channel. The heterosynaptic class of learning rules (e.g. PCA, K_2) show the opposite behavior (see Section 9.2). This dependence on the noise can also be used to make an estimate of the conversion between simulation time and real time, by finding parameter ranges over which the time-dependence of the simulation on deprivation is consistent with the real-time dependence of deprivation. This estimate places an iteration (the time-scale of synaptic modification) at about 200 ms, and the motion of the threshold on the order of 1/2 hour. Further refinements in the experiments, through chronic recording, should be able to improve this estimate.

Finally, many other deprivation protocols can be simulated, including forms of recovery from monocular deprivation such as reverse suture and binocular recovery. Comparisons between these, and their dependence on the noise and other parameters, provide a direct comparison of theory with experiment and show that the BCM theory with a *single set* of parameters is consistent with experimental results.

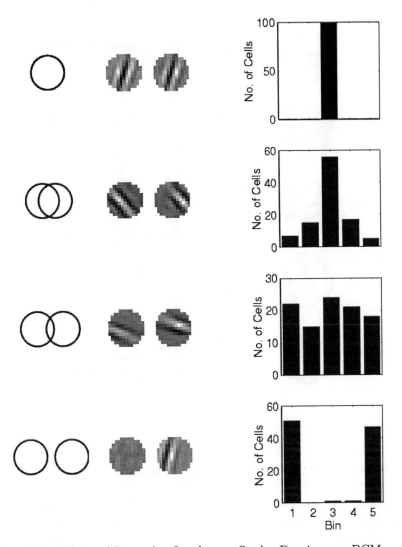

Figure 7.4: Effects of Binocular Overlap on Ocular Dominance. BCM neurons with different overlap values; $O = 1.0, 0.6, 0.2, -0.2$ from top to bottom. The ocular dominance histograms summarize the ocular dominance of 60 cells at each overlap value. The dependence of ocular dominance on visual overlap is evident.

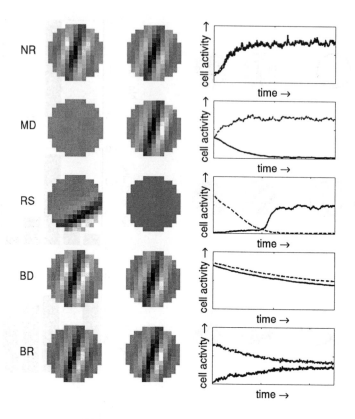

Figure 7.5: BCM Simulations. Left: Final weight configuration. Right: Maximum response to oriented stimuli through the left eye (solid line) and the right eye (dashed line), as a function of time. Simulations from top to bottom are as follows. Normal Rearing (NR): both eyes presented with patterned input. Monocular Deprivation (MD): following NR, one eye is presented with noisy input and the other with patterned input. Reverse Suture: following MD, the eye given noisy input is now given patterned input, and the other eye is given noisy input. Binocular Deprivation (BD): following NR, both eyes are given noisy input. **It is important to note that for BCM if Binocular Deprivation is run longer, selectivity will eventually be lost.** Binocular Recovery: following MD, both eyes presented with patterned input.

A

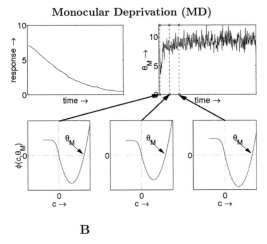

B

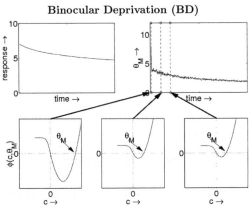

Figure 7.6: Comparison between monocular deprivation and binocular deprivation. **a,** Shown is the response of the closed eye (above left) and the modification threshold, θ_M (upper right), as functions of time, during monocular deprivation. Shown also is the modification function, $\phi(c, \theta_M)$ (below), sampled at three different time steps. During MD, the patterned input into the open eye keeps the threshold, θ_M, high resulting in a larger depression region of the modification function. **b,** Same conventions as (**a**), but for BD. In BD, the unpatterned activity entering both eyes is insufficient to maintain the threshold at a high value, resulting in significantly reduced depression. Thus, the time scale for BD is longer than MD.

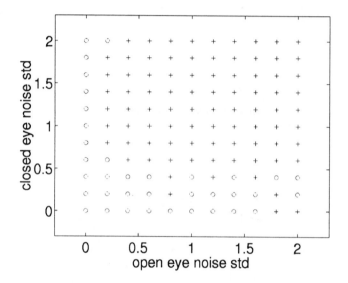

Figure 7.7: Relative speed of recovery of Binocular Recovery (BR) compared to Reverse Suture (RS). Shown are the open and closed eye noise levels where BR is faster than RS (+) and where BR is slower then RS (0). Except for very small open-eye noise (slow BR), and small closed eye noise (slow MD resulting in fast RS), the binocular recovery is faster than reverse suture.

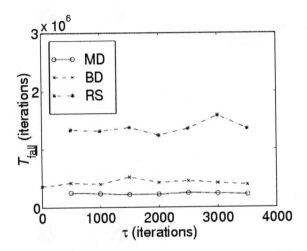

Figure 7.8: The dependence of the half-fall times, $T_{\text{fall}}^{\text{MD}}$, $T_{\text{fall}}^{\text{BD}}$, and $T_{\text{fall}}^{\text{RS}}$ on the memory constant τ.

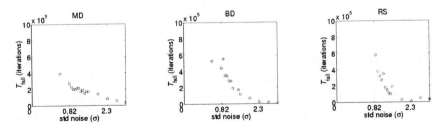

Figure 7.9: The dependence of the half-fall times, $T_{\text{fall}}^{\text{MD}}$, $T_{\text{fall}}^{\text{BD}}$, and $T_{\text{fall}}^{\text{RS}}$ on the standard deviation of the noise, σ. ($\eta = 5e - 6$, $\tau = 1000$).

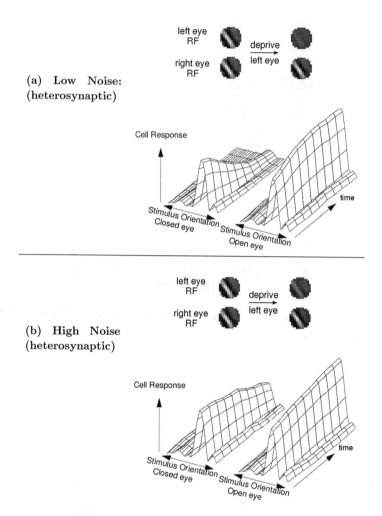

Figure 7.10: The effect of noise from the closed eye on the disconnection of the closed eye in monocular deprivation (MD) using the heterosynaptic rule, K_2. Left and right receptive fields (above), before and after depriving the left eye. The tuning curves versus time are shown in the lower panels. Presented are a low noise environment (a) and a high noise environment (b). Compare to the next figure, with the homosynaptic rule, BCM. The two rules have the opposite dependence on the noise from the closed eye of the rate of disconnection of the closed eye in MD.

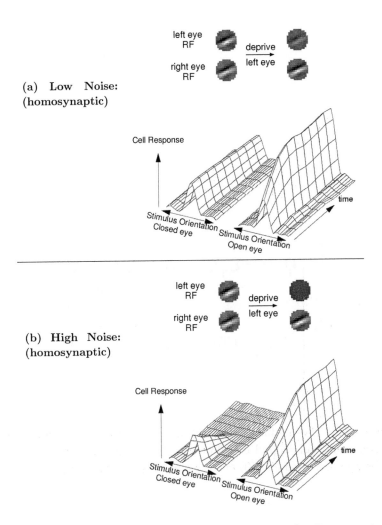

(a) **Low Noise:**
(homosynaptic)

(b) **High Noise:**
(homosynaptic)

Figure 7.11: The effect of noise from the closed eye on the disconnection of the closed eye in monocular deprivation (MD) using the homosynaptic rule, BCM. Left and right receptive fields (above), before and after depriving the left eye. The tuning curves versus time are shown in the lower panels. Presented are a low noise environment (**a**) and a high noise environment (**b**). Compare to the previous figure, with the heterosynaptic rule, K_2. The two rules have the opposite dependence on the noise from the closed eye of the rate of disconnection of the closed eye in MD.

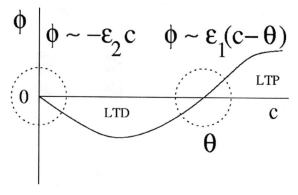

Figure 7.12: The modification function for a selective neuron. The responses would fall around $c \approx 0$ or $c \approx \theta_M$, so the modification function can be approximated as $\phi(0) \approx -\epsilon_2 c$ and $\phi(\theta_M) \approx \epsilon_1(c - \theta_M)$.

Chapter 8

Networks of Interacting BCM Neurons

8.1 Simplified Environments

Even the most reclusive theoretician is aware of the fact that the brain is not just a single cell – that it is a complex network of neurons with interconnections. However, for simplicity, we have so far tried to understand the development of neural properties primarily from the properties of single cells, ignoring most of the possible contributions of lateral connectivity and feedback. In Chapter 4 we did explore a mean-field approximation for network interactions, and in Section 4.3 we explored the effect of the lateral interactions, using a matrix analysis. We summarize the main results of these chapters below:

Network interactions can

1 change the *single-cell* receptive field properties
2 change the organization of receptive fields across the network

The mean-field approximation addresses (1) above, by allowing the effective weights from all-excitatory feed-forward connections to be both positive and negative. In this way, the lateral interaction allows the development of single-cell receptive fields which would not be possible without the lateral connectivity. The mean-field does not address (2) above, because it ignores possible correlations between output neuron responses.

The matrix analysis assumes bi-polar weights or, in other words, weights that can be either positive or negative. The conclusions relate both to (1) and (2) above. The main conclusions of this analysis are

(a) the lateral connectivity does *not* change the number of fixed points *or their stability*

(b) the lateral connectivity does *not* change the values of the fixed points, for the *outputs* of the neurons. The weights adjust to keep these outputs the same as the case without lateral connections, compensating for this connectivity

(c) The lateral connectivity does change the probability that those fixed points are reached, making some fixed points more likely than others

Here we carry out our more detailed network analysis with a simulation of neurons in a simplified input environment, shown in Figure 8.1, with various lateral connectivity organizations. This allows us to understand the effects of the lateral connectivity in an intuitive setting, before we approach the problem of natural images and lateral connectivity. The results in the simplified environment generalize to the natural scene environment, with few modifications.

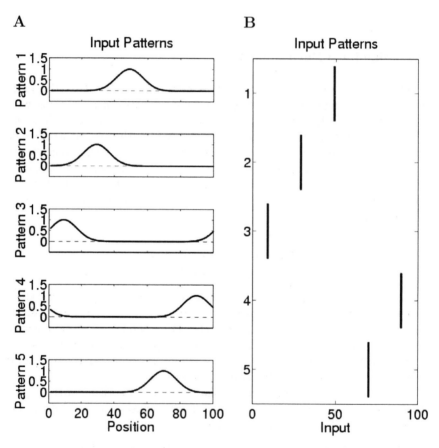

Figure 8.1: Simplified Input Environment of 5 Gaussian Patterns. (A) The 5 input vectors. (B) The positions of the maxima of the 5 input vectors, as a simpler representation.

Each cell's activity is calculated in two stages. First, the activity due to the geniculo-cortical feed-forward component is calculated. Then, activity due to the lateral component is added. Synaptic strength is then modified on the basis of the total activity. The activity of the kth neuron due to feed-forward connectivity is

$$c_k^0 = \sum_l m_{kl} d_l,$$

where d_l represents the activity of the lth input neuron, m_{kl} represents the synaptic weight connecting the lth input neuron to the kth cortical cell. The activation of the ith neuron due to lateral connectivity is

$$c_i = \sum_k L_{ik} \sigma(c_k^0)$$

where c_k^0 represents the feed-forward activity of the kth cortical neuron, as above, σ is a sigmoidal activation function, L_{ik} represents the synaptic weight connecting the kth cortical cell to the ith cortical cell, and the sum is taken over the set of lateral connections described above. In the simplified environment, this function is assumed to be linear over the entire possible activation range. For the natural image environment we will use a sigmoidal activation function with a lower saturation limit of -1 and an upper saturation limit of 50.

Therefore, the total activity of the ith cell in the network is

$$c_i = \sigma \left(\sum_j m_{ij} d_j + \sum_k L_{ik} \sigma(c_k^0) \right) \tag{8.1}$$

where the term on the left represents the activation due to feed-forward input. d_j represents the activity of the jth input neuron, m_{ij} are the synaptic weights connecting cortical neuron i to input neuron j. The sum is taken over all of the inputs. The term on the right represents the combined influence of all the lateral connections. This form is the same as the feed-forward network explored earlier (Equation 4.31).

The effects of the lateral connectivity can be seen in Figures 8.2 and 8.3. When there is no lateral connectivity (Figure 8.2), neurons become independently selective to different input patterns, some neurons to the same pattern. When there is only excitatory connectivity (Figure 8.3A), all neurons become selective to the *same* pattern. When there is only inhibitory connectivity (Figure 8.3B), all neurons become selective to *different* patterns.

In addition to all excitatory and inhibitory, we introduce a simple form for the lateral connectivity consisting of a local excitatory connectivity and medium-range inhibitory connectivity. This "Mexican hat" structure is common in the literature[von der Malsburg, 1973; Shouval et al., 1997b; Erwin and Miller, 1998]. To see the effect of a center-surround connectivity, we extend the environment to 34 vectors. There is no significant difference between the 34 vector and the 5 vector environments, but certain types of structures can be seen only in larger networks. It makes no sense, for example, to speak about continuity of features across a network if the network itself contains only a few neurons.

The results of these simulations, in the 34-dimensional environment with 34 neurons, are shown in Figures 8.5 and 8.6. The same qualitative results from the lower dimensional case are repeated: with all excitatory connections, the neurons mostly respond to similar patterns and with all inhibitory they mostly respond to different patterns (Figure 8.5). With center-surround connectivity, we see nearby neurons responding to nearby patterns, and neurons farther away responding to different patterns (Figure 8.6). This yields continuity across the network. This form of continuity is seen in orientation maps in the visual cortex[Bonhoeffer and Grinvald, 1991].

One necessary condition for continuity to exist is for the input patterns themselves to be wide enough to cause responses in several nearby neurons. If the input patterns are nearly orthogonal, then only the local excitation will have an effect, and the medium-range inhibition will not cause neurons to become different from each other, because only a few neurons will be active simultaneously. In Figure 8.7 we show typical input patterns with various widths. The effect of changing the widths is shown in Figure 8.8. For very narrow patterns, small groups of identically selective neurons form. As the size of the input patterns increases, the spatial extent of the groups becomes more significant, providing continuity across the network. In Figure 8.5 the width is $\sigma = 15$.

8.2   Natural Image Environment

8.2.1   *Orientation Selectivity*

We simulate receptive field development as before, in the natural image environment. The network consists of a monocular, single-layer of striate cortex cells. Each cortical cell receives input from a circular region of diameter 13 pixels. The RF center for each neuron is shifted with respect to its immediate neighbors in both the horizontal and vertical directions by 2 pixels. Initially, all feed-forward synaptic weights are randomly distributed

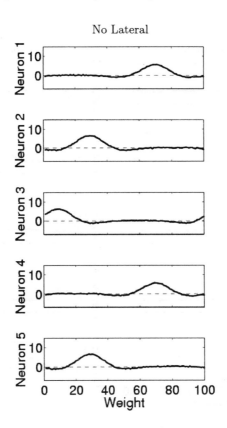

Figure 8.2: BCM Simulations in Environment of 5 Gaussian Patterns, with no lateral connectivity. Neurons become independently selective with no lateral connectivity.

in the range $[-0.1, 0.1]$. The activity of the neurons is calculated as shown above, using Equation 8.1. As above, σ is a sigmoidal activation function with a lower saturation limit of -1 and an upper saturation limit of 50.

The effects of the lateral connectivity can be seen in Figure 8.9. When there is no lateral connectivity, neurons become independently selective to different orientations, and no overall structure is seen. Introducing a local lateral connection, in the form of a center-surround difference of Gaussians, produces maps with some structure. Nearby neurons have similar orientation, and several orientation "patches" exist across the network. Making the lateral connectivity more spread out (higher standard deviation on the center and surround Gaussians) makes the orientation changes smoother, but also increases the size of the orientation patches. Larger networks

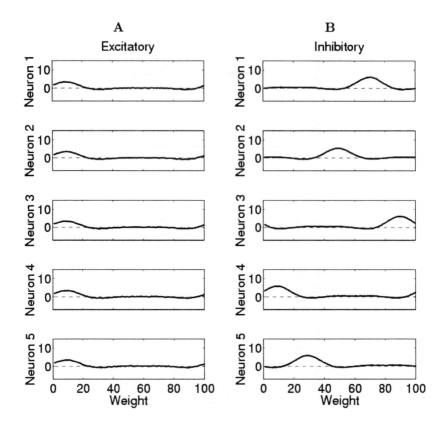

Figure 8.3: BCM Simulations in Environment of 5 Gaussian Patterns. (A) selective to the *same* pattern with excitatory connections and, (B) selective to *different* patterns with inhibitory connections.

need to be run in order to see both large orientation patches and smoothly changing orientation across the network. A common feature observed in models[Erwin et al., 1995] and in experiment[Bonhoeffer and Grinvald, 1991; Obermayer and Blasdel, 1997] is the "pinwheel", a small point on the map around which the orientation changes by a full 180 degrees. This feature can be clearly seen in Figure 8.9.

8.2.2 *Orientation Selectivity and Ocular Dominance*

Analogous to the single cell binocular misalignment simulations (Section 7.1), we simulate a network of neurons with two eyes where the two eyes see partially overlapping areas of the visual field (Figure 8.10). Again, the

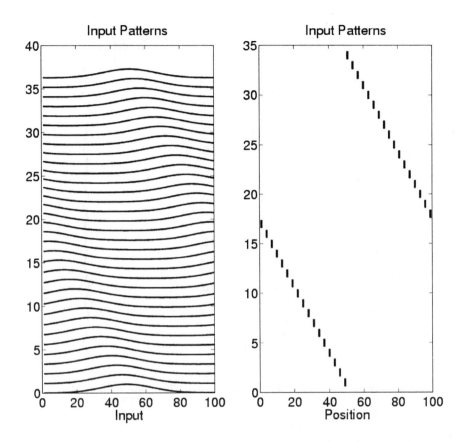

Figure 8.4: Simplified Input Environment of 34 Gaussian Patterns. (A) The 34 input vectors. (B) The positions of the maxima of the 34 input vectors.

network has a difference of Gaussian connectivity, and produces smoothly varying orientation maps. Also, one achieves ocular dominance patches, where a group of cells responds more strongly to one eye. These are similar in some ways to ocular dominance columns in visual cortex[Hubel et al., 1977].

8.2.3 Orientation and Direction Selectivity

Using a straightforward generalization of the single cell direction selectivity simulations (Section 6.5), one can achieve maps of orientation and direction selectivity. We find (Figure 8.11) good agreement with the maps measured

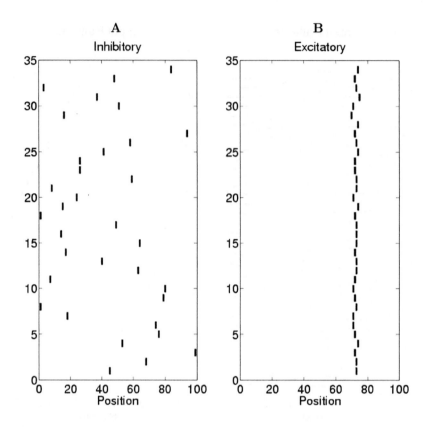

Figure 8.5: BCM Simulations of 34 neurons in an environment of 34 Gaussian Patterns. Shown is the position of the peak of the pattern yielding the peak response. As in the 5-dimensional case, (A) Neurons become selective to *different* patterns with inhibitory connections and, (B) selective to the *same* pattern with excitatory connections.

in experiment[Shmuel and Grinvald, 1996]. Some of the primary properties of the experimental maps, also seen in the simulation maps, are

- direction selectivity (DS) is mostly perpendicular to orientation selectivity (OR)
- DS singularities are line-like
- OR singularities are point-like
- OR patches have two DS patches of opposite direction
- OR singularities are connected to low DS line
- DS singularity endpoints do not match OR singularity points

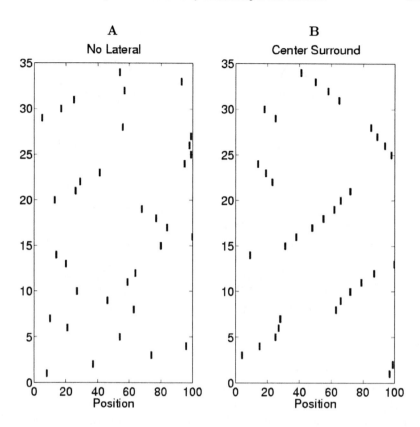

Figure 8.6: BCM Simulations of 34 neurons in an environment of 34 Gaussian Patterns. Shown is the position of the peak of the pattern yielding the peak response. As in the 5-dimensional case, (A) Neurons become independently selective with no lateral connectivity. In (B), with center-surround connectivity, the nearby neurons become selective to *similar* patterns, and a pattern of many neurons responding in a continuous fashion to the input environment.

8.3 Structured Lateral Connectivity

Recently, investigators have shown that orientation maps are present in binocularly deprived animals at eye-opening [Chapman et al., 1996; Gödecke et al., 1997; Crair et al., 1998] and that orientation maps are stable throughout the critical period [Chapman et al., 1996; Gödecke et al., 1997]. Furthermore, a dramatic optical-imaging/reverse-suture experiment [Gödecke and Bonhoeffer, 1996] has shown that two eyes without common

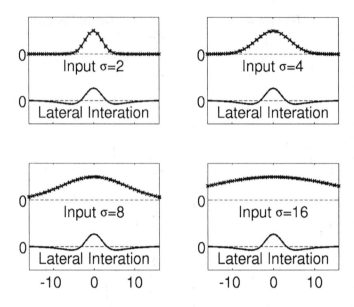

Figure 8.7: Input Patterns and Center-Surround Lateral Interaction for BCM Simulations of 34 neurons in an environment of 34 Gaussian Patterns. The relationship between the input pattern size and the spatial extent of the center-surround lateral connectivity determines, in part, the organizational structure of features found across the network, as shown in the next Figure.

visual experience develop similar orientation maps.

How can we reconcile these two apparently contradictory findings about the plasticity of orientation selectivity in the visual cortex? On one hand, there are strong indications that orientation selectivity shows experience-dependent plasticity. On the other, orientation maps seem stable through-out development and are laid down independent of visual experience.

Our major hypothesis is that a network of lateral connections in the visual cortex forms a *scaffold* that sets the orientation map, produces broadly tuned cells and biases the development of orientation selectivity[Shouval et al., 2000]. Orientation selectivity then develops through experience-dependent modifications of the feed-forward synaptic connections.

To demonstrate how the lateral connectivity can bias the development of a map, we look at a simple example of a 4×4 network of neurons in a natural image environment. We've already demonstrated that excitatory

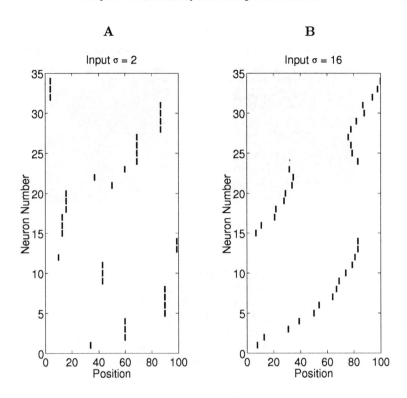

Figure 8.8: BCM Simulations of 34 neurons in an environment of 34 Gaussian Patterns, with center-surround (2:6) lateral connectivity. Shown is the position of the peak of the pattern yielding the peak response, for several different input-pattern widths. (A) shows a small input pattern width and yields groups of neurons with nearly identical feature response properties. (B) shows a large input pattern width and yields more continuous groups of neuron responses across the network.

connections bias the connected neurons to become selective to the same features, and inhibitory connections bias the neurons to become selective to different features. We construct a network where the lateral connectivity is structured in the following way (see Figure 8.12):

- Neurons in Group A (upper left 4 neurons, and lower right 4 neurons) are connected to each other with *excitatory* connections,
- Neurons in Group B (lower left 4 neurons, and upper right 4 neurons) are connected to each other with *excitatory* connections,

A

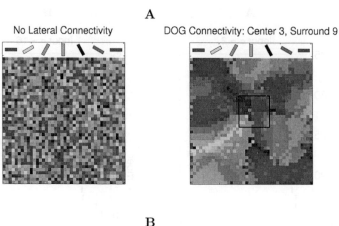

No Lateral Connectivity   DOG Connectivity: Center 3, Surround 9

B

Weights

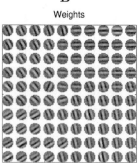

Figure 8.9: Orientation Map of a Network of BCM Neurons. (A) Shown is a pseudo-color orientation map, where each color represents selective response to a particular orientation. No structure in the map is seen when there is no lateral connectivity (above,left). A clear pinwheel structure is seen when there is DOG lateral connectivity (boxed area in plot above, right). (B) The weight vectors around the pinwheel, in the boxed area of the plot above, showing the change in the preferred orientation.

- Neurons in Group A are connected to neurons in Group B with *inhibitory* connections.

This connectivity structure, combined with BCM learning, should produce a network with two groups of neurons with similar orientation responses. The neurons in Group A should all have the same orientation preference. The neurons in Group B should all have the same orientation preference, which should be a *different* preference than the one developed

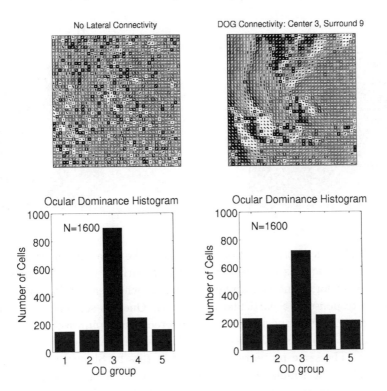

Figure 8.10: Network of BCM neurons develops ocular dominance and orientation selectivity. Same display conventions as Figure 8.9. Gray level on the orientation map (upper left) represents ocular dominance, where white corresponds to a cell dominated by the left eye, black corresponds to a cell dominated by the right eye, and gray corresponds to a binocular cell. Left, is a network without any lateral connectivity. Right, is a network with a center-surround (DOG) lateral connectivity. Patches of orientation and ocular dominance form (all white, or all black patches) in the center-surround case, but not in the case with no lateral connectivity. The ocular dominance histograms below for each case show that most neurons are binocular, but that the center-surround connectivity (right) develops more monocular cells. (1600 total cells).

by Group A neurons (due to the inhibitory connections between the two groups). If this were the entire story, then the orientation map is not biased by the lateral connectivity (other than forming two groups): there is no restriction, or bias, in the development of *which* orientation is found by a particular group. This bias can be easily introduced by adding an offset

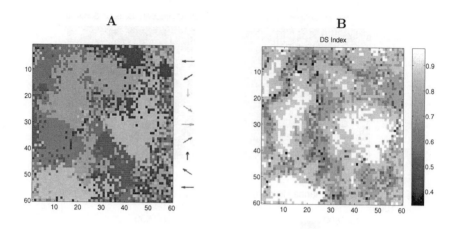

Figure 8.11: The overall relationship between the organization of orientation and direction, as achieved by the BCM learning rule. (A) Shown is the pseudo-color orientation and direction map where each color represents selective response to a particular orientation. One can see regions of similar orientation but opposite direction preference, and pinwheel orientation singularities. (B) Shows the direction index, where clear lines of low-DS are observed. The same properties measured in cats by Shmuel et. al. 1996 are found in the simulated maps. Orientation preference forms patches of similar orientation, often containing two patches of direction preference perpendicular to the orientation preference, but in opposite directions. The singularities of the orientation preference tend to be point-like, and often fall on points of low direction preference. The singularities of the direction preference tend to be line-like, and do not end near the orientation singularities.

between the neurons in their field of view (Figure 8.13). When neurons see slightly shifted versions of the input, then somewhat-distant neurons have correlated inputs when the environment contains long bars or edges.

This added correlation is enough to produce a bias where neurons connected with lateral excitatory connections are more likely to produce orientation preferences in the same direction of their lateral excitatory connections. Sample simulations of this are shown in Figure 8.14 for our simple 4×4 network. The network with offsets in the field of view of the neuron develops similar orientations in the two groups of connected neurons (upper left with lower right, and upper right with lower left). Further, the orientation preference found is along the direction of the lateral connections: approximately 45° for the neurons connected between the upper right and lower left, and approximately 135° for the neurons connected between the upper left and lower right. With the same simulations, but the neurons *do not* have offsets in their field of view, the two groups of neurons develop similar orientations within a group (and different between-group orientations), but from one simulation to another the orientation preference is different. There is no bias in the development of the specific orientation preference when there is no offset in the field of view of the neurons

In order to understand the result of the reverse-suture experiment of [Gödecke and Bonhoeffer, 1996], where it is shown that two eyes without common visual experience develop similar orientation maps, one need only assume a structured lateral connectivity exists before the development. The lateral connectivity must have the same structure as the resulting map, such that two neurons, say Neuron 1 and Neuron 2, are connected if they have similar orientation preference *and* the line connecting the center of the RF of Neuron 1 to Neuron 2 is nearly parallel to the Neuron 2's preferred orientation. The possible mechanisms for the development of this lateral connectivity scaffold, and the theoretical and experimental consequences of it are currently being investigated.

8.4 Conclusions

Addition of network interactions can change both the *single-cell* receptive field properties, and the organization of receptive fields across the network. Many of the properties of BCM neurons can be understood by analyzing a single-cell. We add network interactions to study properties that are network dependent, for example the organization of receptive field properties across the network. Having no lateral connectivity leads to the development of independent receptive fields, with no organization across the network. All excitatory and all inhibitory connection schemes lead to receptive fields across the network that are all similar or all different, respectively. Using a simple difference of Gaussians connectivity, with short-range excitation and medium-range inhibition, we get continuity across the network.

Using the difference of Gaussians connectivity in a natural image environment we obtain networks that develop smooth orientation maps, with pinwheel singularities. As in the single-cell case, adding retinal misalignment leads to ocular dominance. Network interaction leads to patches of similar ocular dominance, consistent with the columnar organization observed in experiment. In the case with lagged and non-lagged LGN cells, the network can develop realistic orientation and direction maps. Lateral connectivity can also serve to bias the development of the maps, if the connectivity map has structure to it. This may explain some of the similarity between maps observed under conditions where the eyes do not have

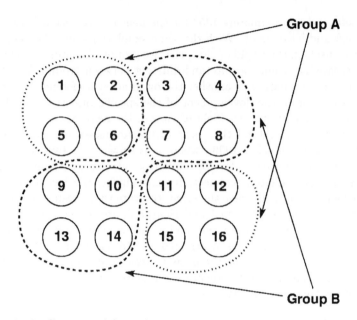

Figure 8.12: Structured lateral connectivity in a 4×4 network. Neurons in Group A (neurons 1,2,5,6,11,12,15, and 16) are connected to each other with *excitatory* connections, and connected to neurons in Group B (neurons 3,4,7,8,9,10,13, and 14) with *inhibitory* connections. The same is true for neurons in Group B: they are connected to each other with *excitatory* connections and to neurons in Group A with *inhibitory* connections.

common experience.

We conclude that it is possible to construct a network of BCM neurons with connectivity in agreement with experimental data, that reproduces observed network properties. This is done with very few additional postulates, none of which affect any of the conclusions found in the single-cell analysis. Thus, with a *single set of parameters*, one can reproduce many different experimental results, including network properties.

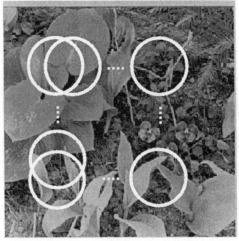

**Neuron Offsets
(highly exaggerated)**

Figure 8.13: Neuron field-of-view offsets (exaggerated for illustration). Adding an offset between the neurons in their field of view produce neurons that see slightly shifted versions of the input. Nearby neurons see similar parts of the image, but distant neurons may see completely different parts of the image. Somewhat-distant neurons have correlated inputs when the environment contains long bars or edges.

A

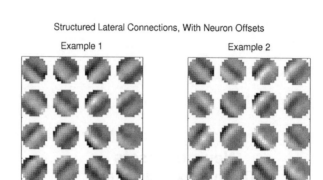

Structured Lateral Connections, With Neuron Offsets

Example 1   Example 2

B

Structured Lateral Connections, No Neuron Offset

Example 1   Example 2

Figure 8.14: Simulations of a 4×4 network with structured lateral connectivity. (A) The neurons have an offset in their field of view, and develop similar orientations in the two groups of connected neurons (upper left with lower right, and upper right with lower left). Further, the orientation preference found is along the direction of the lateral connections: approximately 45° for the neurons connected between the upper right and lower left, and approximately 135° for the neurons connected between the upper left and lower right. (B) The same simulations, but the neurons *do not* have offsets in their field of view. The two groups of neurons develop similar orientations within a group (and different between-group orientations), but from one simulation to another the orientation preference is different. There is no bias in the development of the specific orientation preference when there is no offset in the field of view of the neurons.

Chapter 9

Experimental Evidence for the Assumptions and Consequences of the BCM Theory

In the previous chapters we have described the BCM theory of synaptic plasticity: its key postulates, its analytical properties, particularly those that concern receptive field plasticity and map formation. As said before, a theory can be tested by examining experimentally the validity of its assumptions as well as by comparing its predicted consequences with experimental results. In the next two sections we review some experimental results and compare them to the assumptions and consequences of the BCM theory. In addition, we briefly discuss some evidence for the cellular and molecular bases of this theory.

9.1 Evidence Confirming the Postulates of the BCM Theory

The postulates of BCM a theory of synaptic plasticity are contained in two equations. The first

$$\dot{m}_j = d_j \phi(c, \theta_M), \qquad (9.1)$$

describes how the change in synaptic strength depends on the presynaptic activity d_j the postsynaptic depolarization or activity c, and the modification threshold θ_M. The sign of synaptic change depends on the non-monotonic function ϕ, which is schematically shown in Figure 1.2. This function is multiplied by the local presynaptic variable d_j. Therefore no modification occurs if $d_j = 0$; this is termed synapse specificity or homosynaptic modification. The second equation is:

$$\theta_M(t) = \overline{c^{1+\xi}} = \frac{1}{\tau} \int_{-\infty}^{t} c(t')^{1+\xi} e^{-\frac{(t-t')}{\tau}} dt'. \qquad (9.2)$$

which determines the dependence of the value of the modification threshold, θ_M, on the history of postsynaptic activity. This equation depends on two parameters, τ the time scale of the temporal averaging and $\xi > 0$, that insures insures that this is a super-linear function. We use several variants of this equation as described in Chapter 2. The general requirement for convergence is that θ_M is some temporal average of a super-linear function of c.

We have not yet precisely defined the physiological correlates of the pre- and postsynaptic activity variables d_j and c. In simulations and analysis we allow these to take continuous analog values. However, making a mapping between the variables used in the theory and physiological variables is not trivial; but it is reasonable to believe, given our present understanding, that the relevant molecular variables are presynaptic glutamate and post synaptic Ca^{2+} levels. A natural interpretation is that d_j is proportional to presynptic firing rate and c is proportional to postsynaptic firing rate or to postsynaptic depolarization.

9.1.1 The shape of the plasticity curve

Rate based induction

The most commonly employed method for inducing synaptic plasticity is rate based induction. It is technically the simplest method because only extracellular stimulating and recording electrodes are required. Usually hippocampal or neocortical slices are the preparations used. The recording electrode detects a relatively low frequency signal, that is usually referred to as the field potential. This signal is a spatial integration of EPSP's in many cortical cells. Since the magnitude of EPSP's can change as a result of changes in synaptic strength, changes in the field potential magnitude or slope can indicate synaptic plasticity. The stimulating electrodes (Figure 9.1a) are placed so that they activate afferent axons that make contact with neurons in the vicinity of the recording electrode.

In order to control the level of postsynaptic depolarization, different frequencies of presynaptic stimulation are used. Low frequencies cause little temporal integration in the postsynaptic neuron (Figure 9.1b, top) whereas higher frequencies cause significant postsynaptic depolarization (Fig 9.1b, bottom). Typically high frequency stimulation is delivered to produce a long term potentiation of synaptic strength (LTP) and low frequency stimulation is delivered to produce a long term depression in synaptic strength (LTD).

Typically before this conditioning stimulus is delivered, a baseline is established by stimulating for 15-30 minutes at a very low frequency (< 0.1 Hz). After a stable baseline is established a high frequency conditioning stimulus is delivered. Subsequent to the conditioning stimulus the low frequency baseline protocol is repeated, only now it produces a significantly larger response (Figure 9.1c). In some experiments an independent control pathway is monitored as well; a conditioning stimulus is not delivered to this pathway. Typically, responses to stimulation of this pathway are unchanged, indicating that LTP is synapse specific.

The use of high frequency stimulation to produce LTP, was first described by Bliss and Lomo in 1973 . In contrast to current practice they used an in vivo preparation. Since then LTP has been described in many different cortical structures and in many different animals, from invertebrates [Murphy and Glanzman, 1997] to humans[Chen et al., 1996]. The physiological and molecular substrates of LTP have been extensively studied; this is briefly reviewed below.

As described in the previous sections, the BCM theory requires bidirectional synaptic modification: synaptic strengths can be weakened as well as strengthened. Other theories contain synaptic weakening [von der Malsburg, 1973; Sejnowski, 1977; Oja, 1982]. However, the functional form of this weakening differs. This has motivated many attempts to induce synaptic weakening [Stanton and Sejnowski, 1989; Artola and Singer, 1992]. The pioneering experiments by Dudek and Bear (1992), that first demonstrated the induction of low frequency LTD, were specifically motivated by the BCM theory. These experiments show that low frequency stimulation, from 1-3 Hz produces LTD (Figure 9.1d), and high frequency stimulation produces LTP. These results are shown in Figure 1.4. Like LTP, the induction of LTD is synapse specific. This form of LTD is termed homosynaptic LTD and is consistent with the assumptions of the BCM theory. The induction protocol, used originally by Dudek and Bear (1992), has been reproduced by many others [Mulkey and Malenka, 1992; Mayford et al., 1995] and is now the standard induction protocol for LTD.

The frequency response curve produced by such LTP and LTD experiments in hippocampus [Dudek and Bear, 1992] and neocortex [Kirkwood and Bear, 1994a] reproduce the ϕ function of the BCM theory (as illustrated above), with the assumption that presynaptic frequency is related to postsynaptic potential, due to temporal integration. Synapse specificity (also demonstrated) allows us to write the plasticity equation in the separable form proposed by BCM. These findings have been confirmed in many different regions of neocortex in many species both young and old animals. Of particular interest is recent data showing the same principles of synaptic plasticity apply in the human inferotemporal cortex, a region believed to be a repository of visual memories[Chen et al., 1996]. Together, the data support the idea that very similar principles guide synaptic plasticity in many species in widely different regions of the brain.

Pairing based induction

The rate based induction protocol has produced significant results consistent with the BCM theory. However, there are problems with this method; extracellular recording is not the best way to measure the EPSP. Current intracellular techniques offer a more precise method of measuring the single cell EPSC. There is also the question of the precise mapping between stimulation frequency and postsynaptic potential; it would be better if the postsynaptic potential could be controlled directly. Both of these problems are overcome by the pairing induction protocol. Here a voltage clamp is established on a single postsynaptic cell. This method allows a direct measurement of the EPSC's due to presynaptic stimulation. In this method the presynaptic stimulus is delivered at a low frequency (0.1-2 Hz). Baseline is established at resting membrane potential (≈ -65 mV). LTP is induced if the postsynaptic cell is highly depolarized, to approximately 0 mV, during the presynaptic stimulation, and LTD is produced by a more moderate depolarization. Such protocols have been used in hippocampal[Stevens and Wang, 1994] cells and in different neocortical systems [Feldman et al., 1998; Feldman, 2000; Ngezahayo et al., 2000]. The exact voltages at which LTP and LTD are produced differ among the different systems; however they share the same qualitative features: at baseline no plasticity is induced, moderate depolarization induces LTD and a larger depolarization results in LTP (Figure 9.2). These results (as with the rate dependent results) are consistent with the form of the ϕ function in the BCM theory. Pairing induced plasticity, like rate based plasticity, is synapse specific.

Although evidence from these two different induction paradigms is qualitatively consistent with the form of the ϕ, and with synapse specificity, as proposed by the BCM theory, there is some evidence for forms of plasticity that may be different then those proposed by BCM. For example heterosynaptic plasticity [Abraham, 1996] has been described in vivo preparations of hippocampus. It is not clear if this is really inconsistent with BCM, for example it might be a network effect. Another possible interpretation consistent with BCM is that the presynaptic activity may not be measured with respect to zero, but with respect to spontaneous activity, thus the inactive path might have a negative value of presynaptic activity. Another example is that plasticity might not be perfectly local [Engert and Bonhoeffer, 1997; Fitzsimonds et al., 1997]. Such questions will probably be best addressed with increasing knowledge of the underlying cellular and molecular mechanisms.

Possible physiological bases of synaptic plasticity

The great technological advances in physiological techniques such as the widespread use of intercellular techniques and calcium imaging as well as the great advances in molecular biology have had significant influence on the study of the underlying mechanisms of synaptic plasticity. However the implication of the mechanisms on the functional properties of synaptic plasticity are not always simple. We are currently attempting to bridge the gap between the molecular biology of synaptic plasticity, the resulting physiology and theoretical models such as BCM [Castellani et al., 2001; Shouval et al., 2002a; Shouval et al., 2002b]. The detailed description of these efforts is beyond the scope of this book; however we briefly describe some of the fundamental mechanisms and our contributions to modeling their effect below.

Although there are different paradigms for inducing LTP and LTD, it has become clear that in many cases a key variable is the integrated activity of NMDA receptors. This was first observed for LTP [Collingridge et al., 1983; Harris et al., 1984] and later observed for LTD induction as well [Dudek and Bear, 1992; Mulkey and Malenka, 1992; Dudek and Bear, 1993]. However, there are systems and induction paradigms for which this does not hold, and in which plasticity is NMDAR independent [RA and Nicoll, 1990; Katsuki et al., 1991; Oliet et al., 1997; Huber et al., 2001]. The NMDA receptors have properties that are necessary for implementing Hebbian synaptic plasticity since their activation depends both on presynaptic and on postsynaptic activity. The NMDAR depend on release of glutamate from the presynaptic neurons but they are blocked by magnesium, that is relieved only when the postsynaptic cell is depolarized [Jahr and Stevens, 1990].

There is significant evidence that calcium, flowing in through the calcium permeable NMDAR, is the key mediator of synaptic plasticity [Cummings et al., 1996; Cho et al., 2001; Cormier et al., 2001], and that the influx of calcium ions might be sufficient for inducing bidirectional synaptic plasticity [Neveu and Zucker, 1996; Yang et al., 1999]. But how can calcium influx trigger both LTP and LTD? An important idea is that a moderate rise in intracellular calcium levels triggers LTD whereas a larger increase in calcium results in LTP [Bear et al., 1987; Lisman, 1989]. Lisman (1989) suggested that this could occur if a moderate increase in calcium levels activates phosphatases that somehow reduce synaptic conductance while a larger increase in calcium triggers kinanses that produce an increase in synaptic conductance [Lisman, 1989].

Despite technological advances there is still no consensus about how synaptic plasticity is expressed. There are three dominant, not mutually exclusive, views: synaptic plasticity is produced by (1) changes in presynaptic probability of release [Stevens and Wang, 1994; Goda and Stevens, 1998; Zakharenko et al., 2001] (2) changes in the number of postsynaptic AMPA receptors [Liao et al., 1995; T. et al., 1996; Malinow and Malenka, 2002] (3) changes in the conductance of postsynaptic AMPA receptors due to phosphorylation/dephosphorylation [Lee et al., 2000; Banke et al., 2000]. These different mechanisms might be active in different systems, or possibly even in the same system under different conditions.

Molecular biologists have identified a large number of molecules that are associated with synaptic plasticity, these include the receptors, neurotransmitters, and many different enzymes and associated anchoring proteins [Sanes and Lichtman, 1999; Malenka and Nicoll, 1999]. In particular they have identified many of the steps in the signal transduction cascade; these start with changes in calcium levels and leads eventually to changes in pre- or postsynaptic proteins that control synaptic conductance. We do not yet understand the function of these many different interacting molecules in the induction and expression of synaptic plasticity. There have been however several attempts [Lisman, 1989; Castellani et al., 2001; Shouval et al., 2002b; Bhalla, 2002] to model the physiology of synaptic plasticity on the basis of the molecular mechanisms that are identified as associated with it.

There can be different functional consequences of these different modes of expression; for example, changes in probability of release can also alter the short term dynamics of synaptic transmission, not only their magnitude whereas postsynaptic changes do not have this effect [Tsodyks and Markram, 1997; Artun et al., 1998]. We expect that once the detailed molecular and physiological mechanisms are taken into account this will add complexity to BCM synaptic plasticity; in the same way, as mentioned before, that real gases contain complexities that go beyond the ideal gas equation.

9.1.2 *The sliding modification threshold*

Another key BCM assumption is the sliding modification threshold. The BCM theory requires that the threshold between LTD and LTP move as a super-linear function of the history of cell activity. If activity is high the modification threshold moves to the right favoring LTD over LTP and if activity is low the modification threshold moves to the left (Figure 1.3). This may be regarded as a negative feedback mechanism that stabilizes learning and prevents the runaway positive feedback that is a consequence of Hebbian mechanisms if additional constraints are not imposed. This sliding modification threshold changes the form of synaptic plasticity as a function of the history of the cells activity. Changes in the form of synaptic plasticity function have been called metaplasticity [Abraham and Bear, 1996]. However, not all possible forms of metaplasticity will ensure stability. It has also been proposed that the BCM theory could explain the observation of synaptic scaling [Turrigiano, 1999]. This phenomenon, associated with a mechanism for preserving homeostasis, would then be a consequence of the sliding threshold so that BCM would enforce homeostasis[Yeung et al., 2003].

If activity in a cortical region is reduced, we expect that the modification threshold should slide to the left. Such a shift was observed by Kirkwood et. al. (1996) by dark rearing rats. Dark rearing should reduce neural activity in visual cortex, but not in other brain regions such as hippocampus. In Figure 9.3 we show the plasticity curves obtained from normal and dark reared animals. These results show a significant shift of the threshold to the left in the dark reared animals, consistent with BCM. As a control Kirkwood et al. (1996) also show that this shift is absent in the hippocampus. In addition this effect is reversed with as little as two days of light exposure. Note that although plasticity in this experiment was examined in vitro, metaplasticity took place in vivo.

A similar approach was used to assess synaptic strength and plasticity, in piriform cortex [Lebel et al., 2001] and somatosensory cortex [Rioult-Pedotti et al., 2000] after skill learning. In both cases it was shown that after skill learning the magnitude of LTP was reduced; in the case of piriform cortex the magnitude of LTD was shown to increase. These experiments show metaplasticity due to skill learning. It is not straightforward however to relate them directly to cortical activity as it is not clear that the neural activity increases during skill learning. Further, other changes resulting from skill learning, such as changes in synaptic weights might be the origin of the metaplasticity observed. We therefore conclude that although these results are strongly suggestive of the sliding threshold hypothesis, they do not directly confirm it.

Another approach for inducing a shift in the threshold is to induce meta-plasticity by altering electric activity directly in the slice. This approach is used by J.J. Wagner and co workers in two papers [Holland and Wagner, 1998; Wang and Wagner, 1999]. They use adult hippocampal slices, that exhibit very little 1 Hz LTD. To these slices they delivered a priming stimulus, that consists of two sets of three 1 sec. episodes of 100 Hz stimulation. This stimulation is delivered in the presence of APV in order to block NMDA receptor-dependent synaptic plasticity. After APV is washed out, different conditioning stimuli are delivered, in order to induce synaptic plasticity. In Figure 9.5 we show the plasticity curves they obtain with and without priming. As required by BCM, priming has very significantly shifted the modification threshold to the right. This is a whole cell effect, as priming shifts the threshold in a non-potentiated path as well. Since the priming induced shift occurred in the presence of APV, this indicates that this metaplasticity does not depend on activation of NMDA receptors.

A very different experiment[Mayford et al., 1995] using genetically altered mice has been interpreted as indicating the sliding threshold. Also, recently published results of Tang et. al. (1999) again using genetically altered mice (a different alteration) taken together with results of Quinlan et. al. (1999) that link cellular activity with the ratio of two distinct sub-units of the cortical NMDA receptor support the idea that θ_M is set according to the activation history of the cell (Figure 9.4). Additional experiments in which metaplasticity has been induced in vivo have been carried out by several groups [Ngezahayo et al., 2000; Abraham et al., 2001]. The results of these experiments are more complex. Although they clearly demonstrate meta-plasticity, it is not clear if the conditions that elicit this metaplasticity, are the same as those required in the sliding modification threshold proposed in the BCM theory.

An extensive review of the physiological and molecular mechanisms that underly synaptic plasticity and metaplasticity is beyond the scope of this chapter. However, it is important to note that several possible mechanisms for metaplasticity have been suggested and experimentally observed. They include single cell effects such as changes in the time constants and subunit composition of NMDA receptors [Carmignoto and Vicini, 1992; Quinlan et al., 1999; Philpot et al., 2001; Shouval et al., 2002b], the number of NMDA receptors [Watt et al., 2000; Shouval et al., 2002b], the ratio of α and β isoforms of CaMKII [Thiagarajan et al., 2002], as well as network effect such as plastic changes in the level of inhibition [Steele and Mauk, 1999] .

9.2   Evidence Confirming the Consequences of the BCM Theory

The BCM theory was originally developed to account for receptive field plasticity in visual cortex. In the previous chapters we demonstrated how it can account for both ocular dominance plasticity and the development of orientation plasticity. The existence and robustness of ocular dominance plasticity is not in dispute. However, there is a distinct possibility the organization of ocular dominance columns depends on different mechanisms than those that govern ocular dominance plasticity during the critical period [Crowley and Katz, 2002]. It is possible that activity independent mechanisms as well as mechanisms dependent on spontaneous activity contribute to the organization of ocular dominance across the cortical map. Nevertheless it is well documented that ocular dominance plasticity in the critical period depends on NMDA receptor activity [Kleinschmidt et al., 1987; Roberts et al., 1998], as does synaptic plasticity on the cellular level.

In chapter 1 we reviewed evidence that supports a significant role for synaptic plasticity in the development of orientation selectivity and orientation maps. Although the dependence of orientaton selectivity on experience and synaptic plasticity is a more contentious issue than ocular dominance plasticity, accumulated evidence paints a very similar picture: receptive fields and cortical maps are formed by a combination of experience dependent and experience independent factors. Some fraction of visual cortex neurons are somewhat selective at, or before, eye opening. However, this selectivity requires a patterned visual environment to mature [Buisseret and Imbert, 1976; Chapman et al., 1999], and requires functioning NMDA receptors [A.S. Ramoa et al., 2001]. The shape of the cortical map seems to be set before eye opening [Chapman et al., 1996; Kim and Bonhoeffer, 1994], but its magnitude and final shape depend of the visual experience [Sengpiel et al., 1999; Chapman et al., 1996]. The nomenclature often used to discuss such plasticity, in our opinion, is not very useful. Terms such as instructive and permissive plasticity, do little to elucidate the complex issues and do not point toward a mechanism.

One of the major differences between BCM and many other plasticity models is that BCM is not based on competition between synapses for a limited resource. In Sections 2.7.2 and 7.2.2 we have shown how the rate of ocular dominance plasticity, in the BCM theory, increases as the noise level from closed eye increases. This is in contrast with competitive models, where increased activity from the deprived channel reduces the rate of ocular dominance [Blais et al., 1999]. A prevailing notion in the neuroscience community has been that ocular dominance plasticity is dependent on a competition between synapses, due to the much faster disconnection rate in monocular deprivation when compared to binocular deprivation.

This was put to an experimental test by Rittenhouse et. al. (1999) . In order to control activity levels in the deprived eye, a sodium channel blocker TTX was injected into the deprived eye in one group of animals, and saline was injected into the deprived eye of a control group. This injection abolishes action potentials in the eye and markedly reduces activity in the LGN when compared with controls. The result of this experiment, in agreement with the BCM predictions and at odds with the prevailing view, show that ocular dominance plasticity in the TTX group is significantly reduced in comparison with the control group. This indicates that a homosynaptic model, like BCM, is likely to be responsible for ocular dominance plasticity. The experimenters used quantitative methods to assess the ocular dominance shift and were blind as to whether the animals were from the control or TTX group. Why then is binocular deprivation so much slower than monocular deprivation? In context of the BCM theory this is due to the sliding modification threshold, as explained Section 7.2.2 and in Figure 7.6. More recently the same groups of researchers have shown that other ways of reducing activity in the deprived channel such as using a dark patch in addition to lid suture, or using an opaque patch instead of lid suture have results that are consistent with the BCM theory as well[Rittenhouse et al., 2000] (not yet published results).

In contrast, an experiment performed by Chapman et. al. (1986) has produced an ocular dominance shift in the absence of any visual activity. They produced a shift by injecting TTX into one eye, and suturing the other eye. Cats were either left in the normal environment or kept in the dark. In both cases they observe a shift away from the TTX eye and toward the sutured eye. This is taken as evidence for a competitive (heterosynaptic) mechanism, and is difficult to make consistent with the BCM theory of synaptic plasticity, as implemented in previous chapters. In this experiment the ocular dominance class is determined subjectively using hand held stimuli, and the researchers were not blind as to which eye had lid suture and which had TTX. An attempt to replicate this result by Greuel et. al. (1987) did not produce a significant result. The two sets of experiments are methodologically nearly identical, the age differences are minimal and although somewhat different levels of TTX are used in both experiments, both groups have used similar methods to assess inactivation of retinal responses during the deprivation period and recovery during the recording period. We have no explanation of such different results, this experiment should be repeated.

Even if true, the results by Chapman et. al. described above, do not directly contradict those by Rittenhouse et. al. (1999). These two results differ not only in the experimental paradigm tested, but also in that the animals used by Chapman et. al. were significantly younger, and the deprivation period significantly longer(7 vs. 2 days). Nevertheless, these suggest different mechanisms; synaptic competition in the case of Chapman et. al. versus a homosynaptic BCM-like mechanism in the case of Rittenhouse et. al. (1999). It is conceivable that different mechanisms are indeed employed at these different ages or due to the significantly different period of deprivation.

Two recent experiments provide additional evidence against the competitive view of ocular dominance plasticity [Mitchell et al., 2001; Kind et al., 2002]. Both of these examine the recovery from monocular deprivation, under different conditions, and suggest that there is an important role for cooperativity in ocular dominance plasticity. In one, optical imaging is used to image the fraction of visual cortex dominated by either of the two eyes [Kind et al., 2002]. Here recovery is induced by opening the previously deprived eye, but without suturing the previously open eye. In one group the previously open eye is operated on to induce strabismus. More significant recovery is found in the non-strabismic animals; further, the degree of recovery in the strabismic animals is inversely correlated to the degree of strabismus. These results suggest that when the inputs received by the two eyes are more similar, more recovery is induced. Thus cooperation between the two eyes enhances the degree of recovery. But would the rate of recovery be faster if the previously deprived eye gained a competitive advantage over the dominant eye, as would be expected from a competitive mechanism. To test this the rate of recovery is compared between binocular recovery and reverse suture, using a behavioral assay [Mitchell et al., 2001]. The surprising results are that the initial recovery during binocular recovery is more rapid than during reverse suture. This result is clearly at odds with a competitive mechanism. Although, recovery in the reverse suture case is delayed, after it starts it proceeds at a faster rate than binocular recovery. These results are consistent with BCM, as we show in Chapter 7, Figure 7.5. In contrast to recovery in cats, binocular recovery seems ineffective in monkeys [Blakemore et al., 1981]. This species difference might stem from the much smaller receptive fields in primates in combination with a small misalignment between the eyes after MD, which could imply near strabismus during recovery.

Pharmacological manipulations of activity in the visual cortex also effect the outcome of monocular deprivation. A reversible blockade of action potentials in visual cortex, using an infusion of TTX seems to eliminate ocular dominance plasticity [Reiter et al., 1986], and seems to indicate that action potentials are necessary for inducing synaptic plasticity. However, infusion of muscimol, an agonist of the inhibitory neurotransmitter GABA eliminates postsynaptic action potentials but produces an reverse ocular dominance shift [Reiter and Stryker, 1988]. This reverse shift results in the sutured eye becoming dominant. Surprisingly, a reduction of inhibition with bicuculline produces a reduced ocular dominance shift [Ramoa et al., 1988]. They also show that acute bicuculline infusion reduces orientation selectivity of cortical cells. There are additional indications that neurons with reduced selectivity show less of an ocular dominance shift [Rauschecker and Singer, 1979; Rauschecker and Singer, 1981]. This is consistent with BCM for which, as is Chapter 7, reduced selectivity results in a slower OD shift (Section 2.7.2). We expect that it will be possible to account for such various pharmacological manipulations with BCM but that this will require being more explicit about the physiological basis of the BCM variables such as c, d_j and θ_M as well as including inhibitory neurons. We believe the new generation of more detailed physiological models, which are currently being developed[Castellani et al., 2001; Shouval et al., 2002a] are required to explain these effects.

9.3   Conclusion

We trust this work demonstrates not only that theory is possible but, more important, that the interaction of theory with experiment – so fruitful in the physical sciences – is also fruitful in neuroscience. The BCM theory of cortical plasticity has been extensively compared with experiment. Its consequences are in agreement with observations made in visual cortex over the past 50 years. In patterned environments, the stable fixed points of BCM synaptic modification are selective; the theory produces the Hubel-Wiesel orientation selective, binocular receptive fields for normal rearing in natural image environments. It also accounts for the development of receptive fields in various altered visual environments including monocular deprivation, binocular deprivation, reverse suture and binocular recovery. The theory has various subtle and counter-intuitive consequences such as the noise dependence of the loss of response of the closed eye in monocular deprivation. These have suggested new experiments that have tested and confirmed the theoretical predictions.

Experiments to test the assumptions of the BCM theory have uncovered new phenomena. These include long-term depression (LTD) and bi-directional synaptic modification dependent on the depolarization of the post-synaptic cell, as well as the sliding modification threshold dependent on cell activity. These observations are in agreement with the BCM synaptic modification function and provide experimental verification of the postulates of BCM theory. Further, this theory, as all successful theories, clarifies connections between seemingly unrelated concepts and observations. BCM provides links between very different phenomena in different brain regions such as LTD and LTP in hippocampus and reverse suture results in visual cortex. There is a connection between the BCM unsupervised learning algorithm and projection pursuit-a statistical procedure that seeks interesting projections in high dimensional spaces of data points. This suggests the possibility that the biological neuron has evolved in such a way as to perform sophisticated data analysis.. As mentioned above, BCM might be regarded as a phenomenological theory in the sense that its basic variables and assumptions are expected to be defined and refined when it becomes possible to construct them from underlying cellular and molecular mechanisms. (This is analogous to the ideal gas equation $PV = nRT$, its variables defined from underlying kinetic theory or statistical mechanics and the equation itself modified for real gases by additions such as van der Waals forces and the sizes of real molecules.) For BCM we expect that the proper definition of d and c and spontaneous activity, the behavior of for c near (or even below) zero, the precise form of ϕ and θ_M, as well as a host of other issues, will be clarified when the underlying mechanisms are understood.

Such clarifications will very likely be an outcome of the great effort now being devoted to investigations of the cellular and molecular mechanisms that underlie the synaptic changes and the sliding modification threshold required by the BCM theory. Experiment has revealed dependence of synaptic modification on the influx of calcium into cells when accompanied by activate synapses. One underlying calcium dependent mechanism has been proposed to account for the different methods of inducing synaptic plasticity. It is generally believed that various receptors in the postsynaptic membrane play critical roles and that the modification of some of them through such processes as phosphorylation or changes of subunit ratios are responsible for changes in synaptic strength and the sliding modification threshold. The detailed genetic and molecular events that are responsible for these changes as well as those that control transfer of short or intermediate memories into long-term storage (including the interaction of local signals with global modulatory signals as a probable basis for memory consolidation) are now subjects of intense interest. The implication of LTD mechanisms in such pathologies as the Fragile X Syndrome as well as pathologies that might result if the mechanisms responsible for the sliding threshold or for LTD or LTP were impaired are being explored currently and will, no doubt , be extensively investigated in the future. All of these are likely to lead to a more detailed and realistic understanding of synaptic modification and its involvement in various pathologies as well as in 'normal' learning and memory storage.

When we have progressed, in this manner, from ideal to real BCM, the theory will become more complex as well as richer and more realistic (compare our understanding of the role of DNA at present with earliest conceptions in the fifties). This progression is both natural and usual. Complications that could reasonably be added now or in the future, when indicated by experiment, often would be ridiculous, introduced earlier.

. . . .

We hope this book makes clear both the structure of the BCM theory as well as the role it has played in guiding research, elucidating critical questions and suggesting experiments that have led to a deeper understanding of the mechanisms underlying cortical plasticity: the cellular and molecular basis of learning and memory. We hope, also, that this book, with its accompanying software package, *Plasticity*, will make it possible for readers not only to understand and to replicate our results, but to test refinements of their own. If this leads to a new generation of deeper theoretical structures with further illumination of experimental results our effort will have been worthwhile.

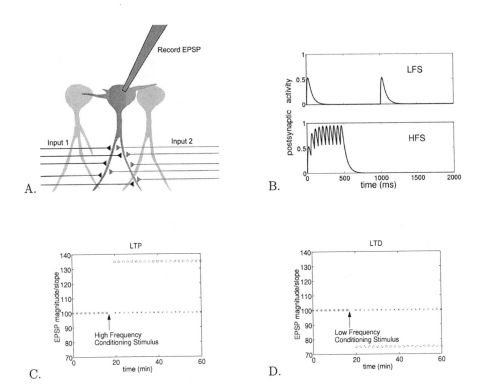

Figure 9.1: Rate based synaptic plasticity. (A) A schematic diagram depicting the arrangement of neurons, stimulating and recording electrodes during rate based induction of synaptic plasticity. (B, top) During low frequency stimulation (LFS) (1 Hz) there is little temporal integration of postsynaptic activity. (b, bottom) A higher frequency (HFS) (50 Hz) produces larger postsynaptic activity due to temporal integration. (C) A schematic description of an LTP experiment. First a baseline is established from two pathways, then a high frequency stimulus is delivered to one pathway. After the conditioning stimulus, the response of the conditioned pathway (o) increases whereas that of the control pathway (x) does not change. (D) A schematic description of an LTD experiment. First a baseline is established from two pathways, then a low frequency stimulus is delivered to one pathway. After the conditioning stimulus, the response of the conditioned pathway (o) decreases whereas that of the control pathway (x) does not change.

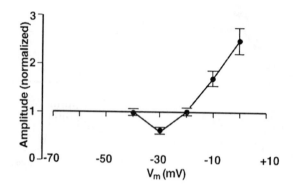

Figure 9.2: Pairing induced synaptic plasticity. Here we show an LTP/LTD curve obtained by Ngezahayo et. al. (2000). The sign and magnitude of synaptic plasticity depends on the level of postsynaptic depolarization. Below a lower threshold no plasticity is induced, above this threshold LTD is induced, and at higher levels of depolarization LTP is induced.

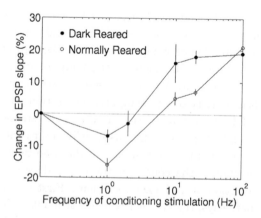

Figure 9.3: The sliding modification threshold (experimental), reproduced from [Kirkwood, et.al. 1996]

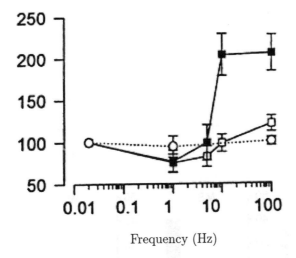

Figure 9.4: Frequency plasticity curves obtained by Tang et.al. 1999. Shown is the selective enhancement of 10-100 Hz-induced potentiation in transgenic mice (filled squares) compared with wild-type mice (open squares).

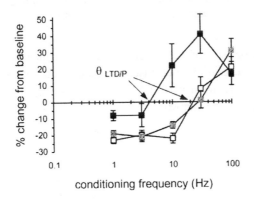

Figure 9.5: Frequency plasticity curves obtained by Wang and Wagner (1999) for naive and prestimulated pathways. The LTP/LTD curves in slices that have been previously stimulated, in both the conditioning (open squares) and control (thatched squares) pathways are shifted to the right in comparison to the control pathway (black squares).

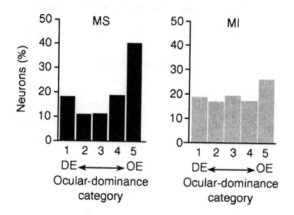

Figure 9.6: Comparison of ocular dominance distribution resulting from two days of MD, in two distinct cases monocular lid suture (MS) on left and monocular inactivation with TTX (MI) on the right. MS produces a significantly larger shift than MI.

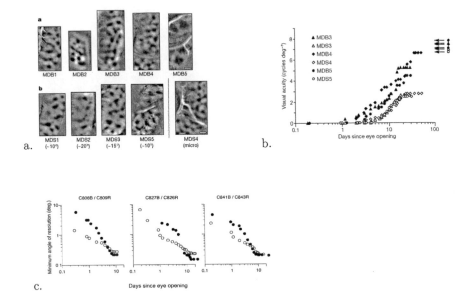

Figure 9.7: Cooperativity in ocular dominance plasticity. (a)Optical imaging of ocular dominance maps during binocular recovery. On the top normal binocular recovery and on the bottom recovery when artificial strabismus is induced prior to recovery. Significantly more recovery is observed in normal binocular recovery. (b) Acuity, examined with a behavioral assay, in deprived eye after binocular recovery for concordant binocular vision (filled symbols) and strabismic recovery (open symbols). (c) Comparison of recovery from monocular deprivation with binocular vision (open symbols) and reverse suture (full symbols), in matched litter mates. Initial recovery for binocular vision is more rapid than during reverse suture.

Bibliography

Abbott, L. F., Varela, J. A., Sen, K., and Nelson, S. B. (1997). Synaptic depression and cortical gain control. *Science*, pages 220–223.

Abeles, M. (1981). *Corticonics*. Cambridge University Press, Boston.

Abraham, W. (1996). Induction of heterosynaptic and homosynaptic ltd in hippocampal sub-regions in vivo. *J Physiol Paris.*, 90:305–6.

Abraham, W., Mason-Parker, S., Bear, M., Webb, S., and Tate, W. (2001). Heterosynaptic metaplasticity in the hippocampus in vivo: a bcm-like modifiable threshold for ltp. *Proc Natl Acad Sci*, 98:10924–9.

Abraham, W. C. and Bear, M. F. (1996). Metaplasticity: the plasticity of synaptic plasticity. *Trends Neurosci.*, 19(4):126–30.

Adelson, E. H. and Bergen, J. R. (1985). Spatiotemporal energy models for the perception of motion. *Science*, 275:220–222.

Alberts, B., Bray, D., Lewis, J., Raff, M., Roberts, K., and Watson, J. D. (1994). *Molecular Biology of the Cell*. Garland Publishers.

Amari, S., Cichocki, A., and Yang, H. H. (1996). A new learning algorithm for blind signal separation. In Tesauro, G., Touretzky, D., and Leen, T., editors, *Advances in Neural Information Processing Systems*, volume 8, pages 757–763. MIT Press.

Artola, A. and Singer, W. (1992). Long-term potentiation and nmda receptors in rat visual cortex. *Nature*, 330:649–652.

Artun, O. B., Shouval, H. Z., and Cooper, L. N. (1998). The effect of dynamic synapses on spatio-temporal receptive fields in visual cortex. *Proc. Natl. Acad. Sci*, 95:11976–11980.

A.S. Ramoa, A. S., Mower, A., Liao, D., and Jafri, S. (2001). Suppression of cortical nmda receptor function prevents development of orientation selectivity in the primary visual cortex. *J. Neurosci.*, 21:4299–309.

Atick, J. J. (1992). Could information theory provide an ecological theory of sensory processing? *Network*, 3:213–251.

Atick, J. J. and Redlich, A. (1992). What does the retina know about natural scenes. *Neural Computation*, 4:196–211.

Banke, T. G., Bowie1, D., Lee, H.-K., Huganir, R. L., Schousboe, A., and Traynelis, S. F. (2000). Control of GluR1 AMPA receptor function by cAMP-Dependent protein kinase. *Journal of Neuroscience*, 20(1):89–102.

Barlow, H. and Levick, R. (1965). The mechanism of direction selectivity in the rabbit's retina. *Journal of Physiology*, 173:477–504.

Barlow, H. B. (1961). Possible principles underlying the transformations of sensory messages. In Rosenblith, W., editor, *Sensory Communication*, pages 217–234. MIT Press, Cambridge, MA.

Barlow, H. B. (1985). Cerebral cortex as model builder. In Rose, D. and Dobson, V. G., editors, *Models of the visual cortex*, pages 37–46. Wiley, New York.

Barlow, H. B. (1989). Unsupervised learning. *Neural Computation*, 1(3):295–311.

Barlow, H. B. (1990). Conditions for versatile learning, helmholtz's unconscious inference, and the task of perception. *Vision Research*, 30:1561–1571.

Barlow, H. B. (1994). What is the computational goal of the neocortex. In Koch, C. and Davis, J. L., editors, *Large Scale Neuronal Theories of the Brain*. MIT Press.

Barlow, H. B., Kaushal, T. P., and Mitchison, G. J. (1989). Finding minimum entropy codes. *Neural Computation*, 1(3):412–423.

Barron, A. R. and Barron, R. L. (1988). Statistical learning networks: A unifying view. In Wegman, E., editor, *Computing Science and Statistics: Proc. 20th Symp. Interface*, pages 192–203. American Statistical Association, Washington, DC.

Bear, M. F., Cooper, L. N., and Ebner, F. F. (1987). A physiological basis for a theory of synapse modification. *Science*, 237:42–48.

Bear, M. F., Gu, Q., Kleinschmidt, A., and Singer, W. (1990). Disruption of experience-dependent synaptic modification in the striate cortex by infusion of an NMDA receptor antagonist. *Journal of Neuroscience*, 10:909–925.

Bear, M. F. and Malenka, R. C. (1994). Synaptic plasticity: LTP and LTD. *Curr. Opin. Neurobiol.*, 4:389–399.

Bell, A. J. and Sejnowski, T. J. (1995). An information-maximization approach to blind separation and blind deconvolution. *Neural Computation*, 7(6):1129–1159.

Bell, A. J. and Sejnowski, T. J. (1997). The independent components of natural scenes are edge filters. *Vision Research*, 37(23):3327–3338.

Bellman, R. E. (1961). *Adaptive Control Processes*. Princeton University Press, Princeton, NJ.

Bhalla, U. S. (2002). Biochemical signaling networks decode temporal patterns of synaptic input. *J. Comput. Neurosci.*, 13:49–62.

Bichsel, M. and Seitz, P. (1989). Minimum class entropy: A maximum information approach to layered networks. *Neural Networks*, 2:133–141.

Bienenstock, E. L., Cooper, L. N., and Munro, P. W. (1982). Theory for the development of neuron selectivity: orientation specificity and binocular interaction in visual cortex. *Journal of Neuroscience*, 2:32–48.

Blais, B., Cooper, L. N., and Shouval, H. (2000). Formation of direction selectivity in natural scene environments. *Neural Computation*, 12(5).

Blais, B., Shouval, H., and Cooper, L. N. (1996). Dynamics of synaptic plasticity: A comparison between models and experimental results in visual cortex. In *The Neurobiology of Computation: Proceedings of the fifth annual Computation and Neural Systems conference*. Plenum Publishing Corporation.

Blais, B., Shouval, H., and Cooper, L. N. (1999). The role of presynaptic activity in monocular deprivation: Comparison of homosynaptic and heterosynaptic mechanisms. *Proc. Natl. Acad. Sci.*, 96:1083–1087.

Blais, B. S. (1998). *The Role of the Environment in Synaptic Plasticity: Towards an Understanding of Learning and Memory*. PhD thesis, Brown University, Institute for Brain and Neural Systems; Dr. Leon N Cooper, Thesis Supervisor.

Blakemore, C. (1976). The conditions required for the maintenance of binocularity in the kitten's visual cortex. *Journal of Physiology*, 261(2):423–44.

Blakemore, C. and Cooper, G. F. (1970). Development of the brain depends on the visual environment. *Nature, Lond.*, 228:477–478.

Blakemore, C. and van Sluyters, R. R. (1974). Reversal of the physiological effects of monocular deprivation in kittens: further evidence for sensitive period. *J. Physiol. Lond.*, 248:663–716.

Blakemore, C. and Van-Sluyters, R. R. (1975). Innate and environmental factors in the development of the kitten's visual cortex. *J. Physiol.*, 248:663–716.

Blakemore, C., vital Durand, F., and Garey, L. (1981). Recovery from monocular deprivation in the monkey. i. reversal of physiological effects in the visual cortex. *Proc. R. Soc. London B*, 213:399–423.

Bliss, T. V. P. and Lømo, T. (1973). Long-lasting potentiation of synaptic transmission in the dentate area of the anesthetized rabbit following stimulation of the perforant path. *J. Physiol. , London*, 232.

Bonhoeffer, T. and Grinvald, A. (1991). Iso-orientation domains in cat visual cortex are arranged in pinwheel-like patterns. *Nature*, 353:429–431.

Bryan, J. G. (1951). The generalized discriminant function: mathematical foundations and computational routines. *Harvard Educational Review*, 21:90–95.

Buisseret, P. and Imbert, M. (1976). Visual cortical cells: their developmental properties in normal and dark reared kittens. *J. Physiol., Lond.*, 255:511–525.

Burr, D. (1981). A dynamic model for image registration. *Computer Graphics and Image Processing*, 15:102–112.

Cardoso, J.-F. and Laheld, B. (1996). Equivariant adaptive source separation.

Carmignoto, G. and Vicini, S. (1992). Activity dependent increase in NMDA receptor responses during development of visual cotex. *Science*, 258:1007–1011.

Carpenter, R. (1977). *Movements of the Eyes*. Pion, London.

Castellani, G. C., Intrator, N., Shouval, H., and Cooper, L. N. (1999). Solutions of the BCM learning rule in a network of lateral interacting linear neurons. *Network: Computation in Neural Systems*, 10:111–121.

Castellani, G. C., Quinlan, E. M., Cooper, L. N., and Shouval, H. Z. (2001). A biophysical model of bidirectional synaptic plasticity: Dependence on ampa and nmda receptors. *Proc. Natal. Acad. Sci.*, 98:12772–77.

Chance, F. S., Nelson, S. B., and Abbott, L. F. (1998). Synaptic depression and the temporal response characteristics of V1 cells. *Journal of Neuroscience*, 18:4785–4799.

Chapman, B., Godecke, I., and Bonhoeffer, T. (1999). Development of orientation preference in the mammalian visual cortex. *J. Neurobiol*, 41:18–24.

Chapman, B., Jacobson, M. D., Reiter, H. O., and Stryker, M. P. (1986). Ocular dominance shift in kitten visual cortex caused by imbalance in retinal electrical activity. *Nature*, 324:154–156.

Chapman, B., Stryker, M. P., and Bonhoeffer, T. (1996). Development of orientation preference maps in ferret primary visual cortex. *Journal of Neuroscience*, 16:6443–6453.

Chen, W. R., Lee, S., Kato, K., Spencer, D. D., Shepherd, G. M., and Williamson, A. (1996). Long-term modifications of synaptic efficacy in the human inferior and middle temporal cortex. *Proceedings of the National Academy of Science*, 93:8011–8015.

Cho, K., Aggelton, J., Brown, M., and Bashir, Z. I. (2001). An experimental test of the role of postsynaptic calcium levels in determining synaptic strength using peririhinal cortex in rat. *J. Physiol.*, 532:459–66.

Clothiaux, E. E., N Cooper, L., and Bear, M. F. (1991). Synaptic plasticity in visual cortex: Comparison of theory with experiment. *Journal of Neurophysiology*, 66:1785–1804.

Collingridge, G., Kehl, S., and McLennan, H. (1983). Excitatory amino acids in synaptic transmission in the schaffer collateral-commissural pathway of the rat hippocampus. *J Physiol.*, 334:33–46.

Comon, P. (1994). Independent component analysis, a new concept? *Signal Processing*, 36:287–314.

Cooper, L. N. (1973). A possible organization of animal memory and learning. In *Proceedings of the Nobel Symposium on Collective Properties of Physical Systems, Aspensagarden, Sweden*, pages 252–264. New York: Academic Press.

Cooper, L. N., Liberman, F., and Oja, E. (1979). A theory for the acquisition and loss of neurons specificity in visual cortex. *Biol. Cyb.*, 33:9–28.

Cooper, L. N. and Scofield, C. L. (1988). Mean-field theory of a neural network. *Proceedings of the National Academy of Science*, 85:1973–1977.

Cormier, R., Greenwood, A. C., and Connor, J. A. (2001). Bidirectional synaptic plasticity correlated with the magnitude of dendritic calcium transients above a threshold. *J. Neurophysiol.*, 85:399–406.

Cover, T. and Thomas, J. (1991). *Elements of Information Theory*. Wiley.

Crair, M. C., Gillespie, D. C., and M.P, M. P. S. (1998). The role of visual experience in the development of columns in cat visual cortex. *Science*, 279:566–70.

Crowley, J. and Katz, L. (2002). Ocular dominance development revisited. *Curr Opin Neurobiol*, 12.

Cummings, J., Mulkey, R., Nicoll, R., and Malenka, R. (1996). Ca2+ signaling requirements for long-term depression in the hippocampus. *Neuron*, 16:825–33.

Cynader, M., Berman, N., and Hein, A. (1973). Cats reared in stroboscopic illumination: effects on receptive fields in visual cortex. *Proceedings of the National Academy of Sciences*, 70:1353–1354.

Cynader, M., Berman, N., and Hein, A. (1975). Cats raised in a one dimensional world:effects on receptive fields in visual cortex and superior colliculus. *Experimental Brain Research*, 22:267–280.

Cynader, M. and Chernenko, G. (1976). Abolition of direction selectivity in the visual cortex of the cat. *Science*, 193:504–505.

Cynader, M. and Mitchell, D. (1977). Monocular astigmatism effects on kitten visual cortical development. *Nature*, 270:177–178.

d'Alché Buc, F. and Nadal, J.-P. (1996). Redundancy reduction and independent component analysis: Conditions on cumulants and adaptive approaches.

Dayan, P. and Abbott, L. F. (2001). *Theoretical Neuroscience: Computatonal and Mathematical Modeling of Neural Systems*. MIT Press, Cambridge, Massachusetts.

Dayan, P. and Goodhill, G. (1992). Perturbing hebbian rules. In *Advances in Neural Information Processing Systems 4*.

Deangelis, G. C., Ohzawa, I., and Freeman, R. C. (1995). Receptive field dynamics in the central visual pathway. *Trends in Neuroscience*, 18:451:458.

Delfosse, N. and Loubaton, P. (1995). Adaptive blind separation of independent sources: a deflation approach. *Signal Processing*, 45:59–83.

Diaconis, P. and Freedman, D. (1984). Asymptotics of graphical projection pursuit. *Annals of Statistics*, 12:793–815.

Dotan, Y. and Intrator, N. (1998). Multimodality exploration in training an unsupervised projection pursuit neural network. *IEEE Transactions on Neural Networks*, 9(3):464–472.

Duda, R. O. and Hart, P. E. (1973). *Pattern Classification and Scene Analysis*. John Wiley, New York.

Dudek, S. M. and Bear, M. F. (1992). Homosynaptic long-term depression in area CA1 of hippocampus and the effects on NMDA receptor blockade. *Proc. Natl. Acad. Sci.*, 89:4363–4367.

Dudek, S. M. and Bear, M. F. (1993). Bidirectional homosynaptic modifications in hippocampus in vitro. *Journal of Neuroscience*, 13:2910–2918.

Duffy, F. H., Sonodgrass, S. R., Burchfiel, J. L., and Conway, J. L. (1976). Biculculine reversal of deprivation amblyopia in the cat. *Nature*, 260:256–257.

Engert, F. and Bonhoeffer, T. (1997). Synapse specificity of long-term potentiation breaks down at short distances. *Nature*, 388:279–84.

Erwin, E. and Miller, K. D. (1995). Modeling joint development of ocular dominance and orientation maps in primary visual cortex. In *Proceedings of the Computation and Neural Systems*.

Erwin, E. and Miller, K. D. (1998). Correlation-based development of ocularly matched orientation and ocular dominance maps: determination of required input activities. *J Neurosci.*, 18(23):9870–95.

Erwin, E., Obermayer, K., and Schulten, K. (1995). Models of orientation and ocular dominace in visual cortex. *Neural Computation*, 7.3:425–468.

Feidler, J. C., Saul, A. B., Murthy, A., and Humphrey, A. L. (1997). Hebbian learning and the development of direction selectivity: the role of geniculate response timings. *Network: Computational Neural Systems*, 8:195–214.

Feldman, D. E. (2000). Timing-based ltp and ltd at vertical inputs to layer ii/iii pyramidal cells in rat barrel cortex. *Neuron*, 27:45–56.

Feldman, D. E., Nicoll, R. A., Malenka, R. C., and Issac, J. T. (1998). Long-term depression at thalamocortical synapses in developing rat somatosensory cortex. *Neuron*, 21:347–57.

Feng, J., Pan, H., and Roychowdhury, V. P. (1996). On neurodynamics with limiter function and linsker's developmental model. *Neural Computation*, 8:1003 – 1021.

Field, D. J. (1987). Relations between the statistics of natural images and the response properties of cortical cells. *Journal of the Optical Society of America*, 4:2379–2394.

Field, D. J. (1994). What is the goal of sensory coding. *Neural Computation*, 6:559–601.

Field, D. J. and Brady, N. (1997). Wavelets, blur and the sources of variability in the amplitude spectra of natural scenes. *Vision Research*, 37:3367–3383.

Fisher, R. A. (1936). The use of multiple measurements in taxonomic problems. *Annals of Eugenics*, 7:179–188.

Fitzsimonds, R., Song, H., and Poo, M. (1997). Propagation of activity-dependent synaptic depression in simple neural networks. *Nature*, 388:439–48.

Foldia, P. (1989). Adaptive network for optimal linear feature extraction. *In Proc. IJCNN, Washington D.C.*, pages 401–406.

Freeman, R., Mallach, R., and Hartley, S. (1981). Responsivity of normal kitten striate cortex deteriorates after brief binocular deprivation. *Journal of Neurophysiology*, 45(6):1074–1084.

Freeman, R. and Olson, C. (1982). Brief periods of monocular deprivation in kittens: Effects of delay prior to physiological study. *Journal of Neurophysiology*, 47(2):139–150.

Frégnac, Y. and Imbert, M. (1978). Early development of visual cortical cells in normal and dark reared kittens: relationship between orientation selectivity and ocular dominance. *J. Physiol., Lond.*, 278:27–44.

Frégnac, Y. and Imbert, M. (1984). Development of neuronal selectivity in the primary visual cortex of the cat. *Physiol. Rev.*, 64:325–434.

Friedman, J. H. (1987). Exploratory projection pursuit. *Journal of the American Statistical Association*, 82:249–266.

Friedman, J. H. and Tukey, J. W. (1974). A projection pursuit algorithm for exploratory data analysis. *IEEE Transactions on Computers*, C(23):881–889.

Fyfe, C. and Baddeley, R. (1995). Finding compact and sparse-distributed representations of visual images. *Network*, 6:333–344.

Geman, S. (1977). Averaging for random differential equations. In Bharucha-Reid, A. T., editor, *Approximate Solution of Random Equations*, pages 49–85. North Holland, New York.

Geman, S. and Bienenstock, E. (1995). Compositional vision. Talk given at the Object Features for Visual Shape Representation workshop, NIPS.

Geman, S., Bienenstock, E., and Doursat, R. (1992). Neural networks and the bias/variance dilemma. *Neural Computation*, 4(1):1–58.

Girolami, M. and Fyfe, C. (1996). Negentropy and kurtosis as projection pursuit indices provide generalised ica algorithms. Preprint.

Goda, Y. and Stevens, C. (1998). Readily releasable pool size changes associated with long term depression. *Proc Natl Acad Sci*, 95:1283–8.

Gödecke, I. and Bonhoeffer, T. (1996). Development of identical orientation maps for two eyes without common visual experience. *Nature*, 379:251–254.

Gödecke, I., Kim, D.-S., Bonhoeffer, T., and Singer, W. (1997). Development of orientation preference maps in area 18 of kitten visual cortex. *European Journal of Neuroscience*, 9:1754–1762.

Goldberg, D. H., Shouval, H. Z., and Cooper, L. N. (1999). Lateral connectivity as a scaffold for developing orientation preference maps. *Neurocomputing*, 26-27:381–387.

Greuel, J. M., Luhmann, H. J., and Singer, W. (1987). Evidence for a threshold in experience-dependent long-term changes of kitten visual cortex. *Devel. Brain Research*, 34:141–149.

Hammond, P. (1978). Directional tuning of complex cells in area 17 of the feline visual cortex. *J. Physiol. (Lond)*, 275:479–491.

Harman, H. H. (1967). *Modern Factor Analysis*. University of Chicago Press, Second Edition, Chicago and London.

Harris, E., Ganong, A., and Cotman, C. (1984). Long-term potentiation in the hippocampus involves activation of n-methyl-d-aspartate receptors. *Brain Res.*, 323:132–7.

Hebb, D. O. (1949). *The Organization of Behavior; a neuropsychological theory*. Wiley, New York.

Hinton, G. and Nowlan, S. (1990). The bootstrap widrow-hoff rule as a cluster formation algorithm. *Neural Computation*, 2(3).

Holland, L. L. and Wagner, J. J. (1998). Primed facilitation of homosynaptic long term depression and depotentiation in rat hippocampus. *Journal of Neuroscience*, 18(3):883–894.

Huang, Y. Y., Colino, A., Selig, D. K., and Malenka, R. C. (1992). The influence of prior synaptic activity on the induction of long-term potentiation. *Science*, 255:730–733.

Hubel, D. H. and Wiesel, T. N. (1959). Receptive fields of single neurons in the cat striate cortex. *J. Physiol. (London)*, 148:509–591.

Hubel, D. H. and Wiesel, T. N. (1962). Receptive fields, binocular interaction and functional architecture in the cat's visual cortex. *J. Physiol*, 160:106–154.

Hubel, D. H. and Wiesel, T. N. (1963). Receptive fields of cells in stiate cortex of very yong, visually inexperienced kittens. *J. Neurophysiol.*, 26:994–1002.

Hubel, D. H. and Wiesel, T. N. (1965). Binocular interactions in striate cortex of kittens reared with artificial squint. *J. Neurophysiol.*, 28:1041–1059.

Hubel, D. H., Wiesel, T. N., and Levay, S. (1977). Plasticity of ocular dominance columns in monkey striate cortex. *Phil. Trans. Roy. Soc. London B.*, 278:377–409.

Huber, K., Roder, J., and Bear, M. (2001). Chemical induction of mglur5- and protein synthesis–dependent long-term depression in hippocampal area ca1. *J Neurophysiol*, 86:321–5.

Huber, P. J. (1985). Projection pursuit. (with discussion). *The Annals of Statistics*, 13:435–475.

Humphrey, A. L. and Saul, A. B. (1998). Strobe rearing reduces direction selectivity in area 17 by altering spatiotemporal receptive-field structure. *Journal of Neurophysiology*, 80:2991–3004.

Humphrey, A. L., Saul, A. B., and Feidler, J. C. (1998). Strobe rearing prevents the convergence of inputs with different response timings onto area 17 simple cells. *Journal of Neurophysiology*, 80:3005–3020.

Huynh, Q., Cooper, L. N., Intrator, N., and Shouval, H. (1996). Classification of underwater mammals using feature extraction based on time-frequency analysis and BCM theory. Technical report, Institute for Brain and Neural Systems, Brown University.

Hyvarinen, A. (1998). Independent component analysis by minimization of mutual information. *?*

Hyvarinen, A. and Oja, E. (1996). A fast fixed-point algorithm for independent component analysis. *Int. Journal of Neural Systems*, 7(6):671–687.

Hyvarinen, A. and Oja, E. (1997). A fast fixed-point algorithm for independent component analysis. *Neural Computation*, 9(7):1483–1492.

Imbert, M. and Buisseret, P. (1975). Receptive field characteristics and plastic properties of visual cortical cells in kittens reared with or without visual experience. *Exp. Brain Res.*, 22:25–36.

Intrator, N. (1990a). An averaging result for random differential equations. Technical Report 54, Center For Neural Science, Brown University.

Intrator, N. (1990b). A neural network for feature extraction. In Touretzky, D. S. and Lippmann, R. P., editors, *Advances in Neural Information Processing Systems*, volume 2, pages 719–726. Morgan Kaufmann, San Mateo, CA.

Intrator, N. (1996). Neuronal goals: Efficient coding and coincidence detection. In Amari, S., Xu, L., Chan, L. W., King, I., and Leung, K. S., editors, *Proceedings of ICONIP Hong Kong. Progress in Neural Information Processing*, volume 1, pages 29–34, Berlin, Germany. Springer.

Intrator, N. and Cooper, L. N. (1992). Objective function formulation of the BCM theory of visual cortical plasticity: Statistical connections, stability conditions. *Neural Networks*, 5:3–17.

Intrator, N., Reisfeld, D., and Yeshurun, Y. (1996). Face recognition using a hybrid supervised/unsupervised neural network. *Pattern Recognition Letters*, 17:67–76.

Jackson, J. D. (1975). *Classical Electrodynamics*. Wiley.

Jacobson, M. D., Reiter, H. O., Chapman, B., and Stryker, M. P. (1985). Ocular dominance shift in kitten area 17 in the absence of patterned visual experience. *Soc. Neurosci. Abstr.*, 11:102.

Jahr, C. E. and Stevens, C. F. (1990). Voltage dependence of nmda-activated macroscopic conductances predicted by single channel kinetics. *The Journal of Neuroscience*, 10:3178–3182.

Jaynes, E. T. (1957a). Information theory and statistical mechanics I. *Phys. Rev.*, 106:620–530.

Jaynes, E. T. (1957b). Information theory and statistical mechanics II. *Phys. Rev.*, 108:171–190.

Jaynes, E. T. (1982). *Papers on probaility, statistics and statistical physics*. Reidel, Dordrecht.

Jones, J. P. and Palmer, L. A. (1987). The two-dimensional spatial structure of simple receptive fields in cat striate cortex. *Journal of Neurophysiology*, 58(6):1187–1258.

Jones, M. C. (1983). The projection pursuit algorithm for exploratory data analysis. Unpublished Ph.D. dissertation, University of Bath, School of Mathematics.

Jones, M. C. and Sibson, R. (1987). What is projection pursuit? (with discussion). *J. Roy. Statist. Soc.*, Ser. A(150):1–36.

Jutten, C. and Herault, J. (1991). Blind separation of sources, part I: An adaptive algorithm based on enuromimetic archtecture. *Signal Processing*, 24:1–10.

Katsuki, H., Kaneko, S., Tajima, A., and Satoh, M. (1991). Separate mechanisms of long-term potentiation in two input systems to ca3 pyramidal neurons of rat hippocampal slices as revealed by the whole-cell patch-clamp technique. *Neurosci Res.*, 12:393–402.

Kendall, M. and Stuart, A. (1977). *The Advanced Theory of Statistics*, volume 1. MacMillan Publishing, New York.

Kim, D.-S. and Bonhoeffer, T. (1994). Reverse occlusion leads to precise restoration of orientation maps in visual cortex. *Nature*, 370:370–372.

Kind, P., Mitchell, D., Ahmed, B., Blakemore, C., Bonhoeffer, T., and F, F. S. (2002). Correlated binocular activity guides recovery from monocular deprivation. *Nature*, 416:430–3.

Kirkwood, A. and Bear, M. F. (1994a). Hebb synapses in visual cortex. *The Journal of Neuroscience*, 14(3):1634–1645.

Kirkwood, A. and Bear, M. F. (1994b). Homosynaptic long-term depression in the visual cortex. *The Journal of Neuroscience*, 14(5):3404–3412.

Kirkwood, A., Rioult, M. G., and Bear, M. F. (1996). Experience-dependent modification of synaptic plasticity in visual cortex. *Nature*, 381:526–528.

Kleinschmidt, A., Bear, M. F., and Singer, W. (1987). Blockade of NMDA receptors disrupts experience-dependent plasticity o f kitten striate cortex. *Science*, 238:355–358.

Kohonen, T. (1982). Self-organization of topologically correct feature maps. *Biological Cybernetics*, 43:59–69.

Kohonen, T. (1984). *Self-Organization and Associative Memory*. Springer-Verlag, Berlin.

Kruskal, J. B. (1969). Toward a practical method which helps uncover the structure of the set of multivariate observations by finding the linear transformation which optimizes a new 'index of condensation'. In Milton, R. C. and Nelder, J. A., editors, *Statistical Computation*, pages 427–440. Academic Press, New York.

Kruskal, J. B. (1972). Linear transformation of multivariate data to reveal clustering. In Shepard, R. N., Romney, A. K., and Nerlove, S. B., editors, *Multidimensional Scaling: Theory and Application in the Behavioral Sciences, I, Theory*, pages 179–191. Seminar Press, New York and London.

Kuffler, S. (1953). Discharge patterns and functional organization of the mamallian retina. *Journal of Physiology*, 16:37–68.

Kullback, S. (1959). *Information Theory and Statistics*. John Wiley, New York.

Law, C. and Cooper, L. (1994). Formation of receptive fields according to the BCM theory in realistic visual environments. *Proceedings National Academy of Sciences*, 91:7797–7801.

Lebel, D., Grossman, Y., and Barkai, E. (2001). Olfactory learning modifies predisposition for long-term potentiation and long-term depression induction in the rat piriform (olfactory) cortex. *Cereb Cortex.*, 11:485–9.

Lee, H.-K., Barbarosie, M., Kameyama, K., Bear, M. F., and Huganir, R. L. (2000). Regulation of distinct AMPA receptor phosphorilation sites during bidirectional synaptic plasticity. *Nature*, 405:955–9.

Levental, A. G. and Hirsh, H. V. B. (1980). Receptive field properties of different classes of neurons in visual cortex of normal and dark-reared cats. *Journal of Neurophysiology*, 43:1111–1132.

Liao, D., Hessler, N. A., and Malinow, R. (1995). Activation of postsynaptically silent synapses during pairing-induced LTP. *Nature*, 375:400–404.

Linsenmeier, R., Frishman, L. J., Jakiela, H. G., and Enroth-Cugell, C. (1982). Receptive field properties of X and Y cells in the cat retina derived from contrast sensitivity measurments. *Vision Research*, 22:1173–1183.

Linsker, R. (1986a). From basic network principles to neural architecture: emergence of orientation columns. *PNAS*, 83:8779–8783.

Linsker, R. (1986b). From basic network principles to neural architecture: Emergence of orientation selective cells. *PNAS*, 83:7508–7512,8390–8394,8779–8783.

Linsker, R. (88). Self-organization in a perceptual network. *Computer*, March 1988:105–117.

Lisman, J. A. (1989). A mechanism for the Hebb and the anti-Hebb processes underlying learning and memory. *Proceedings of the National Academy of Science*, 86:9574–9578.

Liu, Y. and Shouval, H. Z. (1994). Localized principal components of natural images - an analytic solution. *Network*, 5:317–324.

MacKay, D. J. and Miller, K. D. (1990). Analysis of linsker's simulation of Hebbian rules. *Neural Computation*, 1:173–187.

MacKay, D. J. C. and Miller, K. D. (1994). The role of constraints in Hebbian learning. *Neural Computation*, 6:100–126.

Maex, R. and Orban, G. A. (1996). Model circuit of spiking neurons generating directional selectivity in simple cells. *Journal of Neurophysiology*, 75:1515–1545.

Malenka, R. and Nicoll, R. (1999). Long-term potentiation–a decade of progress? *Science*, 285:1870–4.

Malinow, R. and Malenka, R. (2002). AMPA receptor trafficking and synaptic plasticity. *Ann. Rev. Neurosci.*, 25:103–26.

Markram, H., Lübke, J., Frotscher, M., and Sakmann, B. (1997). Regulation of synaptic efficacy by coincidence of postsynaptic aps and epsps. *Science*, 275:213–215.

Mastronarde, D. N. (1987). Two classes of single input X-cells in cat lateral geniculate nucleus. Cat lateral geniculate nucleus. I. Receptive field properties and classification of cells. *Journal of Neurophysiology*, 57:357–380.

Mayford, M., Wang, J., Kandel, E., and O'Dell, T. (1995). CaMKII regulates the frequency-response function of hippocampal synapses for the production of both LTD and LTP. *Cell*, 81:1–20.

McClelland, J., Rumelhart, D., and the PDP Research Group (1986). *Parallel Distributed Processing: Explorations in the Microstructure of Cognition*, volume 2. MIT Press, Cambridge.

Miller, K. D. (1992). Development of orientation columns via competition between on- anf off-center inputs. *NeuroReport*, 3:73–76.

Miller, K. D. (1994). A model for the development of simple cell receptive fields and the orderd arrangement of orientation columns through activity-dependent competition between on- and off-center inputs. *J. Neurosci.*, 14:409–441.

Miller, K. D., Keller, J., and Stryker, M. P. (1989). Ocular dominance column development: Analysis and simulation. *Science*, 240:605–615.

Miller, K. D. and MacKay, D. J. C. (1994). The role of constraints in Hebbian learning. *Neural Computation*, 6:98–124.

Mioche, L. and Singer, W. (1989). Chronic recording from single sites of kitten striate cortex during experience-dependent modification of synaptic receptive-field properties. *J. Neurophysiol.*, 62:185–197.

Mitchell, D., Gingras, G., and Kind, P. (2001). Initial recovery of vision after early monocular deprivation in kittens is faster when both eyes are open. *Proc Natl Acad Sci*, 98:11662–7.

Movshon, J. A. (1976). Reversal of the physiological effects of monocular deprivation in the kitten's visual cortex. *J. Physiol., Lond.*, 261:125–174.

Mulkey, R. and Malenka, R. C. (1992). Mechanisms underlying induction of homosynaptic long-term depression in area ca1 of the hippocampus. *Neuron*, 9:967–75.

Mumford, D. (1995). Thalamus. In Arbib, M., editor, *The Handbook of Brain Theory and Neural Networks*, pages 981–983. MIT Press.

Murphy, G. G. and Glanzman, D. (1997). Mediation of classical conditioning in aplysia californica by long-term potentiation of sensorimotor synapses. *Science*, 278:467–71.

Nass, M. N. and Cooper, L. N. (1975). A theory for the development of feature detecting cells in visual cortex. *Biol. Cyb.*, 19:1–18.

Neveu, D. and Zucker, R. (1996). Long-lasting potentiation and depression without presynaptic activity. *J Neurophysiol*, 75:2157–60.

Ngezahayo, A., Schachner, M., and Artola, A. (2000). Synaptic activity modulates the induction of bidirectional synaptic changes in adult mouse hippocampus. *J Neurosci.*, 20:2451–8.

Obermayer, K. and Blasdel, G. G. (1997). Singularities in primate orientation maps. *Neural Computation*, 9:555–575.

Oja, E. (1982). A simplified neuron model as a principal component analyzer. *Journal of Mathematical Biology*, 15:267–273.

Oja, E. (1992). Principal components, minor components, and linear neural networks. *Neural Networks*, 5:927–935.

Oliet, S., Malenka, R., and Nicoll, R. (1997). Two distinct forms of long-term depression coexist in ca1 hippocampal pyramidal cells. *Neuron*, 18:969–82.

Olshausen, B. A. and Field, D. J. (1996a). Emergence of simple cell receptive field properties by learning a sparse code for natural images. *Nature*, 381:607–609.

Olshausen, B. A. and Field, D. J. (1996b). Emergence of simple cell receptive field properties by learning a sparse code for natural images. *Nature*, 381:607–609.

Olshausen, B. A. and Field, D. J. (1996c). Natural image statistics and efficient coding. *Network*.

Orban, G. A. (1984). *Neuronal Operations in the Visual Cortex*. Springer Verlag.

Papoulis, A. (1984). *Probability, Random Variables, and Stochastic Processes*. McGraw-Hill.

Perez, R., Glass, L., and Shlaer, R. J. (1975). Development of specificity in the cat visual cortex. *J. Math. Biol.*, 1:275.

Pettigerew, J. D. and Freeman, R. D. (1973). Visual experience without lines: effects on developing cortical neurons. *Science*, 182:599–601.

Philpot, B. D., Sekhar, A. K., Shouval, H. Z., and Bear, M. F. (2001). Visual experience and deprivation bidirectionally modify the composition and function of NMDA receptors in visual cortex. *Neuron*, 29:157–69.

Piepenbrock, C., Ritter, H., and Obermayer, K. (1997). The joint development of orientation and ocular dominance: role of constraints. *Neural Computation*, 9(5):959–70.

Quinlan, E. M., Philpot, B., Huganir, R., and Bear, M. (1999). Rapid, experience-dependent expression of synaptic NMDA receptors in visual cortex in vivo. *Nature Neuroscience*, 2(4):352–357.

RA, R. Z. and Nicoll, R. (1990). Comparison of two forms of long-term potentiation in single hippocampal neurons. *Science*, 248:1619–24.

Ramoa, A. S., Paradiso, M. A., and Freeman, R. D. (1988). Blockade of intracortical inhibition in kitten striate cortex: Effects on receptive field properties and associated loss of ocular dominance plasticity. *Experimental Brain Research*, 73:285–296.

Rauschecker, J. P. and Singer, W. (1979). Changes in the circuitry of the kitten visual cortex are gated by postsynaptic activity. *Nature*, 280:58–60.

Rauschecker, J. P. and Singer, W. (1981). The effects of early visual experience on the cat's visual cortex and their possible explaination by hebb synapses. *Journal of Physiology*, 310:215–39.

Reid, R. C. and Alonso, J. (1995). Specificity of monosynaptic connections from thalamus to visual cortex. *Nature*, 378:281–284.

Reid, R. C., Soodak, R. E., and Shapley, R. M. (1991). Directional selectivity and spatiotemporal structure of receptive fields of simple cells in cat striate cortex. *Journal of Neurophysiology*, 66(2).

Reiter, H. O. and Stryker, M. P. (1988). Neural plasticity without action potentials: Less active inputs become dominant when kitten visual cortical cells are pharmacologically inhibited. *Proceedings of the National Academy of Science*, 85:3623–3627.

Reiter, H. O., Waitzman, D., and Stryker, M. (1986). Cortical activity blockade prevents ocular dominance plasticity in the kitten visual cortex. *Exp. Brain Res.*, 65:182–88.

Rioult-Pedotti, M., Friedman, D., and Donoghue, J. (2000). Learning-induced ltp in neocortex. *Science*, 290:533–6.

Rittenhouse, C., Voelker, C., Siegler, B., Paradiso, M., and Bear, M. (2000). Evidence for homosynaptic depression in the superficial layers of visual cortex following brief monocular deprivation. *Society for Neuroscience Abstracts*.

Rittenhouse, C. D., Shouval, H. Z., Paradiso, M. A., and Bear, M. F. (1999). Evidence that monocular deprivation induces homosynaptic long-term depression in visual cortex. *Nature*, 397:347–350.

Roberts, E., Meredith, M., and Ramoa, A. (1998). Suppression of nmda receptor function using antisense dna block ocular dominance plasticity while preserving visual responses. *J Neurophysiol.*, 80:1021–32.

Rochester, N., Holland, J., Haibt, L., and Duda, W. (1956). Tests on a cell assembly theory of the action of the brain, using a large scale digital computer. *IRE Transactions of Information Theory*, IT-2:80–93.

Rubner, J. and Tavan, P. (1989). A self-organizing network for principal component analysis. *Europhysics Letters*, 10(7):693–698.

Ruderman, D. L. (1994). The statistics of natural images. *Network*, 5(4):517–548.

Sanes, J. R. and Lichtman, J. W. (1999). Can molecules explain long-term potentiation? *Nature Neuroscience*, 2(7):597–604.

Sanger, T. D. (1989). Optimal unsupervised learning in a single-layer linear feedforward neural network. *Neural Networks*, 2:459–473.

Saul, A. B. and Humphrey, A. L. (1990). Spatial and temporal properties of lagged and nonlagged cells in the cat lateral geniculate nucleus. *Journal of Neurophysiology*, 68:1190–1208.

Scofield, C. L. and N Cooper, L. (1985). Development and properties of neural networks. *Contemp. Phys.*, 26:125–145.

Sebestyen, G. (1962). *Decision Making Processes in Pattern Recognition.* Macmillan, New York.

Sejnowski, T. J. (1977). Storing covariance with nonlinearly interacting neurons. *Journal of Mathematical Biology*, 4:303–321.

Sengpiel, F., Stawinski, P., and Bonhoeffer, T. (1999). Influence of experience on orientation maps in cat visual cortex. *Nature Neurosci*, 2:727–32.

Shannon, C. E. (1948). A mathematical theory of communication. *Bell Syst. Tech. J.*, 27:379–423 and 623–656.

Sherk, H. and Stryker, M. (1975). Modification of cortical orientation selectivity in cat by restricted visual experience: a reexamination. *Science*, 190:904–6.

Sherman, S. M. and Spear, P. D. (1982). Organization of visual pathways in normal and visually deprived cats. *Physiol. Rev.*, 62:738–855.

Shmuel, A. and Grinvald, A. (1996). Functional organization for direction of motion and its relationship to orienation maps in cat area 18. *Journal of Neuroscience*, 16(21):6945–6964.

Shouval, H., Intrator, N., and Cooper, L. N. (1996a). Effect of binocular misalignment on networks of plastic neurons. In *The Neurobiology of Computation: Proceedings of the fifth annual Computation and Neural Systems conference.*

Shouval, H., Intrator, N., and Cooper, L. N. (1997a). BCM network develops orientation selectivity and ocular dominance in natural scene environment. *Vision Research*, 37:3339–3342.

Shouval, H., Intrator, N., Law, C. C., and Cooper, L. N. (1996b). Effect of binocular cortical misalignment on ocular dominance and orientation selectivity. *Neural Computation*, 8(5):1021–1040.

Shouval, H., Intrator, N., and N Cooper, L. (1997b). BCM network develops orientation selectivity and ocular dominance from natural scenes environment. *Vision Research*, 37(23):3339–3342.

Shouval, H. and Liu, Y. (1996). Principal component neurons in a realistic visual environment. *Network*, 7(3):501–515.

Shouval, H. Z., Bear, M. F., and Cooper, L. N. (2002a). A unified theory of nmda receptor-dependent bidirectional synaptic plasticity. *Proc. Natl. Acad. Sci.*, 99:10831–6.

Shouval, H. Z., Castellani, G. C., Yeung, L., Blais, B. S., and N., C. L. (2002b). Converging evidence for a simplified biophysical model of synaptic plasticity. *Bio. Cyb.*, 87:383–91.

Shouval, H. Z., Goldberg, D. H., Jones, J. P., Beckerman, M., and Cooper, L. N. (2000). Structured long-range connections can provide a scaffold for orientation maps. *Journal of Neuroscience*, 20(3):1119–28.

Sillito, A., Jones, H., Gerstein, G., and West, D. (1994). Feature-linked synchronyzation of thalamic relay cell firing induced by feedback from visual cortex. *Nature*, 369:479–482.

Stanton, P. and Sejnowski, T. J. (1989). Associative long-term depression in the hippocampus induced by Hebbian covariance. *Nature*, 339:215–218.

Steele, P. M. and Mauk, M. D. (1999). Inhibitory control of ltp and ltd: Stability of synapse strength. *J Neurophysiol*, 81:1559–1566.

Stent, G. (1973). A physiological mechanism for hebb's postulate of learning. *Proceedings of the National Academy of Sciences, U.S.A*, 70:997.

Stevens, C. and Wang, Y. (1994). Changes in reliability of synaptic function as a mechanism for plasticity. *Nature*, 371:704–7.

Stryker, M., Sherk, H., Levental, A. G., and Hirsh, H. V. (1978). Physiological consequences for the cat's visual cortex of effectively restricting early visual experience with oriented contours. *Journal of Neurophysiology*, 41(4):896–909.

Stuart, A., Kendall, M., and Ord, J. K. (1987). *Advanced Theory of Statistics 1: Distribution Theory*. Oxford University Press.

Stuart, A. and Ord, J. K. (1994). *Kendall's Advanced Theory of Statistics*. Edward Arnold.

Suarez, H., Koch, C., and Douglas, R. (1995). Modeling direction selectivity of simple cells in striate visual cortex within the frameworkof the canonical microcircuit. *Journal of Neuroscience*, 15:6700–6719.

Switzer, P. (1970). Numerical classification. In Barnett, V., editor, *Geostatistics*. Plenum Press, New York.

T., I. J., G.O., H., A., N. R., and C., M. R. (1996). Silent synapses during development of thalamocortical inputs. *Proceedings of the National Academy of Science*, 93(16):8710–8715.

Tang, Y.-P., Shimizu, E., Dube, G. R., Rampon, C., Kerchner, G. A., Zhuo, M., Liu, G., and Tsien, J. Z. (1999). Genetic enhancement of learning and memory in mice. *Nature*, 401:63 – 69. Doogie.

Tankus, A., Yeshurun, Y., and Intrator, N. (1997). Face detection by direct convexity estimation. *Pattern Recognition Letters*, 18(9):913–922.

Thiagarajan, T., Piedras-Renteria, E., and Tsien, R. (2002). alpha- and betacamkii. inverse regulation by neuronal activity and opposing effects on synaptic strength. *Neuron*, 36:1103–14.

Tretter, F., Cynader, M., and Singer, W. (1975). Modification of direction selectivity in neurons in the visual cortex of kittens. *Brain Research*, 84:143–149.

Tsodyks, M. and Markram, H. (1996). Plasticity in neocortical synapses and extraction of dynamic features of presynaptic network activity. submitted.

Tsodyks, M. V. and Markram, H. (1997). The neural code between neocortical pyramidal neurons depends on neurotransmitter release probability. *Proc. Natl. Acad. Sci.*, 94:719–723.

Turrigiano, G. (1999). Homeostatic plasticity in neuronal networks: the more things change, the more they stay the same. *Trends Neurosci.*, 22::221–7.

van Sluyters, R. (1977). Artificial strabismus in the kitten. *Invest. Ophthalmol. Vis. Sci. Suppl.*, 16:40.

van Sluyters, R. C. and Levitt, F. B. (1980). Experimental strabismus in the kitten. *Journal of Neurophysiology*, 43:689–699.

Viola, P. and Wells, W. M. (1995). Alignment by maximization of mutual information. In *Proceedings of the 1st International Conference on -1z Computer Vision*. IEEE Computer Society.

von der Malsburg, C. (1973). Self-organization of orientation sensitive cells in striate cortex. *Kybernetik*, 14:85–100.

Wand, M. P. (1994). Fast computation of multivariate kernel estimators. *Journal of Computational and Graphical Statistics*, 3:433–445.

Wang, H. and Wagner, J. J. (1999). Priming-induced shift in synaptic plasticity in the rat hippocampus. *Journal of Neurophysiology*, 82(4):2024–2028.

Watson, A. B. and Ahumada, A. J. (1985). Model of human visual-motion sensing. *Journal of the Optics Society of America*, A2:322–342.

Watt, A. J., Rossum, M. V., MacLeod, K. M., Nelson, S. B., and Turrogiano, G. G. (2000). Activity coregulates quantal AMPA and NMDA currents at neocortical synapses. *Neuron*, 26:659–70.

Weliky, M. and Katz, L. C. (1999). Correlational structure of spontaneous neuronal activity in the developing lateral geniculate nucleus in vivo. *Science*, 285:599–604.

Wiesel, T. and Hubel, D. (1962). Comparison of effect of unilateral and bilateral eye closure on cortical unit response in kittens. *Journal of Physiology*, 180(180):106–154.

Wiesel, T. N. and Hubel, D. H. (1963). Single-cell responses in striate cortex of kittens deprived of vision in one eye. *Journal of Neurophysiology*, 26:1003–1017.

Wiesel, T. N. and Hubel, D. H. (1965). Comparison of the effects of unilateral and bilateral eye closure on cortical unit responses in kittens. *J. Neurophysiol.*, 28:1029–1040.

Wyatt, J. L. and Elfadel, I. M. (1995). Time-domain solutions of Oja's equations. *Neural Computation*, 7(5):915–922.

Yang, S.-N., Tang, Y.-G., and Zucker, R. (1999). Selective induction of ltp and ltd by postsynaptic $[ca^{2+}]_i$ elevation. *Journal of Neurophysiology*, 81:781–787.

Yang, X. and Faber, D. S. (1991). Initial synaptic efficacy influences induction and expression of long-term changes in transmission. *Proceedings of the National Academy of Science*, 88(10):4299–4303.

Yeung, L., Shouval, H. Z., Blais, B. S., and N., C. L. (2003). Homeostatic metaplasticity accounts for synaptic scaling. *Society for Neuroscience Abstracts*.

Zakharenko, S. S., Zablow, L., and Siegelbaum, S. (2001). Visualization of changes in presynaptic function during long-term synaptic plasticity. *Nat. Neurosci.*, 4:711–7.